FOOD POISONING, POLICY AND POLITICS

Corned Beef and Typhoid in Britain in the 1960s

The problem of food contamination and poisoning is currently one of vigorous debate, highlighted since the 1980s by numerous outbreaks and scares, involving salmonella in eggs, listeria in cheese, links between vCJD and BSE, and *E. Coli* 0157 in cooked meats. There have also been episodes involving chemical contaminants, such as the recent Sudan I affair. These all raise complex problems regarding food safety monitoring, and the identification, withdrawal and disposal of suspect food. Yet, as this book shows, many of the issues involved were important as early as the 1960s, when there were four typhoid outbreaks in Britain, traced to contaminated corned beef imported from Argentina.

Based upon extensive research, this book analyses the typhoid outbreaks and their aftermath, looking at the roles of politicians, officials, health professionals, business interests, the media and the public. It also considers the difficult issue of weighing food safety against international trade and other business and economic interests; conflicts between government departments; rivalry between professionals; the effects upon and influence of victims and local communities; and the conduct of and responses to an official enquiry. Overall, the 1960s corned beef and typhoid episode offers generic lessons regarding food policy making, adding historical perspectives to contemporary debates.

David F. Smith is a lecturer in the history of medicine, Aberdeen University. He is editor of *Nutrition in Britain: Science, Scientists and Politics in the Twentieth Century* (Routledge, 1997) and joint-editor (with Jim Phillips) of *Food, Science, Policy and Regulation in the Twentieth Century: International and Comparative Perspectives* (Routledge, 2000). **H. Lesley Diack** is now a lecturer in Elearning, School of Pharmacy, Robert Gordon University, Aberdeen. **T. Hugh Pennington** was professor of bacteriology at Aberdeen University until his retirement in 2003. He is author of *When Food Kills: BSE, E. Coli, and Disaster Science* (Oxford University Press, 2003). **Elizabeth M. Russell** was professor of social medicine at Aberdeen University until she retired in 2001.

FOOD POISONING, POLICY AND POLITICS

Corned Beef and Typhoid in Britain in the 1960s

David F. Smith and H. Lesley Diack

with

T. Hugh Pennington and Elizabeth M. Russell

THE BOYDELL PRESS

First published 2005
The Boydell Press, Woodbridge

ISBN 1 84383 138 4

The Boydell Press is an imprint of Boydell & Brewer Ltd
PO Box 9, Woodbridge, Suffolk IP12 3DF, UK
and of Boydell & Brewer Inc.
668 Mt Hope Avenue, Rochester, NY 14620, USA
website: www.boydellandbrewer.com

A CIP catalogue record for this book is available
from the British Library

Library of Congress Cataloging-in-Publication Data
Smith, David F., 1954–
Food poisoning, policy, and politics : corned beef and typhoid in Britain
in the 1960s / David F. Smith and H. Lesley Diack with T. Hugh Pennington
and Elizabeth M. Russell.
p. ; cm.
Includes bibliographical references and index.
Summary: "Study of the 1963/4 typhoid outbreak, highlighting issues and
debates which are strikingly relevant today"—Provided by publisher.
ISBN 1-84383-138-4 (hardback : alk. paper)
1. Typhoid fever—Great Britain—Epidemiology. 2. Food poisoning—
Great Britain. 3. Corned beef—Great Britain. 4. Food contamination—
Government policy—Great Britain.
[DNLM: 1. Salmonella Food Poisoning—history—Great Britain. 2. Typhoid
Fever—history—Great Britain. 3. Food Inspection—history—Great Britain.
4. Food Preservation—history—Great Britain. 5. Health Policy—Great Britain.
6. Meat—poisoning—Great Britain.] I. Diack, H. Lesley. II. Title.
RA644.T8S54 2005
614.5'112'0941—dc22
2005001771

This publication is printed on acid-free paper
Typeset by Keystroke, Jacaranda Lodge, Wolverhampton
Printed in Great Britain by
Athenaeum Press Ltd., Gateshead, Tyne & Wear

Contents

Illustrations

Tables

Figures

Preface and acknowledgements

In May 1964 a typhoid outbreak began in Aberdeen, Scotland which, within a few weeks, led to the hospitalisation of over 500 people. A committee of inquiry appointed during the outbreak and which reported in December concluded that the infection had arisen from canned corned beef that had become contaminated by unchlorinated cooling water during the canning process at a factory in Argentina. Three smaller outbreaks in England during 1963 had been explained in the same way. In contrast to the 1963 outbreaks, the Aberdeen outbreak was very well publicised throughout and beyond the UK, in newspapers, and via radio and television news reports. The incident became notorious in the history of food safety and food poisoning, and is remembered vividly by Aberdonians who lived through it.

This book investigates the four corned beef-associated typhoid outbreaks and sets them in the context of the long-term history of typhoid and food poisoning. The policy-making processes surrounding the outbreaks are explored, including the circumstances that allowed the Aberdeen outbreak to happen following the outbreaks in England, the political handling of the Aberdeen outbreak, the shaping of the report of the committee of inquiry, and the implementation of its findings. There are important international dimensions concerning the hygienic control of Argentine meat and meat products, while local dimensions include the role of the health services, especially the medical officer of health, and the experiences of patients and Aberdeen's population. The interactions between and within government departments, such as the Ministry of Agriculture, Fisheries and Food (MAFF), the Ministry of Health and the Scottish Office are analysed, as well as the interactions between the government departments and local actors. In the final chapter, a way of conceptualising the complex processes of food policy making and implementation during the 1960s is presented.

In view of recent widespread interest in food poisoning and food safety, the analysis presented in this book is not merely of historical interest. Recently, however, there have been some profound changes in the food safety regimes in the UK and Europe. The Food Standards Agency (FSA) was created in 1999, and the European Food Safety Authority came into being in 2002. The FSA took over many of the food safety responsibilities of MAFF, and MAFF was subsequently abolished and replaced by the Department for Environment, Food and Rural Affairs (DEFRA), after the foot-and-mouth disease outbreak of 2001.

The recent reforms of the food safety system were stimulated by a series of problems which arose during and since the 1980s, especially the bovine spongiform encephalopathy (BSE) débâcle, and the *E. coli* 0157 outbreaks. The interest of the press, public and politicians in food-poisoning incidents became intense, and food safety became an election issue in 1997, leading to New Labour's manifesto promises which took shape with the formation of the FSA. The major objective was restoring the trust of the public in the government's food safety machinery, and the new watchword was 'openness', the implementation of which has been facilitated by the rise of the internet.

There are some senses in which much has now changed since the 1960s, and yet much also remains the same. The essential actors involved in food safety problems, policy making and implementation remain unchanged. These include micro-organisms, which will probably always retain their capacity to surprise, the food industries, the key objective of which, as in the 1960s, is still to make profits, and politicians, whose major concerns continue to be re-election. The administration of the food safety system remains in the hands of central government civil servants, and local personnel. Although the latter no longer includes medical officers of health and their teams, since the 1974 reorganisation of the health services, locally based staff of the local authority and health service are largely responsible for the implementation of policies and regulations, and the handling of incidents. And while the creation of the FSA has transferred the civil servants concerned with food safety to a more independent department, other departments, such as the health departments, and the Treasury, Foreign Office and Prime Minister's Office, all retain interests in food safety decision making. Food safety policy making and implementation remain very complex, and among the expert civil servants within and beyond the FSA there is still, inevitably, a variety of departmental, disciplinary and professional commitments, which, as will be seen, were a prominent feature of policy making during the 1960s. Interactions between London and Edinburgh-based departments of government continue to be a feature. The importance of this dimension of food policy making has been enhanced by the creation of the Scottish Parliament in 1999, as well as the existence of a national office of the FSA in Scotland (and also in Wales and Northern Ireland).

To the extent that the nature of food policy making and implementation remain unchanged, the episodes explored in this book provide a window on ongoing processes. But inasmuch as the recent reforms of the food safety regime, and especially the doctrine of openness, have reduced or eliminated some past problems, the analyses presented here will also serve as warnings as to the difficulties that may arise in the future. As public interest in food safety policy making wanes (possibly as concern shifts to other issues such as obesity and nutrition), and as the structure of the FSA develops and its operations become more routine, food safety policy may again become largely the private business of civil servants. The authors therefore hope that this book will not only appeal to historians interested in medicine, disease, food and the 1960s, but also current participants in and commentators upon food safety policy making.

This book is the product of a collaborative project, funded by the Wellcome Trust, the research team consisting of a historian of medicine (David Smith), a historian with experience of local history (Lesley Diack), a microbiologist with historical interests (Hugh Pennington), and a public health academic who was involved, as a young doctor, in some of the action on which the book is based (Elizabeth Russell). The principal grant applicant and grant holder was David Smith, while Hugh Pennington and Elizabeth Russell were the co-applicants. Virginia Berridge, of the London School of Hygiene of Tropical Medicine, was a 'named collaborator'. The grant provided funds to employ a named research assistant, Lesley Diack. On being awarded her doctorate, her post was retitled 'research fellow' by Aberdeen University. The grant ran for three years from February 1999, but the Wellcome Trust kindly allowed us to use contingency funds for a short extension of Lesley Diack's contract, and provided a further small grant for gathering additional material on the 'media' dimensions of the Aberdeen typhoid outbreak. The research team is very grateful to the Wellcome Trust for their support, and especially John Malin, the former co-ordinator of the History of Medicine programme, for all his help and advice. Lesley Diack is now lecturer in Elearning at the School of Pharmacy of the Robert Gordon University. Elizabeth Russell and Hugh Pennington entered active retirement in September 2001 and October 2003 respectively.

The project was supervised on a day-to-day basis by David Smith. Elizabeth Russell, and Hugh Pennington, when he could, attended team meetings. Virginia Berridge joined annual meetings to review progress. Lesley Diack received training in oral history at a course funded by the Wellcome Trust and run by Rob Perks and Paul Thompson, and was responsible for all the oral history interviews. David Smith and Lesley Diack shared the archival research.

During the project, Lesley Diack and David Smith together wrote a number of papers for oral presentation, and, in some cases, publication. A paper on the Milne Committee's recommendation on the involvement of medical officers in overseas meat inspection was given at the 'Animals, Vets and Vermin' conference at the University of East Anglia, in April 2000, and formed the basis for a chapter in an edited collection published later that year.[1] This topic is further developed in Chapter 7 (this volume). A paper on the activities of Ian MacQueen, medical officer of health for Aberdeen, during the Aberdeen typhoid outbreak, given at the March 2001 meeting of the Scottish

---

[1] L. Diack, T. H. Pennington, E. Russell and D. F. Smith, 'Departmental and professional agendas in the implementation of the recommendations of a food crisis enquiry: the Milne report and inspection of overseas meat plants', in D. F. Smith and J. Phillips (eds), *Food, Science, Policy and Regulation in the Twentieth Century: International and Comparative Perspectives*, London, 2000, pp. 189–206.

Society for the History of Medicine, awaits publication in the *Proceedings* of the society.[2] Another paper on MacQueen has already appeared in the *Journal of Public Health Medicine*.[3] A further joint paper was given at the spring 2001 conference of the Society for the Social History of Medicine (SSHM), on the media and the management of the Aberdeen typhoid outbreak. This will be published in 2005.[4] A joint paper given at a symposium at University College, London, in May 2001, has been developed into Chapter 2 of this volume. Lesley Diack gave a paper on the history of the corned beef stockpile at a conference of the SSHM in Aberdeen in October 2001, while, on the same day, David Smith spoke on British efforts to stimulate improvements in Argentine meat hygiene after 1964 at the Wellcome Regional Forum in Glasgow. Besides the joint writing projects mentioned above which have helped to shape the current volume, the rest of this book has been written by David Smith, but some oral history material prepared by Lesley Diack, before she completed her contract, is incorporated into Chapter 3. David Smith prepared the index.

Numerous discussions involving those within and beyond the research team have contributed to the shaping of this volume. These include discussions at the various events mentioned above, but especially at a workshop on 'New Perspectives on the Aberdeen Typhoid Outbreak', supported by the Royal Society of Edinburgh and Wellcome Trust, which was held in Aberdeen in December 2001. It is difficult to produce a definitive list of all those who have contributed ideas and suggestions, but special thanks are due to: Annie Anderson, Pete Atkins, Virginia Berridge, Joanna Bornat, Mark Bufton, Roger Cooter, Anne Hardy, Tim Lang, Kelly Loughlin, George Paterson, Rob Perks, Jim Phillips, Jacqui Reilly, Sally Sheard, Eve Seguin, John Welshman and Abigail Woods. I apologise for any omissions. Thanks are also due to all the interviewees who gave so freely of their time, some of whom also attended the workshop. The interviewees are: E. Maurice Backett, Sheena Blackhall, Roger Blamire, Dodson P. Brunton, Joan Burrell, Mabel Clubb, Wilma Craigmile, Duncan Penny Cummine, Lorna Dewar, Michael Franklin, George Godber, Loudoun P. Hamilton, Alice Hay, Betty Hobbs, James Hogarth, Bob Hughes, Douglas Kay, James Kyle, Sandy Logie, Michael McEntegart, Wilson McIntosh, William Mackie, Joyce McKain, Rona McRoberts, Norma Michie, Fiona Milne, Irene Morrison, Campbell Murray, Margaret Nairn,

---

[2] L. Diack and D. F. Smith, 'Dr Ian MacQueen and the Aberdeen typhoid outbreak of 1964; a variety of perspectives', forthcoming in *Proceedings of the Scottish Society for the History of Medicine*.

[3] L. Diack and D. F. Smith, 'Professional strategies of Medical Officers of Health in the post war period (1): 'innovative traditionalism': the case of Dr Ian MacQueen, MOH for Aberdeen 1952–1974', *Journal of Public Health Medicine*, 2002, vol. 24, pp. 123–9.

[4] L. Diack and D. F. Smith, 'The media and the management of a food crisis: Aberdeen's typhoid outbreak in 1964', in V. Berridge and K. Loughlin (eds), *Medicine, the Mass Media and the Market*, London, forthcoming, 2005.

Aileen Pettit, Aenea Reid, John Rennie, Anne Ritchie, Hilda Robb, Elizabeth Russell, Andrew Semple, Robbie Shepherd, George Sinton, John Smith, Linsey Smith, Robert Smith, Alex Stephen, Rosemary Towler, Douglas E. Walker, Molly Walker, Jim Wallace, Keith Webster, Roy Weir, and Ronnie Williamson. Additional thanks are due to those who made available private papers. Thanks are also due to all the archivists and librarians who have supported the research, especially Fiona Watson of the Northern Health Services Archive, and the staffs of the Aberdeen City Archives, Aberdeen University Department of Special Collections, National Archives of Scotland, and Public Record Office. I also wish to thank my successive heads of department/school at the University of Aberdeen, Allan Macinnes, Jane Ohlmeyer, and David Ditchburn, and the school's research committee, for all their support. Finally, I am grateful for Lorna Smith's careful proof-reading, and for the help and advice provided by Peter Sowden and Sarah Pearsall of Boydell and Brewer.

David F. Smith
University of Aberdeen, 28 October 2004

Abbreviations used in text

BMJ	*British Medical Journal*
BSE	Bovine Spongiform Encephalopathy
CAP	Corporación Argentina de Productores de Carne (Corporation of Argentine Meat Producers Ltd)
CDSC	Communicable Disease Surveillance Centre
CDSU	Communicable Disease (Scotland) Unit
CJD	Creutzfeldt-Jakob disease
CMO	Chief medical officer
CVO	Chief veterinary officer
DEFRA	Department for Environment, Food and Rural Affairs
DHSS	Department of Health and Social Security
EE	*Evening Express* (Aberdeen's daily evening newspaper)
EPHLS	Emergency Public Health Laboratory Service
FAO	Food and Agricultural Organisation
FCO	Foreign and Commonwealth Office
FSA	Food Standards Agency
GP/GPs	General practitioner/general practitioners
MAFF	Ministry of Agriculture, Fisheries and Food
MOH/MOsH	Medical officer of health/medical officers of health
MP	Member of Parliament
MRC	Medical Research Council
NHS	National Health Service
P&J	*Press and Journal* (Aberdeen's daily morning newspaper)
PHLS	Public Health Laboratory Service
SHHD	Scottish Home and Health Department
SSHM	Society for the Social History of Medicine
WHO	World Health Organisation

Abbreviations used in footnotes

Archival references

ACA	Aberdeen City Archives
ATO	Aberdeen typhoid outbreak project oral history tape reference. All interviews conducted by Lesley Diack
AULSCA	Aberdeen University Library Special Collections and Archives
AUSHS	Aberdeen University Student Health Service Typhoid Epidemic 1964/folder supplied by Dr Campbell Murray
DK	Papers supplied by Dennis King, retired businessman
EMR	Miscellaneous papers relating to the Aberdeen typhoid outbreak supplied by Professor Elizabeth M. Russell
GUABRC	Glasgow University Archives and Business Records Centre
NAS	National Archives of Scotland
NHSA	Northern Health Services Archive
PRO	Public Record Office

Journals and series

BMJ	*British Medical Journal*
EE	*Evening Express* (Aberdeen's evening newspaper)
MRCSRS	Medical Research Council Special Report Series
P&J	*Press and Journal* (Aberdeen's daily morning newspaper)
PD(C)	*Parliamentary Debates (Commons)* (note that italic column numbers denote 'written answers' at the back of each volume)
PD(L)	*Parliamentary Debates (Lords)* (note that italic column numbers denote 'written answers' at the back of each volume)
RAHSGB	*Report on the Animal Health Services in Great Britain*
RCMO	*Report of the Chief Medical Office of the Ministry of Health/Report of the Chief Medical Office of the Department of Health and Social Security/Report of the Chief Medical Office of the Department of Health* (also entitled *On the State of Public Health*)
RDHS	*Report of the Department of Health for Scotland*
RDHSS	*Report of the Departmental Health and Social Security*
RMOHA	*Report of the Medical Officer of Health for Aberdeen*

RMH   *Report of the Ministry of Health*
RPHMS   Reports on Public Health and Medical Subjects
RSHHD   *Report of the Scottish Home and Health Department* (also entitled
              Health and Welfare Services in Scotland / Health Services in Scotland/
              Health in Scotland)

1

The earlier history of typhoid and food poisoning

Introduction

Through an exploration of the Aberdeen typhoid outbreak of 1964, and three smaller outbreaks in England in 1963, and related episodes, this book aims to provide insights of potential relevance to matters of current worldwide public, political and medical concern: food poisoning and food safety. In all four incidents, the source of infection was traced to corned beef contaminated during manufacture in Argentina. The handling of the outbreaks, the conduct of the enquiry that followed and its consequences, the disposal of the suspect corned beef, and action in Argentina, together provide a window on the complex processes of food safety policy making.

The notion that historical enquiry might illuminate issues of relevance to current concerns in food and nutrition is by no means original. Food policy making has long been extraordinarily difficult and contentious, in view of the plethora of interests and experts involved. Controversy about the claims and implications of the 'newer knowledge of nutrition' (the discovery of vitamins) during the 'hungry thirties' also stimulated the study of history. Vitamin pioneer Professor Jack Drummond, who was to become wartime chief scientific adviser at the Ministry of Food, started work on a project published at the end of the decade as the classic of food history, *The Englishman's Food*.[1] During the 1960s, in a different context, John Yudkin, first professor of nutrition in Britain, turned to history when faced with scientific controversy (over the role of diet in heart disease) and definitional and practical problems. (What constituted the 'science of nutrition' and its application?)[2] Yudkin's initiative, the 'historians' and nutritionists' seminar' at the nutrition department of Queen Elizabeth (later King's) College, London University, met regularly for three decades. It led to three volumes of papers, but attempted no synthesis, the third volume inviting the reader to make connections between the diverse

---

[1] J. C. Drummond and A. Wilbraham, *The Englishman's Food. A History of Five Centuries of English Diet*, London, 1939.
[2] D. F. Smith, 'The discourse of scientific knowledge of nutrition and dietary change in the twentieth century', in A. Murcott (ed.), *The Nation's Diet*, London, 1998, pp. 311–31.

1

topics discussed.[3] Another example of historian–nutritionist collaboration was a conference of the Society for Social History of Medicine organised by the Wellcome Unit for the History of Medicine and the Nutrition Department of Glasgow University in 1993. A sequel to the latter event took place at Aberdeen University in 1999.

Two volumes of collected papers were developed from the SSHM conferences,[4] and the introduction to the second began the process of drawing out common themes from chapters covering different periods, countries and topics.[5] It was commented that the kind of case studies presented would provide the basis for further 'theoretical' development of this area. But what kind of 'theory' is needed for historical 'food studies' which range, as this book does, from experiences of ordinary people to processes of government policy formation and implementation? This is a question that has exercised the authors, when we have emerged from the absorbing task of collecting and attempting to make sense of archival, oral history and other evidence. It was also a question that exercised participants in a workshop on 'New Perspectives on the Aberdeen typhoid outbreak', sponsored by the Royal Society of Edinburgh and held at Aberdeen University in December 2001. This workshop brought together some actors involved in the Aberdeen typhoid outbreak, professionals with recent experience of food safety, and historians and social scientists from a variety of backgrounds. The team was offered new information about the dynamic of events in the 1960s, alerted to influential aspects of the context of the time, and stimulated by parallels and differences between Aberdeen and other outbreaks. We were also given important and valuable insights from the perspectives of media studies and discourse analysis, and urged to investigate the potential of political science theory. One participant, engaged in a leadership role in the new British food safety machinery, asked whether the aim was to produce a 'model of good practice'. All of this set the team thinking with increased vigour, at an important stage of shaping this volume, about the nature of the 'theory' that we need and wish to offer.

It should be said immediately that we make no attempt to provide any kind of 'model' for future food safety policy making. Nevertheless, we hope that there is much in this book that will be suggestive to current and future participants in the field. The Food Standards Agency, which has a UK headquarters in London, and national offices in Scotland, Wales and Northern

[3] D. J. Oddy and D. S. Miller, *The Making of the Modern British Diet*, London, 1976; D. J. Oddy and D. S. Miller, *Diet and Health in Modern Britain*, London, 1985; C. Geissler and D. J. Oddy, *Food, Diet and Economic Change Past and Present*, Leicester, 1993.

[4] D. F. Smith, (ed.), *Nutrition in Britain: Science, Scientists and Politics in the Twentieth Century*, London, 1997; D. F. Smith and J. Phillips (eds), *Food, Science, Policy and Regulation in the Twentieth Century: International and Comparative Perspectives*, London, 2000.

[5] D. F. Smith and J. Phillips, 'Food policy and regulation: a multiplicity of actors and experts', in Smith and Phillips, *Food, Science, Policy*, pp. 1–16.

Ireland, and which was created in 1999, has already been alluded to. In January 2002, the European Food Safety Authority was also established. We hope that the processes described in this book will alert those working in and watching these agencies to some of the problems of the past, in the hope that this may facilitate the avoidance of similar problems in the future. As for the use of 'theory' from other fields, the authors acknowledge that several perspectives mentioned above, and other strands of contemporary debate, have influenced our interpretations. However, we have come to the conclusion that, fundamentally, our task is to use the typhoid outbreaks of 1963 to 1964, and related events, as a window on the parts of the food safety 'system' during the 1960s that these events illuminate. Through the methods of contemporary history, and original source-based narrative and analysis, we have produced a picture of this system, providing a historical perspective that may sensitise readers to the less visible dimensions of food safety policy making during other eras and in other places.[6]

The longer term context

Before beginning our case study, in the rest of this chapter we will place the 1963 to 1964 typhoid outbreaks in the context of the longer term histories of typhoid and food poisoning in Britain. From the point of view of the health administration, 'enteric fevers' (typhoid and paratyphoid) and 'food poisoning' were distinct entities, discussed in different sections of annual reports. This was a matter of historical accident, since enteric fevers were the subject of concern and statistics long before 'food poisoning' received attention. But the distinction was also rational. Enteric infections are acquired by mouth, via water, milk or food, but the incubation period is prolonged – at least seven and often twenty days – with microbes carried from the gut by the blood to invade and disrupt numerous organs. The symptoms of microbial food poisoning, in contrast, can appear within hours of eating the implicated food, and are usually confined to inflammation and irritation of the gut. In addition, by 1963 to 1964, as a result of improvements in living standards and over a century of sanitary reform, there were other differences. The 1963 to 1964 typhoid outbreaks occurred at a time when enteric fevers had become rare in Britain. Food poisoning, however, had only been recognised as a serious

[6] For a discussion of approaches to the history of health policy, and the ability of contemporary history to produce a 'more comprehensive explanatory framework', see V. Berridge and J. Stanton, 'Science and policy: historical insights', *Social Science and Medicine*, 1999, vol. 49, pp. 1133–8. For a recent discussion of the possible roles of history in current policy making, see V. Berridge, 'Public or policy understanding of history', *Social History of Medicine*, 2003, vol. 16, pp. 511–23.

problem since the Second World War, and had been the subject of comprehensive regulations for less than a decade. But by the early 1960s there was optimism that action to prevent food poisoning was beginning to work. In these circumstances the corned beef-associated typhoid episode served as a signal that food safety and hygiene were not such simple matters as had been imagined. The 1964 committee of enquiry raised questions of food hygiene well beyond that of how corned beef-associated typhoid could be prevented. The affair therefore marks a period of transition from a moment when it seemed that it would not be long before food-borne infectious diseases were vanquished, towards the present widespread anxiety about food safety. The current situation has been created by the experiences and media coverage of such diseases as BSE and *Escherichia coli* O157 poisoning, but, as we shall see, the media also played important roles in conditioning perceptions and decisions during the 1960s.

Part of the aim of the following two sections, which consider in turn the histories of typhoid and food poisoning, is to provide technical knowledge that will make the rest of the book more accessible. The information provided will, for example, help to shed light upon the reactions of professionals and the public to the typhoid outbreaks of 1963 to 1964 and their immediate aftermath. Further background, for example on the machinery of government and the regulation of meat imports, will be introduced at appropriate points in later chapters.

The earlier history of typhoid

By 1963 to 1964, typhoid had been recognised as a distinct disease for little more than a century. During the early nineteenth century, British physicians considered 'continued fever' a general disease with variable manifestations, including those of typhoid and typhus. But by the 1830s, the distinctive characteristics of typhoid had been identified in France and the USA. The illness typically attacked young adults, was uninfluenced by treatment and lasted about twenty-eight days. Characteristic lesions of the small intestine were invariably found in fatal cases. Typhoid affected all classes and occurred sporadically or as small epidemics in villages and towns as well as in cities, arising most regularly during the late summer. Typhus was of faster onset, shorter duration, more highly contagious, and occurred irregularly in larger epidemics among the urban poor.[7] Both diseases were common among combatants during wars, but as urban diseases they were localised problems, and have not received the same attention by historians as cholera, which came

---

[7] L. G. Wilson, 'Fevers', in W. F. Bynum and R. Porter (eds), *Companion Encyclopaedia of the History of Medicine*, London, 1993, pp. 382–411, at pp. 401–3.

from abroad in great spreading waves.[8] It was the work of William Jenner, whose study of fever at the London Hospital was published in 1849, which began to convince the medical world that typhoid and typhus were distinct. Nevertheless, separate statistics for these fevers were not presented in the reports of the Registrar General for Scotland until 1865, the Registrar General for England and Wales following suit in 1869.

Jenner reasoned that if typhoid and typhus were distinct, each must have a specific cause, and the identity of those causes was of great concern in the mid-nineteenth century. According to one estimate, 20,000 people died of typhoid each year in Britain and at least 100,000 survived the disease. William Budd began to argue from 1856 that the means of transmission was drinking water contaminated by sewage containing a specific infective agent, and this idea was repeatedly reinforced by studies of outbreaks during the 1860s and 1870s. Epidemics spread by milk were also described, the infection usually arising from impure water used for washing dairy equipment.[9]

Despite the deepening medical understanding of typhoid, London Fever Hospital statistics suggested that the incidence rose during the 1860s.[10] But the disease began to decline in England and Wales as sanitary reform gathered speed, following the Public Health Act of 1875. The decline in Scotland began about a decade later, probably due to the slower pace of reform. In 1880 there were 261 deaths from typhoid per million of population in England and Wales, but 358 in Scotland. By 1940 there were only three deaths per million in both countries.[11] Much depended upon local initiative and the efforts of MOsH. Anne Hardy argues, however, that improvements in domestic plumbing were also important, following a series of highly publicised cases among the elite.[12] According to pioneer epidemiologist Major Greenwood, there were two main phases in the decline of typhoid in England and Wales: a sharp fall between 1875 and 1885 due to improvements in water supply and drainage, and a renewed decline after 1900 following greater attention to rapid hospitalisation and the role of carriers.[13] Hardy also claims that the reduction in the number of flies in cities, as motor vehicles displaced horses, played an important role.[14] A further factor was the introduction of chlorination of water supplies.

By 1900 there had been important scientific developments. In 1880, three years after Robert Koch demonstrated that anthrax was caused by a micro-organism, a bacillus found consistently in typhoid cases was described by Carl

---

[8] A. Hardy, *The Epidemic Streets: Infectious Disease and the Rise of Preventive Medicine, 1856–1900*, Oxford, 1993, p. 151.

[9] Wilson, 'Fevers', pp. 404–5.

[10] Hardy, *Epidemic Streets*, p. 154.

[11] E. M. Russell, 'Typhoid fever in Aberdeen – a critical analysis', MD thesis, University of Glasgow, 1965, Table 2, following p. 23.

[12] Hardy, *Epidemic Streets*, pp. 165–72.

[13] M. Greenwood, *Epidemics and Crowd-Diseases*, London, 1935, pp. 156–8.

[14] Hardy, *Epidemic Streets*, pp. 184–6.

Eberth, and named *Eberthella typhosa*. (Also known as *Bacillus typhosus* and later as *Salmonella typhi*.) This was obtained in pure culture in 1884, but it was difficult to prove that the bacillus *caused* typhoid in the absence of a susceptible experimental animal. In 1896, however, it was shown that the serum of typhoid patients caused the clumping and precipitation of the bacillus in broth cultures, which was developed into a diagnostic test by Fernand Widal (the Widal test).[15] Around the same time, experiments were conducted on the preparation and use of typhoid anti-sera.[16]

In 1896 a bacillus was isolated which caused an illness similar to typhoid, apart from variations in the clinical signs and source of infection. This disease, paratyphoid, exhibited more diffuse intestinal changes, and larger and more extensive skin eruptions, and was rarely spread by water. Three forms were identified, with varying geographical distributions, paratyphoid B being most common in Europe.[17] Typhoid and paratyphoid were commonly discussed as 'enteric fevers'.

In Britain, Almroth Wright developed an anti-typhoid vaccine in 1897 to 1898, consisting of a suspension of bacilli killed by heat and preserved by phenol. This was tested among inmates of a lunatic asylum near Maidstone, during the largest British outbreak ever reported. Of nearly 2000 cases, 143 died. The outbreak, caused by contaminated mains water, was widely publicised and a public enquiry followed.[18] Another innovation at Maidstone was the chlorination of water with bleaching powder, which encouraged the introduction of continuous chlorination of water supplies during the early twentieth century.[19] Early schemes were introduced before the First World War at Lincoln, Cambridge, Reading and elsewhere. During the war, part of London's water was chlorinated, and from 1920 chlorination using chlorine gas began. However, it was not until after the Croydon outbreak of 1937 that chlorination was routinely employed at all large water undertakings.[20]

Maidstone apart, sanitary reform reduced water-borne typhoid by the end of the nineteenth century. For a time after 1902, epidemiological interest shifted towards typhoid associated with shellfish, following two major incidents

---

[15] C. W. LeBaron and D. W. Taylor, 'Typhoid fever', in K. F. Kiple (ed.), *The Cambridge World History of Disease*, Cambridge, 2003, pp. 1071–7, at p. 1075.

[16] Russell, 'Typhoid fever', p. 18.

[17] R. L. Huckstep, *Typhoid Fever and other Salmonella Infections*, Edinburgh, 1962, pp. 15–16, 21, 36, 43.

[18] Borough of Maidstone, *Epidemic of Typhoid Fever 1897*, London, 1898.

[19] 'The Maidstone typhoid outbreak of 1897: an important centenary', *Eurosurveillance Weekly*, 13 November 1997 (http://www.eurosurveillance.org/ew/1997/971113.asp, accessed 22 October 2003).

[20] W. O. Skeat, *Manual of British Water Engineering Practice*, Cambridge, 1969, p. 34; W. S. Holden, *Water Treatment and Examination*, London, 1970, p. 362.

in which oysters were implicated.[21] But the water-borne disease remained a threat, especially to armies. During the Spanish–American war of 1898 one-fifth of the American army was sick with typhoid. Trials of Wright's vaccine appeared to show that it reduced the attack rate among soldiers in India by 75 per cent, but it was little used in the Boer War, in which typhoid was rife. However, the vaccine was used by the British in the First World War. From 1915 the combined TAB vaccine was used, which also protected against paratyphoid A and B. The typhoid attack rate was reduced to one in 2000, but later doubts were raised about the efficacy of the vaccine.[22]

The carrier state

The existence of diphtheria carriers was postulated in 1884, and by 1900 studies showed that typhoid could also be transmitted by healthy recovered victims of the disease. In 1902 Koch wrote a paper proposing that a person might chronically shed typhoid bacilli and thereby infect others, and began a campaign to investigate and prevent typhoid in South-West Germany. It was found that about 2 per cent of infected individuals became carriers, and that the carrier state was more common among older women. The carriers theory was confirmed dramatically in the USA in 1906, when typhoid occurred in a summer home in Oyster Bay near New York. It was found that shortly before the outbreak a new cook had been hired, Mary Mallon, and a sanitary engineer for the New York health department discovered that over ten years typhoid had occurred among seven of the eight families for whom Mallon had worked. A year later she was associated with another outbreak, and was detained for three years until released on the promise that she would never again handle food. Five years later she was found to be the source of another outbreak, and was then detained for the rest of her life.[23]

'Typhoid Mary' brought the danger of carriers to the attention of the public and health professionals. J. A. Mendolson has argued that the affair had a profound impact upon American public health, shifting the focus from the community and environment towards the identification and control of individuals who posed health risks.[24] Leading public health officials urged health

---

[21] A. Hardy, 'Methods of outbreak investigation in the "Era of Bacteriology" 1880–1920', *Sozial- und Präventivmedizin*, 2001, vol. 46, pp. 355–60.

[22] LeBaron and Taylor, 'Typhoid fever'; Huckstep, *Typhoid Fever*, p. 110.

[23] LeBaron and Taylor, 'Typhoid fever'; J. W. Leavitt, '"Typhoid Mary" strikes back: bacteriological theory and practice in early twentieth-century public health', *ISIS*, 1992, vol. 83, pp. 608–29, at pp. 613–15.

[24] J. A. Mendelson, '"Typhoid Mary" strikes again: the social and the scientific in the making of modern public health', *ISIS*, 1995, vol. 86, pp. 268–77.

departments to concentrate on the search and control of carriers of infectious diseases, and to give up the focus on filth, and control of water and garbage, to public works departments. By the end of 1915, New York health department had examined the urine or faeces and blood of 90,000 cooks, waiters and food handlers, and regulations were introduced to prevent carriers from working in such trades. By 1918, seventy typhoid carriers were under supervision, and numerous American states introduced similar arrangements.[25]

In Britain there were no comparable celebrated cases, but the carrier problem was taken up by the Local Government Board,[26] and the concept deployed in the investigation of outbreaks. Some MOsH became especially interested in the issue, their investigations featuring in *The Carrier Problem in Infectious Diseases*, published in 1912 by bacteriologists of the Lister Institute. However, this work was predominantly based on the German experience.[27] Among the interested MOsH were several in North-East Scotland. Matthew Hay of Aberdeen was invited in 1907 to investigate an outbreak in the nearby town of Peterhead, which involved 423 typhoid cases over four months. The infection, spread through milk, was traced back to the mother of a farm maid-servant, probably the first urinary carrier identified in Scotland.[28] Alexander Ledingham, medical officer of health for Banffshire, co-authored an article in the *BMJ* in 1908 showing that recurrent outbreaks in an asylum could be attributed to the presence of three carriers,[29] and J. P. Watt identified twenty-four carriers in Aberdeenshire between 1908 and 1919.[30] But there were influential voices opposed to strong emphasis upon carriers in practical public health. In particular, William Hamer, MOH of the London County Council, claimed in 1912 that from the perspective of epidemiology rather than bacteriology, the German evidence of the role of carriers in typhoid was not convincing.[31]

In England, Wales and Scotland MOsH were given limited powers to control typhoid carriers by the Public Health (Pneumonia, Malaria, Dysentery, etc.) Regulations, 1919. These allowed them to prevent carriers from entering employment in food handling or preparation for a specified period, provisions

[25] Ibid.; C. H. Browning, *Chronic Enteric Carriers and their Treatment*, MRCSRS, 1933, No. 179, p. 27.

[26] J. C. G. Ledingham, 'Report on the enteric fever "carrier": being a review of current knowledge on the subject', *Report of the Local Government Board*, 1909–10, vol. 39, pp. 250–384.

[27] J. C. G. Ledingham and J. A. Arkwright, *The Carrier Problem in Infectious Diseases*, London, 1912.

[28] M. Hay, *Report on the Origin and Spread of the Epidemic of Typhoid Fever in 1907*, Peterhead, 1908.

[29] A. Ledingham and J. C. G. Ledingham, 'Typhoid carriers', *BMJ*, 1908, vol. 1, pp. 15–17.

[30] J. P. Watt, 'Typhoid carriers in Aberdeenshire', *Journal of Hygiene*, 1924, vol. 22, pp. 417–37.

[31] Hardy, 'Methods'.

subsequently incorporated into the Public Health (Infectious Diseases) Regulations, 1927, covering England and Wales. Under the latter, an MOH would report a suspected carrier to his local authority, which could require medical examination. If carrier status was proven, the local authority could notify the employer. The carrier would also be instructed in personal cleanliness and the safe disposal of excreta, and would remain under the supervision of the local authority.

In Scotland, regulations issued in 1921, and restated in the Public Health (Infectious Diseases) Regulations (Scotland), 1932, gave additional powers. A person judged to be a carrier could be treated as if he or she was actually suffering from the infection according to the Public Health (Scotland) Act 1897. Carriers certified by the MOH and another doctor could be compulsorily removed to hospital or otherwise isolated. The certificate was valid for three months and could be renewed indefinitely, but the carrier could demand re-examination at any time, and had the right of appeal to the Department of Health for Scotland. Following Ledingham's work, which highlighted the carrier problem within asylums, all carriers in Scottish asylums were segregated in a single institution.[32] But in no sense did these arrangements signal a substantial reorientation of public health activity in Britain. During the inter-war period MOsH were busy building their empires which included tuberculosis, venereal disease, and maternal and child welfare services, and former Poor Law institutions.[33] In this context, the control of carriers was a minor role which received little publicity.

Inter-war typhoid

From 1919 to 1935 George Newman was the first CMO of the Ministry of Health, and his writings reinforce the view that the control of typhoid carriers was not a priority in Britain. In his first annual report he remarked that the key factors in the decline of typhoid were improved 'water supply, sanitation, and the protection of food'. In his view, the 'principal vulnerable points' were the 'gathering grounds of water supplies, dairy farms, shell-fish beds' which exerted a 'larger day by day influence than healthy "carriers" or anti-typhoid inoculation'.[34] In Scotland, however, there was rather more emphasis upon carriers. The Scottish Board of Health report for 1920 commented on an outbreak caused by contaminated milk in Stornoway on the Island of Lewis, where typhoid was more or less endemic. Six of fifty cases were fatal, and the report emphasised the importance of eliminating carriers from the milk trade.

[32] Browning, *Chronic Enteric Carriers*, pp. 26–7.
[33] J. Lewis, *What Price Community Medicine?*, Brighton, 1986.
[34] *RCMO 1919–20*, London, 1920, p. 20.

However, because of the cost to public funds of preventing carriers from working as domestic servants, the Board approached the MRC and asked them to investigate possible cures for the carrier state.[35]

In response, the MRC funded a project by Carl Browning and his colleagues at the University and Western Infirmary in Glasgow on the surgical treatment of enteric carriers. This involved operations on the gall bladder, regarded as the main site of continued infection, on one paratyphoid and two typhoid carriers. A report published in 1933 claimed that the operations had been successful in eliminating pathogenic organisms from the faeces. The authors favoured the general application of the technique, arguing that it would be good for the carriers as well as for the community. Carriers were liable to complications arising from gallstones, were frequently depressed by their condition, and were sometimes persecuted by neighbours.[36] But there was never any drive to persuade carriers to subject themselves to operations.

Newman continued to emphasise factors other than carriers in the prevention of enteric fever. In prefaces of reports dealing with outbreaks, he warned about the need for vigilance regarding the maintenance and improvement of water supplies.[37] And in commenting on a paratyphoid outbreak caused by contaminated milk, he condemned the MOH for allowing a suspected case to be nursed at home.[38] Undiagnosed cases, rather than healthy carriers, were a consistent theme, and in connection with a water-borne outbreak in 1932 involving 270 people, Newman emphasised the importance of clinical observation in early diagnosis.[39] In 1933 he commented that the carrier problem could be exaggerated and that it was impractical for central or local government to systematically identify, segregate and treat carriers. Even if such action was taken, it was not certain that it would prove effective. The only feasible approach was to take action only when carriers were identified during the investigation of outbreaks.[40] It was Newman's view that typhoid control could not rest on a single factor and this position was reinforced by an eighteen-year programme of 'experimental epidemiology' supported by the MRC and published in 1936. The authors, led by Major Greenwood, discussed the results of experiments on 'mouse typhoid' in relation to typhoid during the First World War. They concluded that it was the 'whole system of hygienic organisation' that was responsible for the low incidence of typhoid among the

---

[35] *Annual Report of the Scottish Board of Health for 1920*, Edinburgh, 1921, pp. 59–60.

[36] Browning, *Chronic Enteric Carriers*, pp. 20–1.

[37] G. Newman, 'Prefatory note', in W. V. Shaw, *Report to the Minister of Health on an Epidemic of Enteric Fever at Bolton-upon-Dearne*, RPHMS, No. 12, London, 1922.

[38] G. Newman, 'Prefatory note', in W. V. Shaw, *Report on an Outbreak of Paratyphoid Fever in the Borough of Chorley*, RPHMS, No. 30, London, 1925.

[39] G. Newman, 'Prefatory note' in W. V. Shaw, *Report on an Outbreak of Enteric Fever in the Malton Urban District*, RPHMS, No. 69, London, 1933.

[40] *RCMO 1932*, p. 58.

troops.[41] Elsewhere, Greenwood indicated that he thought that existing preventive methods were succeeding. He remarked of enteric fevers:

> I know of no other illnesses in respect of which the evidence of man's theoretical and practical capacity to control them is so cogent. I have little love of the violent metaphors of conquering or stamping out this or that sickness, but they might be applied here with less exaggeration than in many branches of practical epidemiology.[42]

Typhoid was beginning to be considered as a disease of the past. A speaker at the section of hygiene and public health of the 1937 meeting of the British Medical Association remarked that typhoid was now 'almost a clinical curiosity'.[43]

This remark was made shortly after an investigation into a major outbreak in Bournemouth, Poole and Christchurch, and a few months previously an outbreak in Croydon, and a further outbreak in Hawick. These were traced to carriers and showed that optimism about the imminent disappearance of typhoid was misplaced. They also put the Ministry of Health's policy on carriers under strain. It is worth recounting these events, since they raised several issues which emerged during the typhoid outbreaks of 1963 to 1964. These include the responsibilities of MOsH and their relationship with GPs, and the role of the press.

The outbreak on the south coast of England during August and September 1936 became known as the 'Bournemouth' outbreak. The early cases were traced to raw milk from a particular dairy, which was allowed to remain trading on condition that its milk was pasteurised. A farm supplying the dairy was eventually identified where the cows drank from a river containing sewage from a cottage inhabited by a carrier. The milk was believed to have become infected from the exterior of the udders or even from the bacteria passing through the cows. Approximately 718 people contracted the disease, 200 of whom were visitors and 518 residents. Mortality was just over 10 per cent.[44]

The handling of the Bournemouth outbreak was controversial, and an 'Anti-Typhoid League' criticised the local authorities for not announcing the outbreak soon enough and distributing notices giving details of symptoms and prophylactic measures. They were accused of concealing the facts in the hope of protecting the local economy, which was heavily dependent on the holiday

---

[41] M. Greenwood, A. B. Hill, W. W. C. Topley and J. Wilson, *Experimental Epidemiology*, MRCSRS, No. 209, London, 1936, p. 138.

[42] Greenwood, *Epidemics*, p. 138.

[43] J. Ritchie, 'Enteric fever', *BMJ*, 1937, vol. 2, pp. 160–3.

[44] 'Bournemouth typhoid outbreak official report', *BMJ*, 1937, vol. 1, p. 1182; H. G. Smith, 'The Bournemouth, Poole and Christchurch Typhoid Epidemic', *Public Health*, 1937, vol. 50, pp. 295–6.

trade. There were also complaints that patients who could have been nursed at home had been forced to enter isolation hospitals. A judge was appointed to hold an enquiry, which sat for five days in private at Bournemouth Town Hall. He reported in favour of the local authorities. He noted that the early symptoms of typhoid, paratyphoid and food poisoning were difficult to differentiate, and that laboratory tests did not give immediate results. He concluded that officials would have been unwise to sponsor an 'alarmist Press announcement of an existing typhoid epidemic' as soon as the first indications appeared. He thought that the early distribution of notices would have generated public alarm and that there was no attempt to conceal the facts once the situation was established, and he dismissed the allegation of unnecessary hospitalisation, quoting evidence showing that the death rate was highest among those nursed at home.[45]

A *Medical Officer* editorial approved of these findings, commenting that the outbreak had been 'kept quiet', not 'hushed up', and if sensationalised in the press, it would have 'passed out of control completely'. On the other hand, the editorial suggested there should have been a more efficient method of communication with MOsH outside the area and that all MOsH should be informed about outbreaks by the Ministry of Health.[46] However, one doctor writing to the *BMJ* declared that rather than dealing with an outbreak quietly, after the first three notifications, authorities should be 'flaming publicity, with posters on every hoarding and warnings on every cinema screen'. He suggested that detailed advice should be issued, covering the boiling of water and milk, and strict attention to personal hygiene.[47]

The introduction to the official report on the outbreak by Arthur McNalty, Newman's successor, was the first such preface to refer to the carrier issue. Noting that in milk-borne outbreaks an 'unwitting human carrier' was usually involved, McNalty added that there were regulations for dealing with carriers once detected, but that 'it is then too late'. But rather than calling for new measures to detect and control carriers, McNalty remarked that 'the only practical way to reduce the risk of such outbreaks is by pasteurization'.[48] This reflected the ministry's orthodoxy on carriers, and echoed its agenda on pasteurisation. The ministry had been trying to encourage pasteurisation in the face of resistance from other government departments and pressure groups.[49] In his 1936 report, McNalty concluded his remarks on typhoid with comments similar to Newman's first report. He stressed the importance of

---

[45] 'The Bournemouth typhoid outbreak', *BMJ*, 1937, vol. 2, pp. 825–6.

[46] 'The south coast typhoid epidemic', *Medical Officer*, 1937, vol. 1, p. 185.

[47] W. M. Penny, 'Typhoid precautions', *BMJ*, 1937, vol. 2, pp. 1092–3.

[48] A. S. McNalty, 'Prefatory note', in W. V. Shaw, *Report on an Outbreak of Enteric Fever in the County Borough of Bournemouth and in the Boroughs of Poole and Christchurch*, RPHMS, No. 81, London, 1937.

[49] P. J. Atkins, 'The pasteurisation of England: the science, culture and health implications of food processing, 1900–1950', in Smith and Phillips, *Food, Science, Policy*, pp. 37–52.

hygiene in food preparation and spoke of the abolition of extensive typhoid outbreaks as 'one of the greatest triumphs of the nineteenth century'. He warned, however, that a 'constant watch must be maintained against neglect of those sanitary precautions which achieved that success and has since maintained it'.[50]

Bournemouth was followed by a water-borne outbreak in Croydon in late 1937, which led to a public enquiry, underlined the importance of maintaining a 'constant watch', and shook the confidence of public health doctors. The 310 cases and forty-two fatalities were almost certainly caused by a carrier among workmen repairing a well, from which untreated water was fed into the town's water supply. The carrier had suffered typhoid during the First World War, but was unaware of his status. During the outbreak, the press levelled numerous criticisms against Croydon's MOH. *Medical Officer* put this down to lack of understanding of epidemiology among the public and medical profession. The MOH was condemned for not tracing the source with certainty immediately after the initial notifications, and for blaming a well, although typhoid organisms could not be detected in the water. He allegedly failed to give local doctors sufficient warning of what was happening, and to enlist their full co-operation. *Medical Officer* was also highly critical of a speech on the co-ordination of the health services by Lord Dawson, President of the Royal College of Physicians. He suggested that committees of GPs could provide a new channel of communication between MOsH and local doctors, and that such committees would be useful during epidemics. *Medical Officer* declared such machinery useless: faster communication could be achieved by telephone calls and letters.[51]

As in Bournemouth, a committee of concerned citizens was formed, the South Croydon Typhoid Outbreak Committee, and it was their representations that led to the public enquiry. The enquiry was held before Harold Murphy, KC, with expert assessors representing medical and engineering expertise, and sat for seventeen days. The report, published in February 1938, found that lack of communication between the council's officers responsible for water supply and the MOH played a part in the outbreak. The borough engineer had not realised that the repairs would interrupt chlorination, and the workmen had not undergone medical examination. There was little direct criticism of the MOH, apart from the finding that he had not immediately suspected water as the source. However, in observing that there had been a delay in some cases coming to the MOH's attention, Murphy commented that closer GP–MOH communication was desirable, and he suggested that in large centres of population committees of GPs could assist such communication.[52] The BMJ favoured

[50] *RCMO 1936*, pp. 33–4.

[51] 'The Croydon epidemic', *Medical Officer*, 1937, vol. 59, pp. 222–3.

[52] H. L. Murphy, *Report on a Public Local Enquiry into an Outbreak of Typhoid Fever at Croydon*, London, 1939.

the creation of local medical committees to 'take the burden of local medical uneasiness and the interchange of information and opinion' from MOsH during outbreaks, but where no such committee existed, it would be better for the MOH to communicate directly with practitioners. And, although unsatisfactory, doctors should not regard the discovery of an epidemic through the press as an offence, since press publicity was much more rapid than correspondence or meetings.[53]

The Ministry of Health responded with an open letter which advised Croydon Town Council to appoint a specialised water engineer, and to ensure improved communication between their officers, and between the MOH and GPs.[54] The MOH complained in his report for 1937 that the enquiry 'placed heavy additional burdens' upon his department, since it started while the outbreak was ongoing. He warned that 'If this procedure is to form a precedent, then Medical Officers of Health will in future, when called upon to tackle an outbreak of epidemic disease, also have to take steps to protect themselves at the public enquiry held thereinto'.[55] The ministry also issued *Memorandum on Safeguards to be Adopted in the Administration of Water Undertakings*. This stated that clinical histories of workmen should be taken and Widal tests conducted, with bacteriological examination of excreta in the case of positive results. Workers should be suspended from work if suffering from diarrhoea, and detailed arrangements for urination and defecation by workmen were specified.[56]

A third outbreak occurred in Hawick in the South of Scotland, involving 107 cases and five deaths. After extensive investigations it was thought to have been caused by the contamination of cream by an employee who suffered a mild unrecognised attack of typhoid. A detailed analysis in the report of the Department of Health for Scotland for 1938 referred to the employee as 'a "carrier"', emphasising the uncertainty as to the precise cause of the outbreak. In comparison with his colleagues in Bournemouth and Croydon, the MOH for Hawick handled the local press and medical practitioners effectively. The press was used to advise householders of hygienic precautions, and to reassure visitors that there was little risk of infection. And the regular meetings maintained 'close and harmonious co-operation between all the medical men concerned' which 'greatly facilitated the handling of the epidemic and helped to reassure the public that everything possible was being done'.[57]

Although the three large outbreaks were attributed certainly or probably to carriers, proposals for new arrangements for their control were tentative.

---

[53] 'Considerations from Croydon', *BMJ*, 1938, vol. 1, pp. 394–5.

[54] 'Croydon typhoid report: The minister's views', *BMJ*, 1938, vol. 1, pp. 530–1.

[55] 'Croydon epidemic of typhoid', *BMJ*, 1938, vol. 2, p. 1059.

[56] Ministry of Health, *Memorandum on Safeguards to be Adopted in the Administration of Water Undertakings*, London, 1939.

[57] *RDHS 1938*, Edinburgh, 1939, pp. 207–27.

At a meeting of the fever hospitals group of the Society of Medical Officers of Health in January 1938, one speaker suggested that the powers of MOsH to control carriers might need reviewing.[58] However, McNalty's report for 1938, which included a thirteen-page chapter on enteric fevers, made it clear that no changes to the policies set out by Newman were envisaged. McNalty stated:

> It is hardly practical for central or local authorities to take action with a view to the systematic identification, segregation and treatment of chronic carriers, and it is by no means certain that even if practicable, such action would be effective. It is, moreover, not possible to take a census of all the typhoid and paratyphoid carriers in a population, or, if ascertained, to compel them to undergo the various treatments suggested, some of which involve very serious operative measures.[59]

But when the ministry reiterated these policies in a *Memorandum on Typhoid Fever*[60] in November 1939, *Medical Officer* responded with sharp criticisms. Referring to an obituary of Typhoid Mary, who died in 1938, the journal compared the American and British legislation, commenting that the Public Health Regulations 1927 'prescribes a complicated process for obtaining powers to do nothing'. Abroad, and a few places in Britain, carriers were systematically identified and scheduled,[61] and the journal claimed that they could be controlled if powers were created to compel carriers 'to submit to such supervision as the safety of the public health demands'.[62]

The ministry's *Memorandum* also drew comment from Arthur Felix of the Lister Institute. Felix had devised a modified Widal test for an antibody to a particular *Salmonella typhi* antigen, the V_i or 'virulence' antigen, which he had discovered. He regarded this as more reliable as a screening test for the identification of suspected carriers, who might then be subjected to further investigation. The *Memorandum* remarked that the new test was not yet available for routine testing, but Felix complained that this was out of date: the reagents were now available from the Oxford Standards Laboratory of the MRC.[63]

All in all, typhoid declined in inter-war Britain, but it could still give pause for thought, as shown by the outbreaks of 1936 to 1938. These outbreaks, and the enquiries into them, soon featured in public health and water engineering textbooks, and probably conditioned the thinking of public health professionals, especially those in training, such as Ian MacQueen, MOH for

---

[58] 'Prevention and treatment of the enteric diseases', *BMJ*, 1938, vol. 1, pp. 252–3.

[59] *RCMO 1938*, pp. 43–56, at p. 53.

[60] Ministry of Health, *Memorandum on Typhoid Fever*, London, 1939.

[61] Glasgow was one place where a register was maintained. At the end of 1938 there were twenty-six carriers on the list, all women. 'Typhoid in Glasgow', *Medical Officer*, 1939, vol. 62, p. 253.

[62] 'Typhoid carriers', *Medical Officer*, 1939, vol. 62, pp. 252–3.

[63] A. Felix, 'Test for V_i antibody', *BMJ*, 1939, vol. 2, p. 1253.

Aberdeen in 1964. In terms of policy outcomes, the most significant change was the introduction of near-universal chlorination, and other procedures to ensure water safety. However, the three outbreaks were localised affairs and were not followed up by widespread, intensive and prolonged publicity or health education campaigns, which might have created a strong and widespread awareness of typhoid and its causes. Locally, the events of 1936 to 1938 did create strong memories of the disease. In Croydon, for example, the local press took a special interest in the Aberdeen outbreak twenty-three years later.[64] But there was nothing on the scale of Bournemouth, Croydon or Hawick in the recent experiences of Aberdeen and the three English towns that experienced the outbreaks of 1963 and 1964. In Aberdeen, for example, after a milk-borne outbreak in 1918 involving 101 cases and fourteen deaths, the worst outbreak occurred in 1935 when six died out of thirty-nine cases. Twenty-eight of the patients had eaten cold meats – cooked tripe or 'potted head' – from the same small shop. In the counties of Aberdeen and Kincardine, the worst outbreaks occurred in 1939 in Old Deer and Peterhead, where there were eight and twelve cases respectively.[65] But none of these events approached anything like the disasters that had visited Bournemouth and Croydon, or even the less dramatic outbreak in Hawick.

Typhoid and the Second World War

When the Emergency Medical Service was established in June 1938, medical scientists were presented with opportunities to pursue their ambitions for the development of their disciplines' infrastructures. Bacteriologists argued that the expected aerial bombing would disrupt water supplies and sewerage, resulting in epidemics of diseases such as typhoid, leading to the creation of a network of public health laboratories. Since the epidemics failed to materialise, however, the scientists seconded to the service were able to devote time to the development and application of new microbiological techniques.[66] Studies of *Salmonella typhi* had already led to the technique of phage typing, which relied upon the work of Felix at the Lister Institute, but was devised by James Craigie and a colleague in Canada.[67] Felix had discovered the V_i antigen in 1934, and besides an improved diagnostic test, this also led to what was claimed to be an improved vaccine and an improved anti-serum, as well as

---

[64] Leslie Hadfield, 'Take heart from Croydon', *P&J*, 5 June 1964, p. 1a.

[65] Russell, 'Typhoid fever', pp. 31–2.

[66] G. S. Wilson, 'The Public Health Laboratory Service', *BMJ*, 1948, vol. 1, pp. 627–31, 677–82.

[67] J. Craigie and C. H. Yen, 'Demonstration of types of B. typhosus by means of preparations of Type II V_i phage: stability and epidemiological significance', *Canadian Journal of Public Health*, 1938, vol. 29, p. 484; A. Felix, 'Experiences with typing of typhoid bacilli by means of V_i bacteriophage', *BMJ*, 1943, vol. 1, pp. 435–8.

phage typing. In 1939 Felix was seconded to the Emergency Public Health Laboratory Service (EPHLS) and during the war the value of phage typing in field studies was demonstrated. For example, in 1943, W. H. Bradley of the Ministry of Health described how he traced the origin of some sporadic cases over two years to a farm a hundred miles away. He concluded his paper by encouraging a more vigorous approach to the control of carriers. According to Bradley, while it was understandable that, during outbreaks, efforts should focus on limiting spread through sanitary engineering, he thought that the 'final objective – the elimination of the usual reservoir, the undetected persistent human carrier – must . . . be pursued no less vigorously'. Using phage typing, the chronic carrier could be identified:

> . . . no less precisely than can the criminal by his finger-print. Moreover, like the criminal, he is apt to leave this 'finger-print' at the scene of his crimes, where it may provide a specific clue leading to his detection . . . Since infection, like the criminal, does not respect administrative boundaries, there is clearly a need for the equivalent of the Central Criminal Investigation Department.[68]

The EPHLS was beginning to establish a 'finger-print bureau' for typhoid carriers. Bradley noted, however, that the observations and deductions of fieldworkers and the assistance of practitioners and MOsH were also required if the kinds of mysteries as those described in his paper were to be solved. The 'criminal investigation' metaphor seems to have been an aspect of the initial enthusiasm for and celebration of the potential of the new technique, but this way of demonising the typhoid carrier was an uncommon and transitory phenomenon.

Wilson Jameson, McNalty's successor as CMO from 1940, initially gave little encouragement to those in favour of closer monitoring of carriers. According to Jameson, in areas suffering outbreaks, which might be expected to produce new carriers, the incidence of the disease in successive years was typically unexceptional. The risk of allowing carriers to handle food supplies had led American cities to introduce routine examination and certification of food workers, but Jameson commented that 'no such powers will compel personal cleanliness which is a day to day, if not hour to hour, matter. It is not surprising, therefore, that the [American] requirements proved comparatively valueless.' In accordance with this viewpoint, an official circular sent by the ministry to local authorities in November 1940, after a rise in the number of notifications of enteric fever (especially paratyphoid which is usually food-borne), emphasised the importance of caterers and food handlers maintaining a high standard of personal cleanliness.[69]

---

[68] W. H. Bradley, 'An epidemiological study of bact. typhosum D4', *BMJ*, 1943, vol. 1, pp. 438–41.
[69] *RCMO 1939–45*, pp. 38–40.

Jameson commented that for practical purposes the experience of the war served merely to emphasise what was already known, that:

> . . . for infection to take place, excreta must be conveyed to some article of food either by the hands which have themselves been fouled . . . or by sewage by its access to a water supply. The former is entirely a matter of a decent standard of personal cleanliness which cannot be ensured by legislation but only by education; the latter is a communal affair of a purely impersonal kind and therefore susceptible to easier treatment.[70]

Jameson emphasised personal cleanliness to a greater extent than his predecessors, and during the war food hygiene messages were delivered to the public along with propaganda concerning rationing and nutrition. These messages reflected not only anxiety about enteric fevers, but also concern about the increasing incidence of food poisoning.

Phage typing, antibiotics and the achievement of control 1945 to 1954

In 1945 the EPHLS was transformed into the PHLS, and Felix joined the staff, becoming Director of the Central Enteric Reference Laboratory at Colindale. Despite Jameson's views, the momentum generated by the development and deployment of phage typing soon led to proposals for an ongoing programme to identify carriers that won Ministry of Health support. Phage typing, as a powerful but complicated procedure not easily devolved to peripheral laboratories, encouraged the centralisation of this form of bacteriological surveillance. The PHLS placed its facilities at the service of MOsH in the interests of investigating victims of typhoid or paratyphoid, and identifying persistent carriers. Jameson was fully behind these moves, commenting in his report for 1946 that a register of enteric carriers would allow their employment in the food trade to be avoided. As an example he referred to a recent typhoid outbreak in Aberystwyth traced to ice-cream sold by a carrier. It involved 210 cases and four deaths.[71] During 1947, Felix and Craigie published a standardised method of phage typing, and the International Congress for Microbiology recommended that it be adopted universally. An International Committee for Enteric Phage Typing was formed, and Felix's laboratory became the international reference laboratory.[72] In his report for 1947,

---

[70] Ibid., p. 40.

[71] RCMO 1946, pp. 35–6. See also D. J. Evans, 'An account of an outbreak of typhoid fever due to infected ice-cream in the Aberystwyth Borough during the summer of 1946', *Medical Officer*, 1947, vol. 77, pp. 39–44.

[72] J. Craigie, 'Arthur Felix', *Biographical Memoirs of Fellows of the Royal Society*, 1957,

Jameson declared that the laboratory was playing an indispensable part in enteric control, and emphasised that phage typing depended upon the efforts of clinicians and bacteriologists in isolating bacteria and submitting samples. MOsH could encourage these efforts and would be rewarded by a greater knowledge of enteric fever in their districts.[73]

Although Jameson was convinced of the value of a national register of carriers, he remained ambivalent about large-scale screening. He discussed the problem of carriers among immigrants, but suggested that screening them would involve a huge operation, out of proportion to the benefits. In addition, when he discussed the powers of MOsH, he was less concerned with long-term carriers than with the management of recovering but contagious patients. This was highlighted by an outbreak of paratyphoid in which, in view of a bed shortage, twelve hospitals were used, some patients being accommodated at considerable distances from their homes. In these circumstances, nine patients walked out before they were declared free from infection.[74]

As we have seen, Jameson encouraged submission of samples to the PHLS, but the national register was not developed through a systematic campaign to encourage MOsH to obtain samples from known or suspected carriers, regardless of outbreaks.[75] Instead, elements of the inter-war approach remained: efforts to phage type the organisms in the bodies of carriers were concentrated upon those responsible for, and generated by, outbreaks. The PHLS was most concerned to ensure that MOsH attempted to identify such carriers after outbreaks using the V_i test.[76] But some MOsH were even unaware of the existence of the register, since in 1957, in a paper on 'The future of notification of infectious disease', one remarked that 'A national register of typhoid carriers would be useful'.[77] Certainly, the construction of the register was undertaken in such a way that it did nothing to raise awareness of typhoid and the carrier problem among the public.

Doctors studying the CMO's reports could not fail to be impressed by the work carried out using the Enteric Reference Laboratory's services. The report for 1948, for example, outlined how the source of a series of sporadic paratyphoid cases in a north Devon town had been identified. It showed that there was also room for innovation by the peripheral laboratories. The Exeter Public Health Laboratory devised a method of tracing a source of infection through

---

vol. 3, pp. 53–82; C. Andrews, 'James Craigie', *Biographical Memoirs of Fellows of the Royal Society*, 1979, vol. 25, pp. 233–40.

[73] *RCMO 1947*, p. 50.

[74] Ibid., pp. 49–50. See also 'Compulsory segregation of carriers?', *Lancet*, 1947, vol. 2, p. 474.

[75] A. Felix, 'Laboratory control of the enteric fevers', *British Medical Bulletin*, 1951, vol. 7, pp. 153–62.

[76] *RCMO 1951*, p. 69.

[77] J. L. Patton, 'The future of notification of infectious disease', *Public Health*, 1958, vol. 72, pp. 7–16, at p. 14.

sewers by means of swabs dangled down manholes, and examination of the swabs for enteric organisms, using new selective culture media. Jameson reached an ambitious conclusion:

> The object of every enteric investigation should be to find and render innocuous the source, be it patient or carrier, and this should be attempted not only in relation to outbreaks but also in every sporadic case of enteric fever.[78]

Year on year, the CMO's report included remarkable detective stories relying upon phage typing and sewer swabs.[79] Such stories continued after Felix's retirement in 1953, when he was succeeded by a co-worker, E. S. Anderson.

Some outbreaks singled out by the CMO were not as successfully explained as those in north Devon. One involved 122 cases at a special hospital at Oswestry, Shropshire. Thirty-two patients and eighty-eight staff were involved, and there were seven fatalities. Despite extensive investigations of food handlers, staff, patients, and water and milk supplies, the origin of the outbreak was not discovered, although phage typing allowed a local carrier to be ruled out. Besides milk, other foods were considered, but dismissed on the grounds that they could not account for the high attack rate among nurses and the absence of typhoid among other local consumers.[80]

The Oswestry outbreak was reconsidered in the light of the 1963 to 1964 typhoid outbreaks, as was an outbreak centred on the village of Crowthorne in Berkshire, which was described in Jameson's report for 1949. During the investigations in Crowthorne, suspicion fell upon a butcher, and the corned beef he supplied appeared to be the common factor. Some of those involved in the investigation were sceptical about corned beef as the vehicle of infection, until it emerged that a woman contracted the disease after sharing corned beef sandwiches brought to her from the village. A total of forty-two people were infected. The outbreak provided an opportunity to test the antibiotic chloromycetin, which had been shown to be effective against typhoid in 1948,[81] but, nevertheless, two patients died. The corned beef was understood to have originated from a number of tins, and in most cases had been cut with a knife. This suggested that the knife was the immediate source of contamination. As for the remote source, this was not discovered. No member of staff was a carrier, and known local carriers harboured organisms of a different phage type. Jameson noted, however, that the shop used coverings from imported mutton carcasses as wiping cloths and thought it possible that these could have

---

78 *RCMO 1948*, p. 82.

79 *RCMO 1950*, pp. 66–7.

80 *RCMO 1948*, pp. 74–80.

81 T. E. Woodward, J. E. Woodward, H. L. Ley, R. Green and D. S. Mankikar, 'Preliminary report on the beneficial effect of chloromycetin in treatment of typhoid fever', *Annals of Internal Medicine*, 1948, vol. 29, pp. 131–4.

become infected with *Salmonella typhi* in transit. The lesson he drew was that the incident illustrated the hazards of selling loose corned beef with raw meat.[82]

A paper by the MOH for Crowthorne suggests that the criticisms faced by his counterparts during 1936 and 1937 had not gone unnoticed. Early on in the outbreak, although corned beef was under suspicion, the population was advised, by means of a loudspeaker van, to boil water and milk. Every evening the MOH or a colleague phoned each local doctor, and they, in turn, went to some lengths to explain to their patients what was going on.[83] Yet in neither Jameson's nor in the MOH's accounts of the incident is there any discussion of the possibility that the corned beef was already contaminated when it arrived at the shop. One member of staff of the local public health laboratory speculated on the source of infection in the same way as Jameson, adding: 'It was certain that the corned beef was not infected in the tin.'[84]

Despite loose ends such as those left by the Oswestry and Crowthorne investigations, by 1953, the CMO, now John Charles, was celebrating the achievement of control over enteric fever. In his report for 1952 he reproduced a graph showing trends in typhoid mortality, demonstrating that mortality rates in England and Wales were now well below those in other European countries. He declared that the favourable results 'reflect the close investigation of each case of enteric fever in the field and the laboratory', and heaped praise upon Felix and his staff. Inspection of the graph, however, suggests that the role of the new techniques was, at best, to accelerate a well-established downward trend. Furthermore, the widening gap between England and Wales and the other countries during the 1940s may have been largely a result of their slight social disruption compared with war-torn Europe.[85]

As for notifications of typhoid between 1948 and 1952, in England they declined from 369 to 135 and dropped to 101 during the following year. In Scotland, there was a sharp decline from an average of ninety-five notifications per year from 1941 to 1945 to only thirty-five cases in 1949. Aberdeen and the North-East contributed few cases to these totals except in 1947, when six cases occurred at the Royal Mental Hospital in Aberdeen. In the report of the Department of Health for Scotland for 1949, typhoid was described as 'rare'.[86] Declining further to only thirteen cases in 1952 and remaining low, the report for 1954 commented that 'apart from the accidental contamination of foodstuffs by carriers or excretors, an event which is apparently becoming rare as the years go by, the prevalence . . . is likely to diminish'.[87]

[82] *RCMO 1949*, pp. 69–72.
[83] W. B. Moore, 'Typhoid fever, with particular reference to the Crowthorne epidemic, 1949', *Journal of the Royal Sanitary Institute*, 1950, vol. lxx, pp. 93–101.
[84] Ibid., p. 100.
[85] *RCMO 1952*, pp. 53–4.
[86] *RDHS 1949*, p. 14.
[87] *RDHS 1954*, p. 28.

For the remaining cases, chloramphenicol, a synthetic form of chloromycetin, had become available since 1950, and it was soon suggested that the antibiotic might be used to treat carriers. To this end experiments were conducted on carriers in mental hospitals, but the results were inconclusive.[88] During the 1950s there was also a new research effort into the effectiveness of vaccines, including a series of field trials carried out by the WHO. These showed that the 'improved' vaccine developed by Felix conferred no obvious protection, while the traditional heat-phenolised vaccine was 70 per cent effective.[89]

New threats

During the 1940s and 1950s, with chlorination of drinking water and pasteurisation of milk now almost universal, the incidence of water- and milk-borne enteric fever declined and threats from other sources became more visible. In 1949, Bradley commented upon risks associated with an increase in communal eating, and the mass production and wide distribution of food.[90] But how some novel vehicles of infection became contaminated remained unknown, as in the Crowthorne case. Another example was paratyphoid associated with synthetic cream bakery products, which became apparent after the number of cases in England and Wales increased from 291 in 1950 to 1094 in 1951, remaining at 1038 in 1952.[91] The incidents included a series of outbreaks in South Wales, connected with products from several bakeries, which accounted for nearly half of the notifications in 1952. No evidence could be found that the synthetic cream was infected when it arrived at the bakers.[92] The only common factor was the mill supplying flour, and the outbreaks were provisionally attributed to a paratyphoid carrier among the mill workers. There was much scepticism as to whether flour could really act as a vehicle, but experiments seemed to indicate that this was possible.[93] In 1953, the number of paratyphoid cases in England and Wales dropped to 353, but the incidence remained variable, rising to 876 in 1958. Bakery products were again implicated, but this time the source was attributed to frozen bulked egg from China. Imported egg now seemed a possible cause of the earlier outbreaks and others associated with synthetic cream and bakery products dating to 1940.[94] The incidence of paratyphoid remained higher than

---

88 *RCMO 1950*, p. 40; *RCMO 1952*, p. 53; *RCMO 1954*, p. 53; *RCMO 1956*, p. 50.
89 Russell, 'Typhoid fever', p. 16.
90 W. H. Bradley, 'The control of typhoid fever', *Public Health*, 1949, vol. 62, pp. 159–63.
91 *RCMO 1952*, p. 55.
92 Ibid., p. 56. See also A. R. Culley, 'An account of paratyphoid fever in South Wales, 1952', *Medical Officer*, 1953, vol. 89, pp. 243–9, 257–62.
93 *RCMO 1953*, p. 80.
94 *RCMO 1955*, pp. 56, 86–7.

that of typhoid in England and Wales for every year up to and including 1963, except for 1962, when there were 130 cases of typhoid and 126 cases of paratyphoid. In Scotland, the incidence of paratyphoid was consistently higher than typhoid. Total notifications of typhoid were as low as twelve in 1951, and exceeded twenty during only three years in the 1950s. The report of the Department of Health for Scotland described typhoid as 'under control' in 1960, and 'very rare' in 1963.[95] Annual cases of paratyphoid during the 1950s, in contrast, varied between thirty-nine in 1950 to 155 in 1955. And in 1963 there was an outbreak in Edinburgh amounting to around 200 notifications, associated with imported bulked egg.[96]

As for novel sources of typhoid, Charles pointed to a possible new source when he devoted several paragraphs of his 1954 report to a 'curious incident' in Birmingham. A can of foul-smelling imported sterilised cream was found to be contaminated with *Salmonella typhi*. On investigation, 17 per cent of 1955 cans were shown to contain living bacteria, although the typhoid bacillus was not recovered from any further cans. The British Food Manufacturing Industries Research Association advised that the cans were of a type liable to imperfect sealing, and the factory revealed that at the time of processing the batch in question, the usual cooling water supply was not available, and so water from a well and stream was used. The CMO conjectured that the typhoid organism must have entered the can during cooling, and had probably entered other cans too, but as the contents seemed unwholesome, many were probably thrown away without consumption. Only 'one suggestive case of sub-clinical typhoid' was traced among the people who had consumed the cream.[97]

The tinned cream incident was referred to again in the next annual report. Typhoid notifications increased from 122 in 1954 to 193 in 1955, due to an unusually large number of small outbreaks, the most significant involving twenty-eight cases in Pickering, Yorkshire. The common factor was cold meat purchased from the same grocer. Twenty of the twenty-one primary cases had purchased sliced canned tongue, while one purchased ham cut with the knife used for the tongue. The CMO remarked that the manufacturer of the tongue was 'of the highest repute', and that examinations of other cans were all negative. The most reasonable explanation was that 'the contents of one particular can . . . had been infected, either at the time of canning or subsequently, conceivably from the entry of infected material through a temporary pin-hole perforation'.[98] A paper on the outbreak was published in 1956 by the

---

95 *RDHS 1960*, p. 28.
96 *RDHS 1950–62*; *RSHHD 1963*, p. 17. The problem of contaminated egg products had received less attention in Scotland prior to this point. The topic was mentioned in *RDHS 1956*, but the problem was stated to be under control the following year (*RDHS 1956*, p. 23; *RDHS 1957*, p. 27; J. C. Sharp, P. P. Brown and G. Sangster, 'Outbreak of Paratyphoid in the Edinburgh area', *British Medical Journal*, 1964, vol. 1, pp. 1282–5.
97 *RCMO 1954*, pp. 53, 71.
98 *RCMO 1955*, pp. 54–5.

MOH for the area, W. R. Couper, with members of staff of the local public health laboratory and the PHLS epidemiological research laboratory. This included a detailed discussion of the canning process. The suspect can was one of 35,000 produced during 1954, but the factory's owners had not received any other complaints. The factory was next to a fast-flowing river from which its water supplies were drawn. The cooling water was not chlorinated and the factory was situated downstream from a sewage works outlet. It was therefore surmised that the infection had entered the can from the cooling water through a temporary self-sealing seam defect. Since *Salmonella typhi* is a non-gas-producing organism, the problem would not be revealed by the usual fifteen-day incubation period that tested for defective cans.[99] The authors discussed several other outbreaks that may have been caused by contaminated canned meat, including the Crowthorne outbreak and others in 1938 and 1943.

Despite the efforts of Couper and his colleagues to link the Pickering and previous outbreaks, the affair remained an epidemiological curiosity. Compared to the highly publicised Croydon outbreak, it was a small affair which led to no policy response from the Ministry of Health. There were no similar incidents in the late 1950s to stimulate action. In England and Wales, as the annual notifications of typhoid hovered between 123 and 150, the CMO began to refer to the number of cases contracted through overseas travel. Such comments first appeared in the report for 1953, when Charles drew attention to cases occurring in late summer as a result of European holiday travel. He advised travellers to consult their general practitioner or MOH before travelling,[100] and emphasised this point annually for both typhoid and paratyphoid. During 1956, twenty-two out of 136 cases and during 1959 one-third of 123 cases of typhoid were acquired abroad. By this time a pamphlet, *Notice to Travellers*, issued by the Ministry of Health and the Department of Health for Scotland, advised travellers to be inoculated with the TAB vaccine.[101] Besides the cases contracted abroad, the remaining outbreaks were mostly sporadic, caused by a carrier through a lapse of domestic hygiene and confined to a single household, but there were occasional larger outbreaks traced to other sources of infection. For example, Charles' report for 1958 mentioned an outbreak associated with oysters, which involved twelve people.[102]

With a decline of typhoid notifications in England and Wales to only ninety in 1960, the lowest figure on record, there was a strong indication of the

99   W. R. M. Couper, K. W. Newell and D. J. H. Payne, 'An outbreak of typhoid fever associated with canned ox-tongue', BMJ, 1956, vol. 1, pp. 1057–9.
100   *RCMO 1953*, p. 54.
101   *RCMO 1959*, p. 53.
102   *RCMO 1958*, pp. 50–1.

infection being contracted abroad in 43 per cent of cases.[103] The figures were much the same for 1961, but the CMO, now George Godber, reminded readers of his annual report of the continuing threat from carriers. He mentioned an outbreak involving four children from one family and a playmate infected by a grandmother who had suffered typhoid fifty-four years earlier.[104] In 1962, with a jump in the total notifications to 130, half of which were contracted abroad, the threat of the importation of typhoid by travellers appeared to be increasing.[105] This trend was dramatically illustrated in 1963 by the impact in Britain of the large water-borne outbreak in Zermatt, Switzerland. In England and Wales a total of sixty-nine cases of typhoid associated with Zermatt were confirmed bacteriologically, among whom there was one death. Sixty-eight people, all of whom had visited Zermatt, became sick within about a month from 21 February, with one secondary case occurring in April. Only three had been given a TAB inoculation within the previous twelve months, and Godber drew attention to *Notice to Travellers*.[106]

It seems that on the eve of the outbreaks of 1963 to 1964, typhoid was largely a historical disease in Britain. Any continuing threat came either from abroad or from carriers, but most outbreaks were confined to single families. Techniques for identifying sources, and the treatment of cases, were well developed. By 1962, seventy-two phage types of the bacillus had been identified,[107] and antibiotics had reduced the death rate to about 1 per cent. As for the threat from abroad, the conveyance of infection by people rather than by foodstuffs received the greatest publicity, and in Aberdeen there had been little stimulus to public awareness of typhoid in the post-war period. There had been no cases notified in Aberdeen between 1953 and 1964, and only a handful of cases in the surrounding districts. Prior to the 1964 outbreak there were only two known carriers in the city.[108]

The prediction of the report for the Department of Health for Scotland 1954, that the prevalence of typhoid was 'likely to diminish',[109] proved broadly correct, the Aberdeen outbreak being the last major typhoid outbreak in Britain. By 1970 there were only eleven notifications of typhoid in Scotland, six of which were imported, and 159 in England, 122 of which originated abroad.[110] Since then, the total number of cases has increased, the proportion associated with overseas travel also increasing. In 1994, for example, of 227 cases in England, 221 were associated with travel abroad, most commonly to

---

[103] *RCMO 1960*, p. 44.
[104] *RCMO 1961*, p. 48.
[105] *RCMO 1962*, p. 36.
[106] *RCMO 1963*, pp. 42–5. *RDHS 1963* did not mention Zermatt.
[107] Huckstep, *Typhoid Fever*, p. 223.
[108] Russell, 'Typhoid fever', p. 33.
[109] *RDHS 1954*, p. 28.
[110] *RSHHD 1970*, p. 8; *RCMO 1970*, p. 45.

the Indian subcontinent.[111] In Scotland in 1994 there were twelve cases.[112] Occasional reminders of past problems have brought to mind the Zermatt episode rather than the corned beef outbreaks, for example, the thirty-two cases among British visitors to the Greek Island of Kos in 1983.[113] However, in spite of that incident, in 1984 the Joint Committee on Vaccination and Immunisation recommended that vaccination was not now needed for travellers to countries bordering the Mediterranean.[114]

The experience of paratyphoid has been similar. Following the major outbreak in Edinburgh associated with bulked egg during 1963, there was one in Clackmannan in 1964 involving seventy-nine cases. This was traced to a factory canteen, and probably a worker who had become infected while on holiday on the Continent.[115] There was a large milk-borne outbreak in Lancashire involving 750 people in 1965, and a water-borne outbreak in North Riding affecting eighty-nine people in 1970.[116] After this, large paratyphoid incidents became much rarer, but one involved thirty-eight people who attended the Indian Independence Day celebrations in Birmingham in 1988.[117] In 1994, 195 of the 217 cases of paratyphoid A and B in England were associated with travel abroad,[118] and there were only six cases of paratyphoid in Scotland.[119]

Arguably, by 1963, public awareness of and attitudes towards serious infectious diseases were conditioned more by publicity and experience of diseases such as pulmonary tuberculosis, poliomyelitis and smallpox than the enteric fevers. Pulmonary tuberculosis, like typhoid, was a disease in decline, but there had been recent mass screening campaigns for tuberculosis with a view to detecting and treating early cases.[120] There had been several large polio epidemics in Britain in the 1940s and 1950s, and many people knew a child disabled by the condition. Everyone had been exposed to the vaccination drives of the late 1950s and early 1960s. In 1961, an outbreak of poliomyelitis in Kingston-upon-Hull and the East Riding of Yorkshire was halted by a well-

[111] RCMO 1994, p. 190.
[112] *Scottish Health Statistics* 1997, p. 42, internet, http://www.show.scot.nhs.uk/isdonline/ Scottish_Health_Statistics/shs97/Sections/C2.PDF, accessed 1 April 2004.
[113] RCMO 1983, p. 49.
[114] RCMO 1984, p. 46.
[115] RSHHD 1964, pp. 17–18.
[116] RCMO 1970, pp. 46–9.
[117] 'Curry meal blamed for 38 food poisoning cases', *The Times*, 5 March 1988, p. 2b.
[118] RCMO 1965, pp. 128–9; RCMO 1994, p. 190.
[119] Information and Statistics Division, Common Services Agency, *Scottish Health Statistics* 1997, internet http://www.show.scot.nhs.uk/isdonline/Scottish_Health_Statistics/shs97/ Sections/C2.PDF, accessed 5 April 2004.
[120] I. M. Macgregor, *The Two-year Mass Radiography Campaign in Scotland 1957–1958: A Study of Tuberculosis Case-finding by Community Action*, Edinburgh, 1961; Office of Health Economics, *Progress against Tuberculosis*, London, 1962.

publicised emergency mass vaccination campaign.[121] Smallpox was rare in Britain, but wide publicity surrounded an outbreak in England and Wales in 1961 introduced by travellers from Pakistan.[122] These events may help to explain certain aspects of public reaction to the typhoid outbreaks of 1963 to 1964.

Unlike poliomyelitis, tuberculosis and smallpox, the typhoid outbreaks of 1963 to 1964 were associated with food. As mentioned above, however, they were generally regarded as food 'infections', systemic infections introduced via the mouth. Microbial 'food poisoning', in contrast, consisted mainly of irritation of the intestines caused by toxins produced by pathogenic organisms. The toxins might be in the food when consumed, or might be produced in the gut by organisms introduced by contaminated food.[123] These were tenuous distinctions, because some food poisoning organisms, especially in susceptible individuals such as the young or elderly, could invade the blood and organs. In addition, some strains of enteric organisms, especially of paratyphoid, produced only mild symptoms in some individuals. But no matter how typhoid was classified technically, the outbreaks of 1963 to 1964 raised questions of food hygiene. The historical contextualisation of these outbreaks would therefore be incomplete without considering the history of food poisoning and its prevention, and it is to this that we will now turn.

The history of food poisoning

Anne Hardy cites a Local Government Board investigation of an incident in Wellbeck, Nottinghamshire, in 1880 as an important episode in the history of food microbiology, and the creation of 'food poisoning' as a public health problem. For the first time in Britain, vomiting and diarrhoea were associated with living microbes in undercooked hams. Following Wellbeck, the Board began compiling a list of food poisoning outbreaks. Research was then stimulated by the discovery in 1888 of a bacillus named *B. enteritidis* (later *Salmonella enteritidis*) by Gustav Gaertner, which encouraged the expansion of public health into the area. In 1905 the Local Government Board created a food inspectorate as a subdivision of the health department, and commissioned research by William Savage, MOH for Colchester.[124] Savage spent the rest of

---

[121] Ministry of Health, *Report on the Outbreak of Poliomyelitis during 1961 in Kingston-upon-Hull*, RPHMS, No. 107, London, 1963.

[122] Ministry of Health, Scottish Health Service Advisory Council, *Memorandum on the Control of Outbreaks of Smallpox*, London, 1964.

[123] W. G. Savage, 'Acute Food Poisoning', *Public Health*, 1957, vol. 71, pp. 323–35, at p. 325.

[124] A. Hardy, 'Food, hygiene and the laboratory: a short history of food poisoning in Britain, circa 1850–1959', *Social History of Medicine*, 1999, vol. 12, pp. 293–331.

his life working on food poisoning. He published five reports prior to 1913, and *Food Poisoning and Food Infections* in 1920.[125] By this time, it was well known that most food poisoning was associated with meat and other animal products. Savage worked on the distribution of *Salmonellae* in the animal gut and the bacterial contamination of milk, and co-authored two MRC reports in 1925.[126] The recognition of 'animal reservoirs' of infection highlighted the complexity of food poisoning and the need for a multi-dimensional preventative policy addressing animal health, meat hygiene, the control of vermin, and personal and domestic habits.[127]

In 1921, the Ministry of Health issued a memorandum to MOsH on the procedures to be undertaken when investigating food poisoning, which was superseded by a further memorandum in 1935.[128] However, few outbreaks were thoroughly investigated, since in many areas laboratory facilities were not easily available. MOsH could send specimens to the ministry's laboratory, but few did so. Legislation covering hygiene in food trade premises was non-existent, and so concerned MOsH had to rely upon educational efforts aimed at improving personal hygiene and fly and vermin control.[129]

Worldwide, many scientists worked on *Salmonellae*, and the International Society of Microbiologists established a committee on nomenclature and taxonomy. By 1939, thirty-seven countries were engaged in intensive study of the organism, constituting what Hardy refers to as an 'international salmonella research industry', which, along with social changes accompanying the Second World War, decisively raised the profile of food poisoning as a public health problem.[130] But awareness of food poisoning was also boosted by the stimulus given to local action and data collection by legislation. The Public Health (London) Act, 1936, made food poisoning notifiable in the County of London, and from October 1939 notification was extended to England and Wales by the Food and Drugs Act, 1938.[131] Doctors were required to inform MOsH of food poisoning cases, allowing MOsH to investigate. There was no requirement for the information to be passed on to central authorities, but

---

[125] Savage, 'Acute food poisoning', p. 323; idem, *Food Poisoning and Food Infections*, Cambridge, 1920.

[126] W. G. Savage and P. Bruce White, *An Investigation of the Salmonella Group, with Special Reference to Food Poisoning*, MRCSRS, No. 91, London 1925; W. G. Savage and P. Bruce White, *Food Poisoning: A Study of 100 Recent Outbreaks*, MRCSRS, No. 92, London, 1925.

[127] A. Hardy, 'Food, hygiene', p. 302.

[128] E. B. Dewberry, *Food Poisoning, its Nature, History and Causation Measure for its Prevention and Control*, London, 1950, p. 12.

[129] Hardy, 'Food, hygiene', pp. 305, 308.

[130] Ibid., pp. 308–9.

[131] Dewberry, *Food Poisoning*, p. 70. Some background to the act is given in M. French and J. Phillips, *Cheated not Poisoned? Food Regulation in the United Kingdom 1875–1938*, Manchester, 2000, pp. 143–5.

information was collected by the EPHLS, an arrangement continued by the PHLS after 1945.

Educational efforts in the 1940s and early 1950s

The CMO's report for 1939 to 1945 reviewed the outbreaks in England and Wales during this period. The total declined from eighty-three in 1939 to forty-seven in 1940, and then increased, reaching 550 in 1944, and the CMO commented that the rise in communal feeding was probably responsible.[132] In the 1930s, school meals were confined to the poorest pupils, but the school meals service expanded during the war and from 1945 it was the Labour government's policy to make cheap or free meals available to all.[133] Likewise, prior to the war, most workers took food to work, but by the end of the war, in larger workplaces, they were eating in the work's canteen. For workers in smaller workplaces and the general public, the government had supported the establishment of 'British Restaurants'. These began to close soon after the war but the encouragement given to the eating-out habit benefited commercial establishments.[134]

During the second half of the 1940s, the number of outbreaks reported to the PHLS rose to 964 in 1948. *Salmonella* infections were by far the largest category in 1948, the *Salmonellae* accounting for 94 per cent of reported outbreaks.[135] During that year, in order to provide more accurate information, it was decided to instruct MOsH to include food poisoning cases in their weekly returns to the General Register Office, and to make quarterly returns of the total cases amended by reason of corrected diagnoses. This began from 1949.[136] Because of the impossibility of defining food poisoning precisely, the statistics generated would be far from perfect, but it was nevertheless thought desirable to collect additional information. A revised version of the ministry's memorandum gave details of the clinical features of different types of food poisoning, and detailed the field and laboratory investigations to be undertaken.[137]

Jameson's report for 1949 included precise definitions of the data presented. An 'outbreak' involved two or more related cases in different families (later referred to as a 'general outbreak'), and a 'family outbreak', two or more cases within the same family. A 'sporadic case' was, as far as was known, unrelated to other cases. The outbreaks, family outbreaks and sporadic cases were added

---

[132] *RCMO 1939–45*, p. 42.

[133] C. Webster, 'Government policy on school meals and welfare foods 1939–1970', in Smith, *Nutrition*, pp. 190–213.

[134] R. J. Hammond, *Food Volume II: Studies in Administration and Control*, London, 1956, pp. 351–423.

[135] *RCMO 1948*, pp. 48, 54.

[136] *RMH 31 March 1949*, London, 1950, p. 316.

[137] *RCMO 1948*, p. 54.

to give the number of 'incidents'. In 1949 there were 410 outbreaks, 265 family outbreaks and 1753 sporadic cases, or 2428 incidents. According to the 1949 report this amounted to an increase of 1467 incidents over 1948. The high number of sporadic cases recorded in 1949 largely accounts for the increase, which was partly due to the new reporting procedures. As Hardy suggests, the jump between 1948 and 1949 was also due to more patients consulting their doctors, now that they could do so for free under the NHS.[138] As for the total cases, according to the General Register Office figures, this amounted to 6111, but the reports received by the Ministry of Health suggested a figure nearer 11,000.[139] The apparent increase in food poisoning received press publicity and prompted the Ministry of Health and local authorities to intensify their educational activities. The ministry commissioned a film, *Another Case of Food Poisoning*, which was primarily for food industry operatives, but was also used at meetings organised by women's organisations. Between December 1949 and March 1950, there were 432 screenings.[140]

Compared to the Ministry of Health reports, much less space was devoted to food poisoning in the reports of the Department of Health for Scotland. Food poisoning was not notifiable in Scotland, but short paragraphs on the subject were included. Most incidents that came to the attention of the department were of a minor nature, affecting one or two people.[141] However, a few larger outbreaks were mentioned. In 1947, for example, there were two such incidents. In Perthshire, a hundred people were infected by contaminated artificial cream, and in Aberdeenshire a similar number of people were made ill by infected milk.[142] From 1949, the larger outbreaks were often associated with communal eating, such as school and factory canteens and restaurants. One involved contaminated reheated gravy served in several Glasgow schools.[143] Each year comments were made about the apparent increase or decrease in the number of outbreaks, but there was no indication of an overall upward trend in Scotland.

Like the Ministry of Health, the Department of Health for Scotland observed that public concern with food hygiene increased during 1949. The press was 'helping to form a well-informed public opinion on the subject', and the department encouraged local food hygiene education. Some authorities showed films at school meal centres, and issued notices stressing the need for personal hygiene to restaurants and shops. Talks for traders, women's guilds and other organisations were arranged.[144] *Another Case of Food Poisoning*

---

138 Hardy, 'Food, hygiene', p. 310.
139 *RCMO 1949*, p. 48.
140 *RMH 1950*, pp. 108–9.
141 *RDHS 1946*, p. 52.
142 *RDHS 1947*, p. 43.
143 *RDHS 1949*, pp. 56–7.
144 Ibid., pp. 50, 56.

was well used in Scotland, being screened 255 times between January and November 1950, and reaching 15,500 people. The department also produced posters that were distributed to local authorities and factories.[145]

In England, despite the educational efforts and publicity, the number of incidents reported in 1950 increased by 64 per cent, and the CMO thought it unlikely that this was all due to better ascertainment.[146] The ministry analysed outbreaks in terms of the places where the contaminated food was bought or eaten. Few outbreaks were associated with foods bought in shops, but 90 per cent were associated with communal eating. In 41 per cent of outbreaks, the food had been eaten in a canteen (school, works, municipal, service, other) while the corresponding figures for hospitals and institutions, and restaurants and hotels, were 33 per cent and 16 per cent.[147]

Regulations and trends in the 1950s and early 1960s

During the late 1940s three committees were appointed to consider meat inspection arrangements, and how sanitary conditions could be achieved within the meat manufacturing and catering trades. Their deliberations led to reports published in 1950 and 1951,[148] which paved the way for new legislation: in England and Wales the Food and Drugs (Amendment) Act 1954 and the Food and Drugs Act 1955, and, in Scotland, the Food and Drugs (Scotland) Act 1956.[149] During 1955, the new legislation, and the amalgamation of the Food and Agriculture ministries to form MAFF, began to create new arrangements for the preparation and implementation of food safety regulations in England and Wales. A Food Hygiene Advisory Council was created in May 1955, appointed by the Minister of Health and Minister of Agriculture, Fisheries and Food. This consisted of a chairman and representatives of the public, food trades and food trade workers. From 6 July 1955, the primary responsibilities for most food hygiene functions were transferred to the Ministry of Health. Only provisions concerning milk, and meat hygiene in slaughterhouses and in the course of importation remained the primary responsibility of MAFF. The main role of the Food Hygiene Advisory Council was to advise on draft regulations and codes of practice, and the first set of regulations, designed to strengthen local authorities in securing proper

---

145 *RDHS 1950*, pp. 57–8.

146 *RCMO 1950*, pp. 42–3.

147 Ibid., p. 47.

148 Ministry of Food, *Hygiene in Catering Establishments*, London, 1951; Ministry of Food, *Report of the Manufactured Meat Products Working Party*, London 1950; Ministry of Food, *Report of the Inter-departmental Committee on Meat Inspection*, London, 1950.

149 For a detailed study of the role of the catering establishments working party see M. French and J. Phillips, 'Windows and barriers in policy-making: food poisoning in Britain, 1945–56', *Social History of Medicine*, 2004, vol. 14, pp. 269–84.

standards, were issued on 16 December 1955.[150] The operative date was 1 January 1956, except for regulations involving substantial changes in premises, equipment or practices, which came into effect on 1 July 1956.

In England and Wales, the reported numbers of outbreaks and sporadic cases climbed to a peak in 1955. In his report for 1960, however, the CMO included some mildly hopeful remarks about a more recently apparent downward trend. He commented that there was a reduction in incidents during 1960 of 18 per cent compared with 1959 and 12 per cent compared with 1958. He noted that salmonellosis was the 'only serious food-poisoning problem in England and Wales', and pointed out that in 1960 there was a considerable reduction in the number of patients infected with *Salmonella* types normally associated with imported foods. During the 1950s there had been many reports of poisoning caused by contaminated imported egg, and detailed accounts of investigations by the PHLS. These showed that such products frequently contained many strains of *Salmonella*, including paratyphoid.[151] Previously, there was little evidence that the publicity or control measures had made much impact, but the decrease in 1960 suggested that the ministry's efforts were beginning to take effect.[152] The report for 1962 was similarly optimistic, commenting that for thirty-three weeks of the year, the incidence of food poisoning was the lowest since 1955 and in only twelve weeks was the figure above the median for the week in the period 1955 to 1961.[153] Dr Ross, who was responsible for food hygiene at the Ministry of Health, commented at a Food Hygiene Advisory Council meeting that recent statistics signalled 'a shift from large outbreaks to smaller incidents and sporadic cases showing . . . that the Food Hygiene Regulations had been mainly effective in their attack on the central sources of infection'.[154]

As for Scotland, after several false starts due to shortage of parliamentary time, a bill for the consolidation of food and drugs legislation reached the statute books in 1956, coming into force on 1 August 1957. This authorised the Secretary of State for Scotland to issue hygiene regulations prescribing food preparation and handling methods. It also introduced compulsory notification of food poisoning to MOsH from 1957. A Scottish Food Hygiene Council was appointed which helped prepare the Food Hygiene (Scotland) Regulations, 1959. The clauses dealing with hygienic practices and personal cleanliness came into force on 1 May 1959, which was declared 'Clean Food Day', and received widespread publicity. Over 30,000 copies of a guide to the

---

[150] *RMH 1955*, pp. 144–5.
[151] *RCMO 1955*, pp. 56, 61–2, 86–7; *RCMO 1956*, pp. 5, 53; *RCMO 1957*, pp. 58, 92–3, 165–7.
[152] *RCMO 1960*, p. 49.
[153] *RCMO 1962*, p. 57.
[154] Minutes of the seventeenth meeting of the Food Hygiene Advisory Council, 24 July 1962, PRO MAF 260/102.

regulations were sold, as were large numbers of notices to food workers and customers. Regulations dealing with the construction of premises became effective on 1 October 1959.[155] Following the introduction of the Scottish regulations, the food hygiene activities of local authorities shifted towards the inspection and improvement of commercial premises, and facilities in institutions, and away from the education of the public.[156] Courses were arranged for professionals such as sanitary inspectors,[157] but the responses of public health departments to the new legislation depended upon local initiative. In Aberdeen, attempts to organise food hygiene education met with mixed success. The Aberdeen department's innovative health education section, staffed by health visitors, produced two editions of an illustrated fifty-page *Clean Food Guide* published in 1957 and 1961.[158] However, there were insufficient staff to organise a campaign in connection with the introduction of the Scottish Food Hygiene Regulations, and a successful course for food handlers in 1961 was not repeated during 1963 and 1964 due to lack of interest.[159] In Aberdeen, between the introduction of notification and 1963, the number of notified cases varied from five to twenty-nine per year, the highest number occurring in 1961 when there was an incident involving contaminated food at a wedding party.[160]

Nationally, during 1957, the first year of official notification, 114 outbreaks involving 1332 cases were reported in Scotland.[161] The total number of outbreaks in 1958 was about the same, but in 1959 the figure dropped by about 30 per cent, prompting a comment that this may have been due to the introduction of the Food Hygiene (Scotland) Regulations. The decline was not sustained, however, and the figure for 1960 was similar to that for 1958. The report for 1960 admitted there was no obvious explanation, but suggested that it could be due to an increase in communal feeding.[162] The number of cases dropped to 800 the following year, but the hazards of communal eating were again emphasised:

The increase in communal feeding in restaurants, canteens and social gatherings of one kind and another, does increase risk: it is obvious that lapses in hygiene, careless handling of food, leading to infection, will produce more widespread and

---

[155] *RDHS 1959*, pp. 91, 94.

[156] *RDHS 1960*, p. 44; *RDHS 1961*, p. 36.

[157] *RDHS 1962*, p. 81; *RDHS 1961*, p. 37.

[158] *RMOHA 1956*, pp. 155–6; *RMOHA 1961*, p. 54.

[159] *RMOHA 1958*, p. 170; *RMOHA 1961*, p. 90; *RMOHA 1963*, p. 71; *RMOHA 1964*, p. 76.

[160] These data are taken from *RMOHA* for the relevant years; I. N. Sutherland, 'Food poisoning occurrence', Aberdeen City, 9 March 1961, NAS HH 64/211.

[161] *RDHS 1957*, p. 87.

[162] *RDHS 1960*, pp. 27, 45.

spectacular effects in such circumstance than the same sins against hygiene in the household.[163]

After a further drop in the number of cases in 1962, the report for that year commented that the encouraging trend indicated the 'improving state of food hygiene in many parts of Scotland'. This suggests that in Scotland, as in England and Wales, there was a current of optimism about food hygiene on the eve of the typhoid outbreaks of 1963 to 1964: the new regulations were apparently beginning to have an effect.

Despite the optimistic tone about overall trends, there were also signs of some new problems during the early 1960s. The Scottish report for 1962 explained that, immediately following the war, the *Salmonellae* had been the main group of organisms involved in outbreaks, but now *Clostridium welchii* was increasingly important. This was a form of food poisoning that tended to be associated with mass catering,[164] usually due to meat being cooked inadequately the day before serving.[165] The report for 1963 of the CMO of the Ministry of Health commented upon similar trends. Although the number of incidents again declined, this had been due to a reduction in sporadic cases, while the total number of people involved in incidents had increased, the most disturbing feature being a rise in incidents of *Clostridium welchii* poisoning. During 1963, *Clostridium welchii* was responsible for nearly half of the total general outbreaks and more than two-hirds of the cases involved. Of the 3292 cases of *Clostridium welchii* poisoning involved in general outbreaks, 75 per cent were associated with schools, hospitals and canteens.[166]

Canned food as a source of food poisoning

We referred earlier to the Birmingham canned cream incident of 1954, and the typhoid outbreak at Pickering in 1955, which was associated with canned tongue. But there were many other incidents caused by canned food, and, since canned corned beef caused the 1963 and 1964 typhoid outbreaks, we will now consider the accumulated knowledge of canned food-associated food poisoning. A useful analysis covering the period 1949 to 1960 is provided in a paper by W. C. Cockburn, director of the epidemiological research laboratory of the PHLS, published in 1962.

Cockburn's analysis was based upon 3100 general and family outbreaks between 1949 and 1960 in England and Wales, in which there was reasonable certainty that the contaminated food had been identified. This represented

---

[163] *RDHS 1961*, p. 14.
[164] *RDHS 1962*, p. 14.
[165] *RDHS 1963*, p. 17.
[166] *RCMO 1963*, p. 58.

28 per cent of these outbreaks during the period and 5.29 per cent of the total incidents, including the sporadic cases. Of the 3100 outbreaks, 73 per cent were associated with meat. Of these, only 1.5 per cent were associated with fresh meat, 86 per cent with 'processed and made up meat', and 8 per cent with canned meat. Thus some 190 general and family outbreaks had been connected with canned meat. Extrapolating to the total 11,256 general and family outbreaks, this would amount to 690 outbreaks.

Canned foods generally accounted for 321 outbreaks, or about 10 per cent of the outbreaks in which the foods involved were identified. Of these, 59 per cent were associated with meat, 24 per cent with fish, 15 per cent with vegetables and 2 per cent with fruit. Two-thirds of the outbreaks associated with canned meat and larger proportions of the outbreaks associated with the other canned foods were caused by staphylococcal poisoning, which normally arises from human sources. In around 20 per cent of the canned meat and fish outbreaks, and in about 35 per cent of the canned vegetable outbreaks, the contents of the cans were consumed shortly after opening. In Cockburn's view, the possibility of infective agents surviving heating during canning could be ruled out. He suggested that it must therefore be assumed that contamination occurred after heating, explaining this point in the same way that the Pickering typhoid outbreak had been explained. He suggested that pathogens could enter a can through 'a minute momentary leak' during cooling. He concluded:

> It is not suggested that the risk is large, but there is some risk. In this connection it is interesting to note that, of the 30 outbreaks associated with corned beef originating from named packaging plants, 15 came from one plant. The inference is that at least in this plant the hygiene and the process require investigation.[167]

He also commented that 'Canned foods, though generally very safe, are occasionally liable to contamination at the packing plant and a careful watch for break-downs in the normal safeguards is necessary'. It seems, then, that at the PHLS, Britain's foremost centre of expertise on food poisoning, there was, by 1962, clear awareness of the hazards involved in canned meat production. In Chapter 2, however, we will see that awareness of the issue was apparently lacking on the part of MAFF's front-line officer responsible for keeping a 'careful watch' on the South American meat packing industry.

Old and new problems

To conclude, the account of the history of typhoid in Britain in the earlier part of this chapter showed that by 1963 to 1964 the disease was largely

---

167 W. C. Cockburn, 'Reporting and incidence of food poisoning', in W. C. Cockburn, J. Taylor, E. S. Anderson and Betty C. Hobbs, *Food Poisoning Symposium*, London, 1962, pp. 3–14, at pp. 8–12.

regarded as a historical problem. There was, however, some awareness of risks of typhoid from abroad, underlined by the Zermatt outbreak. In contrast, there had been widespread awareness of an apparent rising tide of food poisoning during the 1950s, and by the early 1960s there were concerns about the changing pattern of food poisoning signalled by the rise in *Clostridium welchii* poisoning. Nevertheless, optimism seems to have prevailed about the ability of regulations and education to counteract the threat. There were certainly gaps in knowledge of food poisoning, illustrated by the high proportion of outbreaks in which the causative organism or associated food was unidentified. However, in view of the investigation of the Pickering typhoid outbreak, and knowledge of the risk of contamination of canned food during production, in some quarters understanding of the problem that was to give rise to the typhoid outbreaks of 1963 to 1964 was well advanced.

The typhoid outbreaks of the late 1930s had raised questions concerning relationships between the MOsH and GPs, and the role of the central health administration, but such issues were not very visible in the public documentation of post-war enteric and food poisoning outbreaks prior to 1964. But the NHS had certainly not abolished tensions between MOsH and general practitioners, or between the centre and the periphery, and some features of the new system enhanced the potential for problems. The MOsH remained responsible for outbreak control, but whereas prior to 1948 they controlled the infectious diseases hospitals, upon the establishment of the NHS these hospitals were taken away from the local authorities and were then administered by the local hospital boards. Likewise, the public health laboratories in Scotland (where the PHLS did not operate), formerly part of the public health departments, were now the responsibility of hospital authorities. The efficient functioning of services during outbreaks therefore involved co-ordination between MOsH, hospital boards and GPs. As we shall see, the relationships between the MOsH and the GPs, hospital authorities, laboratory and central authorities all became problematic during the Aberdeen outbreak.

As in the pre-war period, within the NHS there was competition between MOsH and GPs in connection with some services, and the loss of the municipal hospitals and general decline in infectious diseases challenged MOsH to develop new strategies. One innovative MOH was I. A. G. MacQueen, MOH for Aberdeen from 1952, who championed health visiting. By the 1960s, Aberdeen's seventy-strong health visitor team surpassed that of other Scottish cities. MacQueen claimed that they could perform some functions of GPs, leading to tension prior to the Aberdeen typhoid outbreak. He also pioneered local authority health education, and was attracted by the potential of the mass media for health education purposes.[168] This latter enthusiasm may be

---

[168] L. Diack and D. F. Smith, 'Professional strategies of Medical Officers of Health in the post war period (1): "innovative traditionalism": the case of Dr Ian MacQueen, MOH for Aberdeen 1952–1974', *Journal of Public Health Medicine*, 2002, vol. 24, pp. 123–9.

illustrated by MacQueen's strategy during the 'wedding party' food poisoning incident of 1961. After a conversation with MacQueen, Ian Sutherland, epidemiologist at the Scottish Home and Health Department (formerly Department of Health for Scotland), prepared a memorandum for his colleagues remarking on 'an interesting side-light on the way Dr MacQueen uses events'. MacQueen told Sutherland that he thought the incident:

> a good opportunity to warn the City of food poisoning and the methods of avoiding it. Therefore . . . he took the opportunity of referring in general terms to this outbreak and making it the theme for a homily on the prevention of food poisoning. He said that this achieved front-page publicity in at least one of the local papers and was favourably mentioned by them all.[169]

Since the Bournemouth, Croydon and Hawick outbreaks, problems of handling the press had not been an important theme of the documentation of enteric and food poisoning outbreaks. Press activity surrounding the apparent rise in food poisoning in the later 1940s and early 1950s also seems to have been welcomed by the Department of Health for Scotland, and the press was enlisted in support of the launch of the food hygiene regulations in the late 1950s. But in the early 1960s press relations were identified as a problem in connection with the smallpox outbreak in Yorkshire,[170] and, as we shall see in later chapters, the intense publicity given to the Aberdeen typhoid outbreak, and the role of the MOH in this connection, became a major feature of the official enquiry that followed. We will first proceed, however, to a study of the three corned beef-associated typhoid outbreaks of 1963, in which we will begin to examine policy formation and implementation processes much more closely than in this chapter.

---

[169] I. N. Sutherland, 'Food poisoning occurrence', Aberdeen City, 9 March 1961, National Archives of Scotland, HH 64/211.
[170] Ministry of Health, Scottish Health Service Advisory Council, *Smallpox*.

2

The 1963 corned beef-associated typhoid outbreaks in Harlow, South Shields and Bedford

Introduction

In Chapter 1, we learned that during 1949 in Crowthorne there had been an outbreak of typhoid that had been definitely connected with canned corned beef as the vehicle of infection, although it appears that no one thought at that time that the infection could have been in the can before opening. In 1955, however, the investigation that followed an outbreak of typhoid associated with tongue in Pickering suggested that canned meat could be contaminated during manufacture by impure cooling water entering the can through a temporary leak. In addition, in 1962, a published review of food poisoning in England and Wales made it clear that through accumulated experience of food poisoning associated with corned beef, expert opinion at the PHLS was convinced that the explanation offered for the 1955 outbreak was viable. The review even mentioned that several food poisoning incidents associated with corned beef had been found to involve produce from a single factory, and recommended that in such cases the hygiene of the factory concerned should be investigated.[1] In this chapter, however, it will be shown through an examination of the archival records of MAFF that policy makers were slow to take decisive action when evidence began to accumulate of typhoid associated with the corned beef from a specific factory in Argentina which used unchlorinated cooling water. It will be argued that the tardiness of the response was largely the result of an overriding concern to take decisions in secret as far as possible. The wish to avoid publicity was not simply a matter of traditional civil service methods of operation. It also arose from a desire not to offend the Argentine government at a time of delicate negotiations that had been taking place regarding the regulation of the volume of Argentine chilled beef exports to Britain. It is therefore to the background history of the meat trade with Argentina that we will first turn.

[1] See pp. 20–1, 23–4, 35.

38

Britain's beef supply problems in the 1960s

Since the nineteenth century, the import of food from countries where production costs were less than in Britain meant cheaper food and a better diet for the British population, but because of the impact of food imports on British farming, this trade presented a continuous challenge for politicians and officials concerned with food policy. In addition, as British production, processing and shipping companies became entrenched in ventures to exploit the potential of agriculture overseas, a further set of interest groups was created that needed to be considered. Furthermore, as British producers of manufactured goods came to depend upon trade with countries supplying agricultural products, possible trade retaliation by the governments concerned also needed to be considered whenever measures to regulate the flow of food imports to Britain were under discussion. Britain had long been tied to Argentina in this kind of relationship, with Argentina providing 43 per cent of total British meat imports before the Second World War, and 28 per cent in 1950.[2]

The importance of the South American meat supply, and South American markets for manufactured goods, was such that Britain allowed less stringent animal health regulations with regard to the South American countries, as compared with other countries such as France. Meat imports from South America were allowed into Britain even though foot-and-mouth disease was endemic in South America. But some safeguards were provided by the Bledisloe agreement of 1928, which required that herds of origin be certified free of contagious diseases, that animals be examined and found healthy before removal, and that the vehicles used for transporting animals be properly cleansed. In addition, veterinary inspection before and after slaughter, the prohibition of meat exports from herds in which infectious diseases were found, and thorough cleansing of all pens and slaughterhouses were required. A veterinary attaché was stationed at the British Embassy in Buenos Aires to monitor the animal health risks and the implementation of the Bledisloe agreement.[3] Despite the agreement and the efforts of the veterinary attaché, the problem of the importation of foot-and-mouth disease from South America continued. There was an average of about 150 outbreaks per year from 1956

---

[2] C. Lewis, 'Anglo–Argentine Trade 1945–1965', in D. Rock (ed.), *Argentina in the Twentieth Century*, London, 1975, pp. 114–34, at p. 129. For a history of the South American export meat industry up until the 1910s see J. T. Critchell and J. Raymond, *A History of the Frozen Meat Trade*, London, 1969 (first published 1912), and R. Perren, *The Meat Trade in Britain*, London, 1978, pp. 176–96, 205–15; for the twentieth century see R. C. Gebhardt, 'The River Plate meat industry since c. 1900: technology, ownership, international trade regime and domestic policy', Ph.D. thesis, London School of Economics, 2000.

[3] Ministry of Agriculture, Fisheries and Food, *Animal Health A Centenary 1865–1964*, London, 1965, pp. 277–8; J. Winnifrith, *The Minister of Agriculture, Fisheries and Food* (New Whitehall Series No. 11), London, 1962, p. 212.

to 1961, and a peak of 298 in 1960, many of these cases being attributed to the importation of infections from South America.[4]

During the post-war period the British government sought to improve the economic viability of home agriculture by encouraging research and the adoption of modern farming methods, and attempting to stimulate and stabilise the market by means of price guarantees.[5] The possibility of further supporting British farming by reducing the reliance on Argentine meat was discussed in Cabinet in early 1958. The Chancellor of the Exchequer was invited to consider the matter, in consultation with the President of the Board of Trade and the Minister of Agriculture, Fisheries and Food, soon after an adjournment debate on foot-and-mouth disease.[6] An interdepartmental working party subsequently advised that the animal health problem could be used only to justify a ban on Argentine meat imports, not a gradual reduction, but due to Britain's heavy dependence on Argentine beef this was thought impractical. In addition, it considered that repercussions on UK exports to Argentina would reduce or outweigh any benefit of reducing imports.[7] The Minister of Agriculture was convinced that ways could be found to better meet the needs of home agriculture and to enhance trade with the Commonwealth, and he argued for steady reductions in Argentinian beef imports over a ten-year period.[8] But the working party argued that such a scheme would expose the government to severe criticism if the forecasts turned out to be wrong.[9]

In the event, meat exports from Argentina to Britain declined in the late 1950s, due partly to decreasing production and increasing consumption of meat in Argentina. But Argentina remained an important source of beef, and the volume of Argentine beef exports to Britain was still sufficient to disrupt the British beef market should unexpected fluctuations occur in the arrival of consignments. This was because the bulk of Argentine beef was transported chilled rather then frozen, and needed to be marketed immediately upon arrival. In early 1963 such disruption occurred as a consequence of an unanticipated increase in Argentine chilled beef shipments. There were a variety of reasons for this, including a recent devaluation of the peso, a heavy slaughter due to a drought that had struck the country, and the release of supplies following a strike in the packing industry. As a result, beef prices in Britain became depressed at a time when home production was buoyant. As

---

[4] Ministry of Agriculture, Fisheries and Food, *Report of the Committee of Inquiry on Foot-and-Mouth Disease 1968, part one* (Northumberland report), London, 1968, p. 34.

[5] Winnifrith, *Minister of Agriculture*, ch. 4; M. J. Smith, *The Politics of Agricultural Support in Britain*, London, 1990, ch. 4.

[6] PD(C), vol. 583, cols 1297–308 (4 March 1958).

[7] 'Argentine beef', 31 March 1958, PRO MAF 246/195.

[8] 'Argentine beef. Memorandum by the Minister of Agriculture, Fisheries and Food', May 1958, PRO MAF 246/195.

[9] J. Graham to Mr Tame, 15 October 1958; Tame to Mr Hardman, 16 October 1958, PRO MAF 246/198.

the price of beef dropped, the incentive scheme that guaranteed the price paid for beef to British farmers became much more expensive to operate for the British government.[10]

In February 1963, the Minister of Agriculture, Fisheries and Food sent an *aide-mémoire* to the Argentine Embassy, pointing out that low prices in the UK market were not in the interests of either country, and asking for an indication of the level which Argentine supplies of beef to the UK were likely to reach during 1963.[11] The response suggested that from the Argentine point of view it was not their level of beef exports to Britain that was causing problems, because in earlier talks between the two countries, the period 1955 to 1959 had been considered a period indicative of normal levels of trade. From this perspective Argentine beef exports to Britain were still low, having dropped from 22 per cent of the UK's supplies in 1958 to about 14 per cent. While Argentina shared Britain's concern about prices in the UK beef market, they declined to state the intended level of exports during 1963. Nevertheless, a willingness was expressed to enter discussions 'within the framework of the reciprocal cordial trade relations traditionally existing between our two countries, with the purpose of achieving the objective of maintaining and expanding the trade existing between us'.[12]

The Minister of Agriculture, Fisheries and Food, Christopher Soames, was sceptical as to whether the voluntary limitation of beef imports could be achieved, and was convinced that sooner or later enforceable import controls would be necessary.[13] MAFF officials warned, however, that there would be objections from the Board of Trade on general policy grounds and from the Treasury and Foreign Office on the grounds of 'our political and financial relationships with Argentina'.[14] British industrialists with interests in Argentina also began to lobby against limiting Argentine beef imports.[15]

Nevertheless, following talks with the Argentine representative, Soames was able to announce, by the end of April, that they had agreed that their beef exports to Britain for 1963 would not exceed 203,500 tons. In view of the high level of trade in early 1963, this represented a significant restriction during the second half of the year. But the arrangement was informal, and Soames was not convinced it would lead to actual restraint. Pressure for an

[10] Ministry of Agriculture, Fisheries and Food Press Notice, 'Beef supplies', 26 May 1964, PRO MAF 246/217.

[11] '*Aide-mémoire* to the Government of the Argentine Republic Meat Supplies', 1 February 1963, PRO MAF 246/107.

[12] '*Aide-mémoire*', 14 March 1963, PRO MAF 246/107.

[13] Minister of Agriculture, Fisheries and Food to Prime Minister, 19 March 1963, PRO MAF 246/209.

[14] Meat and Livestock Division, 'UK meat supplies brief for the Minister', 26 March 1963, PRO MAF 246/209.

[15] 'Brief for the Minister of State's meeting with Sir Derek Vestey', 14 March 1963, PRO MAF 246/107.

increase in Argentine shipments began soon after the limit had been agreed. Soames had already warned colleagues in a confidential memorandum of the possible consequences of the Argentines reneging on their undertaking. If a further peak in Argentine supplies was to coincide with a peak in home production, then the 'market situation and resulting political pressure at home could be serious'.[16] Such were the concerns of Soames and MAFF officials when the first typhoid outbreak was connected with Argentine corned beef in early June.

The Harlow outbreak: May/June 1963

The first items on the Harlow outbreak appeared in the press shortly after the long-running series of reports on the Zermatt outbreak had subsided. The latter had begun in mid-March. Initial documentation of the increasing incidence of typhoid among British tourists returning from Zermatt, had given way to stories of neglect of sanitation and water supply on the part of the town's authorities, and attempts to avoid publicity and safeguard tourism, the life-blood of the resort.[17] The final stories, in mid-May, covered the efforts of the Swiss national tourist office to repair the damage by offering free holidays and compensation to visitors who had contracted typhoid. There was also a typhoid scare in another Swiss town caused by a relapse of a hotel worker who had been one of the Zermatt cases.[18] In view of recent press reporting of the Zermatt outbreak and its repercussions, press interest in the Harlow outbreak was especially high, and the first reports, in early June, emphasised that there was no link with Zermatt.[19]

An account of the Harlow outbreak by H. L. Hughes, the town's chief public health inspector, appeared in *Municipal Engineering* in August 1963, and referred to the problems caused by media interest. The public health department was 'besieged' by the press, and Hughes suggested that 'special arrangements' were required 'from the outset of such an outbreak if chaos is to be avoided'. According to Hughes' account, the first evidence of typhoid at Harlow appeared on 1 June, when tests confirmed the disease in four patients. Local officials immediately investigated the local sewerage system, water and milk supplies, and interviewed all patients, suspected cases and contacts.

---

[16] 'Meat imports from France and Belgium. Note by the Minister of Agriculture, Fisheries and Food', 17 May 1963, PRO 246/209.

[17] 'Ten British typhoid cases after visits to Zermatt', *Glasgow Herald*, 18 March 1963, p. 1c; '30 typhoid cases', *The Times*, 21 March 1963, p. 12f.; 'Outcry against authorities in Zermatt "Bid to hush up typhoid epidemic"', *The Times*, 29 March 1963, p. 11a.

[18] 'Swiss try to repair damage caused by typhoid. Details of free holiday offers', *The Times*, 14 May 1963, p. 11d; 'New typhoid cases in Switzerland', *The Times*, 16 May 1963, p. 12a.

[19] 'Seven cases of typhoid at Harlow', *The Times*, 5 June 1963, p. 12g; 'Nine typhoid cases at Harlow Link with Zermatt ruled out', *The Times*, 6 June 1963, p. 6a.

It was soon clear that the cases were concentrated in an area that was served by a particular shopping centre, and the shops at this centre were then investigated. All the shop workers were invited to submit themselves for rectal swabs. The police also rounded up itinerant vendors who had entered Harlow to sell their wares over the previous six weeks and further swabs were taken. Only one of the tests was positive, and the whole process was then repeated for blood samples. From the patient interview data, suspicion began to centre on a butcher's shop where one of the staff had contracted typhoid – but who, from the date of his illness, was clearly a victim rather than the source of the outbreak. Further testing of visitors to the shop failed to find a carrier, but suspicion began to fall upon corned beef as the common factor among the patients.[20]

The Times reported on 12 June that there were eighteen cases, and that Isodore Ash, MOH for Harlow, had said that there was 'strong circumstantial evidence' that South American corned beef was involved.[21] As a result, the outbreak came to the attention of MAFF.[22] As mentioned in Chapter 1, when responsibilities for food safety were rearranged in 1955, and the Ministry of Food merged with the Ministry of Agriculture and Fisheries to form MAFF, MAFF had retained the primary responsibility for monitoring the safety of imported meat prior to its arrival in Britain. This duty fell to MAFF's Food Standards, Hygiene and Slaughterhouse Policy division, and it was accomplished by means of the 'official certificate procedure'. This system had begun in 1908, when imported pig meat first required a certificate showing that ante- and post-mortem inspections of animals had been carried out, and that meat was prepared under hygienic conditions.[23] The actual certificates took the form of a document, label, mark or stamp fixed to the merchandise, and applied by the government authority in the exporting country rather than by the exporting firm. Any goods arriving without valid certificates were stopped by port health inspectors.[24]

By 1963, the official certification procedure was based on the Public Health (Imported Food) Regulations 1937 and 1948 and covered most meat or meat products (including canned meat). At first, certificates were recognised for major meat exporting countries without stringent enquiries, but after the publication of the report of the Interdepartmental Committee on Meat Inspection in 1951, it became standard practice for officials (veterinarians) to visit the country before approval was granted. The programme of visits

---

[20] H. L. Hughes, 'How Harlow tackled its Whitsun typhoid outbreak', *Municipal Engineering*, 1963, vol. 140, p. 1176.

[21] 'Tinned meat chief Harlow suspect', *The Times*, 12 June 1963, p. 6e.

[22] 'Events relating to Establishment 25', 5 June 1964, PRO MAF 282/87.

[23] R. V. Blamire, 'Meat hygiene: the changing years', *Journal of the Royal Society of Health*, 1984, vol. 5, pp. 180–5.

[24] 'Imported meat and meat products', 24 June 1964, PRO MAF 282/90.

included both countries applying for and some already holding official certificates, the aim being to establish whether meat inspection was carried out properly and was supervised by qualified staff, and to inspect the standard of hygiene of slaughterhouses and processing plants. If the standards observed were high, and the meat inspection service inspired 'confidence', a certificate could be granted to a country as a whole, but if not all plants were satisfactory, as in South America, unsatisfactory establishments could be excluded from the certificate. Argentina was granted an official certificate for meat in 1938 and visited in 1952 and again in 1955, when the concern was with *frigorificos* (slaughterhouses with freezing/chilling plants), rather than canning. These were the only visits in connection with public health safeguards prior to early 1964.[25] From the establishment of the policy until the 1960s, the veterinary officers concerned were L. B. A. Grace and R. V. Blamire, Grace, as chief technical adviser on meat inspection, being the senior officer. Both Grace and Blamire were former inspectors at London meat markets. Grace had worked at Smithfield, while Blamire had worked at Islington, and both held the Diploma in Veterinary State Medicine.[26]

On 12 June 1963, after consulting the Ministry of Health, Ken Bird, the chief executive officer of MAFF's Food Standards, Hygiene and Slaughterhouse Policy division, recorded that the corned beef apparently involved in the Harlow outbreak had been produced by the Argentine national meat packing company, Corporación Argentina de Productores de Carne (CAP). He also noted that the possibility of typhoid surviving the high temperatures involved in the corned beef production process could be ruled out. More possible, 'but still very unlikely', was 'the introduction, through a minute fault in a can seam, of the germ from water used to cool the cans'.[27] From the start of the 1963 corned beef-associated typhoid outbreaks, there was clearly awareness among officials of the possible mechanism for the contamination of canned food after heating that had been recently outlined in the review by Cockburn.[28]

A few days later, when the *Guardian* reported that the MOH for Harlow thought that the evidence against corned beef was hardening,[29] Bird was surprised that he had been so forthright, because according to the advice of the Ministry of Health the evidence was only tentative. The Ministry of Health had advised that action was not justified against cans bearing the same manufacturer's code as the one involved in Harlow. The code indicated that the date of manufacture was 30 May 1962, and the plant in question was

[25] Ibid.; Table showing countries, products for which it was recognised, date of recognition and date of visit, PRO MAF 282/75.

[26] R.V. Blamire, interview, 12 January 2000, Place, ATO/37.

[27] K. A. Bird to Mr Hensley, 12 June 1963, PRO MAF 282/75.

[28] See p. 35.

[29] Correspondent, 'Typhoid: test on tin of meat', *Guardian*, 13 June 1963, cutting in PRO MAF 282/75.

Frigorifico Yuqueri, Concordia, Province of Entre Rios, Argentina, also known as Establishment 25.[30] At this stage, MAFF officials regarded the outbreak as a matter for the Ministry of Health, since the safety of imported food was their responsibility once it had passed through the ports in Britain. MAFF would become involved only if it were necessary to call for the help of the veterinary attaché in Buenos Aires, Basil Claxton.[31] However, Peter Humphreys-Davies, MAFF's deputy secretary, realised that there was another dimension to this problem of relevance to MAFF: there could be additional repercussions in view of the stockpile of corned beef managed by MAFF as part of Britain's food reserves in case of nuclear war or other emergencies.[32]

The nuclear stockpile dated from the early post-war period, and consisted of sugar, flour, wheat, biscuits, yeast and canned meat. The canned meat was made up almost entirely of corned beef, with a very small proportion of mutton and stewed steak (the latter was bought in 1960/1961, when MAFF was unable to find sufficient supplies of corned beef).[33] The canned meat was located at warehouses throughout Britain. Contracts for the purchase of batches of corned beef were arranged by agents appointed by MAFF and the condition of the material in the warehouses was continuously monitored by a firm of surveyors employed for the purpose. As soon as any deterioration in the condition of the cans was apparent, batches were disposed of through commercial channels to the distributive trade, usually after about ten years. Humphreys-Davies was therefore concerned that the corned beef associated with the Harlow outbreak may have passed through the stockpile, or that within the stockpile there might be stocks from the same canning factory. On enquiry, he was reassured on the first point, but discovered that there was a considerable quantity of Establishment 25 material within the stockpile. It was therefore decided to test samples in the stockpile produced on the same day as the Harlow can. Twelve randomly selected cans and twelve cans with suspected seam defects all tested negative.[34]

The idea of the infection arising from cooling water was publicised by the *Sunday Telegraph* on 16 June. Under the headline 'Typhoid germ is traced' the newspaper stated that experts believed the germ responsible for the Harlow incident may have come from Argentina. The Harlow outbreak was said to parallel one in Yorkshire where Argentine canned meat had been the suspected source.[35] This was clearly a reference to the Pickering outbreak and the conclusions of the investigation into that outbreak which involved the

---

[30] K. A. Bird to Mr Hensley, 13 June 1963, PRO MAF 282/75.

[31] J. Hensley to P. Humphreys-Davies, 13 June 1963, PRO MAF 282/75.

[32] P. Humphreys-Davies to R. J. E. Taylor, 13 June 1963, PRO MAF 282/75.

[33] 'Canned meat', doc 123, PRO MAF 246/178.

[34] R. J. E. Taylor to J. R. Reynolds, 13 June 1963; J. R. Reynolds to R. J. E. Taylor, 14 June 1963; K. A. Bird to Mr Hensley, 4 July 1963, PRO MAF 282/75.

[35] 'Typhoid germ is traced', *Sunday Telegraph*, 16 June 1963, cutting in PRO MAF 282/75.

PHLS, although no mention of the country of origin of the canned tongue involved had been included in either the CMO's report for 1955, or the article on the outbreak published in the *BMJ* in 1956.[36] The source of the newspaper's information is not given, but it could have been obtained either through direct contact with PHLS staff, of from the MOH, Ash, who was himself certainly in contact with the PHLS by this time in connection with the outbreak.

Following this publicity, Leo Grace, MAFF's chief technical adviser on meat inspection, wrote to Claxton in Buenos Aires enclosing the *Sunday Telegraph* article and asking him to visit Establishment 25 to check hygiene standards. Grace thought it important to 'follow the matter up at the production end as discreetly and as quickly as possible'.[37] Claxton, however, found Grace's letter embarrassing, and he informed Grace that CAP were 'very responsible' and that he worked 'very closely' with them. In addition, the hygiene of meat for export was the responsibility of further close 'colleagues' in the Argentine Ministry of Agriculture and Livestock. Claxton's term of service in Buenos Aires was about to end and he could not 'discreetly' visit a factory far from the capital.[38] The impression given here is that Claxton had become so well integrated into the local community while in Argentina that the social dimension of international diplomacy rather overshadowed his role as Britain's policeman of meat hygiene in South America. Claxton reported that he had discussed the question of visiting Establishment 25 with the ambassador and had decided to call at CAP headquarters with Argentine officials to 'lay his cards on the table'. The outcome of the meeting was that CAP provided Claxton with a plane to visit Concordia, to which he travelled accompanied by a senior manager and the government's director of meat inspection. Claxton found that the hygiene standards were good but reported that untreated river water was used for cooling. This, he said, was 'customary in practically all the canning plants in this country'. No epidemic had occurred at the plant for several years, but there had been one in 1962 at Concordia barracks, 35 km north of the factory and 10 km from the river. Claxton's report also noted that the plant would shortly complete a contract for 35,000 cases for the corned beef stockpile.[39] Claxton commented that CAP's management were very co-operative during the visit and 'understood that in a matter of Public health, no stone should be left unturned to eliminate possible doubt regarding the source of infection, and at the same time avoid unnecessary publicity'.[40]

[36] *RCMO 1955*, pp. 54–5; W. R. M. Couper, K. W. Newell and D. J. H. Payne, 'An outbreak of typhoid fever associated with canned ox-tongue', *BMJ*, 1956, vol. 1, pp. 1057–9.

[37] L. B. A. Grace to B. A. Claxton, 17 June 1963, PRO MAF 276/195.

[38] B. A. Claxton to L. B. A. Grace, 27 June 1963, PRO MAF 276/195.

[39] B. A. Claxton, 'Preparation of corned beef at Frigorifico Yuquerí', 27 June 1963, PRO MAF 276/195.

[40] B. A. Claxton to L. B. A. Grace, 27 June 1963, PRO MAF 276/195.

South Shields: June/July 1963

While Claxton's investigations were underway, reports of another typhoid outbreak began to appear in the press. By 24 June, *The Times* reported that there were seventeen cases in South Shields.[41] Initially there seemed to be no similarities to the Harlow outbreak as the newspaper quoted Ash, the MOH for Harlow, stating that the clues which had led to corned beef in Harlow were not apparent in South Shields.[42] On 1 July, however, before Claxton's report had been discussed, Dr John Ross, a medical officer of the Ministry of Health who was responsible for food hygiene matters, telephoned Grace. It was now clear that the South Shields outbreak had been associated with corned beef purchased from a 'Fine Fare' supermarket.[43] Two days later, a meeting was held between representatives of MAFF divisions. Comments by R. E. J. Goodman, principal scientific officer of the Food Science and Plant Health Division, seemed to suggest that the likelihood of the involvement of contaminated cooling water was very small. Apparently, the phage types of the organisms involved in the two outbreaks were different, and this was taken as reducing the likelihood that the two outbreaks were caused in the same way. This assumption was based on the principles for linking different outbreaks with an individual carrier that had become established since the development of the powerful technology of phage typing.[44] No consideration seems to have been given at this stage to the possibility that if meat plant cooling water was contaminated with sewage it might contain multiple pathogenic organisms including more than one phage type of *Salmonella typhi*, which could contaminate different cans. In addition, Goodman added that experience suggested that fewer than two out of 100,000 cans were likely to be 'leakers'. Nevertheless, the meeting agreed to consider requiring plants exporting to Britain to chlorinate cooling water. The safety of the stockpiled corned beef was also discussed, but it was agreed that no special precautions were necessary pending discussion with the Ministry of Health.[45] Grace was far from convinced that corned beef was the source of the outbreaks and a conversation with Ross tended to confirm this view. Ross told Grace that the Ministry of Health currently had no intention of asking suppliers to withdraw corned beef that had already been distributed.[46]

The Times reported that the MOH for South Shields had merely announced that the source of the outbreak had been narrowed to 'tinned meat – corned beef, ham or tongue', and that the possibility of the food being contaminated

---

[41] '17 involved in outbreak of typhoid', *Times*, 24 June 1963, p. 10e.

[42] 'Five more typhoid suspects', *Times*, 26 June 1963, p. 8f.

[43] L. B. A. Grace to Mr Bird, 1 July 1963. PRO MAF 282/75.

[44] See pp. 19–20.

[45] 'Note of meeting held on 3rd July', 4 July 1963, PRO MAF 276/195.

[46] L. B. A. Grace, 4 July 1963, PRO MAF 282/75.

before reaching the shop 'could not be excluded'.[47] However, as a result of the more explicit press publicity associated with the Harlow outbreak, MAFF had received an enquiry from the American Embassy, which requested details about the source of the outbreak for the information of the US Food and Drugs Administration. MAFF officials had not treated the enquiry with any sense of urgency, but now that there was a second outbreak they felt under pressure to respond. However, Under-secretary John Hensley was greatly concerned that if information was given to the Americans about the enquiries that MAFF had been making in Argentina, this might be made public. It would offend the Argentine government if British concerns about hygiene in Argentine meat plants were to reach them via the press or a third country. Hensley suggested that information might be given to the Americans, but that they should be asked to keep it confidential for the time being.[48] He also suggested that his colleagues should consider how to respond to questions that might be expected from the press about the steps being taken to check the source of the canned meat apparently involved in the recent outbreaks. However, these problems were greatly alleviated on 10 July, when the Minister of Health, Enoch Powell, answered a parliamentary question on the typhoid outbreaks. Kenneth Robinson asked:

> How many of the recent outbreaks of typhoid fever have been traced to a particular consignment of corned beef; whether the importer has now recalled all unsold deliveries; and what steps have been taken to warn members of the public who have purchased but not yet consumed corned beef?

Enoch Powell replied simply in writing: 'None. The other questions do not arise.'[49] After this, the expected press enquiries did not materialise and Powell's statement also reduced the urgency of replying to the American Embassy.[50]

Powell's statement was justified by the fact that no corned beef had been recovered that had been contaminated with the typhoid germ, but concerns within the ministries were increasing about the safety of Establishment 25 corned beef. It had become clear that the South Shields stock was also from Establishment 25,[51] and Claxton now reported his suggestion that untreated cooling water was used widely was incorrect.[52] It now appeared that the practice was confined to Establishment 25. He also reported that the outbreak at the Concordia army barracks took place between 1 May and 10 June 1962,

---

[47] 'Food shop shut in typhoid town', *The Times*, 3 July 1963, p. 10e.

[48] J. Hensley to Mr Nield, 8 July 1963, PRO MAF 282/75.

[49] *PD(C)*, vol. 601, col. 150 (10 July 1963).

[50] J. Hensley to Mr Lace, 18 July 1963, PRO MAF 282/75.

[51] R. V. Blamire to Mr Bird, 12 July 1963, PRO MAF 282/75.

[52] L. B. A. Grace to B. A. Claxton, 8 July 1963, PRO MAF 276/195.

covering the date of production of the suspect can at Harlow.[53] Nevertheless, the Ministry of Health still remained convinced that there was no need for any special action to be taken.

Avoiding offending Argentina

Throughout the course of the outbreaks in mid-1963, officials were anxious not to publicly blame Argentine produce for the outbreaks, before an approach about the cooling water could be made through diplomatic channels. In preparation for the approach, it was thought advisable to consult W. C. Tame, an Under-secretary who had been involved in the negotiations over meat imports, on how the Argentinians might react. On past form, they were especially 'touchy' when they were 'asked to bear the burden and other countries are not'.[54] It was therefore thought best to present the matter as part of a 'concerted approach to all countries where there has been no modern check', and Bird subsequently prepared a list of sixteen countries that should be considered for inspections.[55] With only two inspectors, such a programme of visits would clearly take some considerable time. However, there was no immediate action, and at the end of August Bird suggested that since Claxton had now reported that Establishment 25 would chlorinate water from the start of the next canning season, there was no urgency. Claxton was on his way home, and Bird advised that discussion with him should take place before deciding upon the next step.[56]

Additional evidence of a desire to avoid upsetting the Argentinians was provided in the discussion between MAFF and the Ministry of Health concerning a letter from Harlow's MP about the prevention of further outbreaks. On 2 July 1963, the Harlow Chamber of Trade wrote to Graeme Finlay, MP for the Epping Division of Essex, complaining that since the outbreak in Harlow their town was no longer thought of as a 'bright town with attractive and competitive shops'. Now there was 'suspicion – that perhaps there was a danger of catching something here'. The Chamber had gathered from the press that the corned beef responsible may have come from 'small canners using the River Plate for cooling purposes'. In the context of the new outbreak in South Shields the Chamber wanted assurance that the government was taking action to 'pinpoint the infected food' and to 'prevent further outbreaks'.[57] Finlay subsequently wrote to the Ministry of Health, and MAFF

[53] B. A. Claxton to L. B. A. Grace, 16 July 1963, PRO MAF 282/75.

[54] W. A. Nield to Mr Tame, 11 July 1963, PRO MAF 282/75.

[55] N. J. P. Hutchison to W. C. Tame, 15 July; K. A. Bird to Mr Lace, 24 July 1963; PRO MAF 282/75.

[56] K. A. Bird to Mr Hearne, 28 August 1963, PRO MAF 282/75.

[57] R. Blanks to G. Finley [sic], 2 July 1963, PRO MAF 282/75.

were consulted about the wording of the reply. Miss H. J. Morey, senior executive officer of Food Standards, Hygiene and Slaughterhouse Policy Division, expressed doubts about releasing any information beyond bare details of the official certification procedures prior to the impending diplomatic approach to the Argentine authorities. According to Morey's understanding of the situation the source of the outbreak had not been definitely established, and therefore the steps taken by the ministries with regard to corned beef should be regarded as confidential, 'and must remain so since we are anxious not to offend the Argentine authorities'. She also suggested that the letter to Finlay must 'emphasise the fact that we are not certain that the blame attaches to corned beef'. In addition, they should be careful not to imply that the corned beef causing the outbreaks must have come from different batches, since this could mean that 'all corned beef is a possible source of danger'.[58]

Despite the official line of the Ministry of Health, the safety of Establishment 25 corned beef needed further consideration due to the impending delivery for the stockpile. On 22 July, MAFF's Meat and Livestock Division reported that 4056 cases of a 35,000-case contract had reached London. They would be taking delivery unless directed otherwise.[59] In Bird's view, there was still no need for action while the Ministry of Health was prepared to leave Establishment 25 corned beef held in commercial hands in circulation.[60] At the end of August he further suggested that the typhoid outbreak at Concordia barracks, upstream from establishment 25, need have no bearing on any decision making. The barracks was far from the river and the evidence linking the Harlow cases and corned beef was not conclusive anyway.[61] At this point, however, R. E. J. Goodman of the Food Science and Plant Health Division of MAFF disrupted the consensus. He suggested that the Concordia outbreak should not be dismissed as its sewage could have reached the river, and argued that the evidence was strengthened by the new information that Establishment 25 was the only plant using untreated water. Goodman proposed additional investigations in Argentina, and suggested that in the meantime MAFF's stocks of Establishment 25 corned beef produced during and for some time after the Concordia outbreak should be withheld.[62] Grace, returning from leave on 2 September, was now inclined to agree with Goodman. However, there was no immediate danger, since the 1962 Establishment 25 corned beef in the stockpile would not be turned over for some time and there was no need to worry the public.[63]

<hr>

[58] J. Morey to G. O. Lace 1 August 1963, J. Morey to Mr O'Mara, 6 August 1963, PRO MAF 282/75.
[59] A. R. Parselle to K. A. Bird, 22 July 1963, PRO MAF 282/75.
[60] K. A. Bird to Mr Lace, 24 July 1963, PRO MAF 282/75.
[61] K. A. Bird to Mr Hearne, 28 August 1963, PRO MAF 282/75.
[62] R. E. J. Goodman to Mr Bird, 29 August 1963, PRO MAF 282/75.
[63] K. A. Bird to Mr Hensley, 2 September 1963, PRO MAF 282/75.

In mid-September, Ross of the Ministry of Health agreed that there should be additional investigations, but doubted whether it would be possible to get answers to all the relevant questions concerning the outbreak at Concordia and possible ways in which the typhoid organisms could have reached the canning plant.[64] Grace agreed, but suggested that the situation could be further explored with Claxton, who had now returned from Buenos Aires, but who had been taken ill.[65] This was the position when the next outbreak began.

Bedford and action: October/November 1963

The outbreak in Bedford began between 10 and 14 October, and the association with corned beef from Safeway, a new supermarket, was soon realised.[66] Reports about the outbreak appeared in the press on 24 October, and on 28 October they mentioned that contaminated corned beef was believed to be the cause.[67] That day the Ministry of Health told MAFF that the corned beef involved had been produced by CAP.[68] G. O. Lace, the assistant secretary responsible for Food Standards, Hygiene and Slaughterhouse Policy division, advised Hensley, his immediate superior, that if Establishment 25 produce was involved the Ministry of Health would consider the withdrawal of suspect stocks. It was now important to arrange for a MAFF inspector to visit Argentina for, until then, 'the Minister cannot say that he is fully satisfied as to the precautions which are being taken by the Argentine Government'.[69]

Ministry of Health medical officers visited Bedford and reported that the corned beef involved in the outbreak there had originated from Establishment 25.[70] On 4 November, a meeting was held at the Ministry of Health attended by representatives of MAFF. It was agreed that the Ministry of Health would request the recall of Establishment 25 corned beef canned on or after 30 May 1962. The health officials felt that MAFF should withdraw the official certificate from Establishment 25 until a chlorination plant was installed, but Grace and Bird pointed out that this could only be done through diplomatic channels and would take time. The procedure involved framing a recommendation to the Foreign Office, the Foreign Office forwarding an instruction to the embassy in Buenos Aires, the embassy informing the Argentine

<hr>

64 J. M. Ross to K. A. Bird, 17 September 1963, PRO MAF 282/75.

65 Grace to Bird, 25 September 1963, PRO MAF 282/75; 'Corned beef and typhoid fever', 6 June 1964, PRO MAF.282/87.

66 J. F. E. Bloss to J. M. Ross, 4 November 1963, 276/195.

67 '7 typhoid cases in Bedford area', *The Times*, 24 October 1963 p. 12e; 'One more typhoid suspect held', *The Times*, 28 October 1963 p. 6d.

68 R. V. Blamire to J. Hensley, 28 October 1963, PRO MAF 282/75.

69 G. O. Lace to J. Hensley, 31 October 1963, PRO MAF 276/195.

70 J. F. E. Bloss to J. M. Ross, 4 November 1963, 276/195.

government, a notice being published in the government newspaper the *London Gazette*, and local authorities and port health authorities in Britain being notified. In the view of Grace and Bird all this could be avoided since CAP had undertaken to introduce chlorination from 1 January 1964.[71] The MAFF representatives also expressed doubts about the rationale for the date of 30 May 1962. However, Ross argued that as there was no evidence of an outbreak associated with earlier production, there must have been some change in circumstances at around that time. As for the stockpile, it was agreed that MAFF would stall on the acceptance of further shipments from Establishment 25.[72] On 5 November, the importers agreed to the stock recall, and the following day the company met with representatives of the two ministries. Although sceptical about the link between the outbreaks and their corned beef, the company were already recalling stocks, a process they said would take a month.[73]

MAFF now faced the problem of what to do with their suspect stock.[74] It was believed that Establishment 25 had always used untreated river water and so any of the stockpile's 2,409,276 cases of Establishment 25 corned beef dating from 1953 to 1954 might be contaminated.[75] Stockpiled canned meat was normally sold after eight to ten years, and MAFF feared 'We should . . . be open to justifiable censure if a future outbreak of disease could be attributed to food sold by the Government'.[76] Possible solutions were still under discussion when this problem was exacerbated, since the suspect stock in government and private hands multiplied as a result of the Aberdeen outbreak, and took some years to be resolved, as will be discussed in Chapter 8.

As in the earlier handling of enquiries concerning the Harlow and South Shields outbreaks, great care was taken, following the decision to withdraw suspect stock after the Bedford outbreak, to avoid publicity as far as possible. Ross explained to the CAP representatives that the method of implementing the recall through the trade had been chosen to avoid publicity: the alternative was warning 1500 MOsH and naming the brand.[77] Later, the following statement was released:

> Corned beef is one the safest forms of meat, having been highly processed during manufacture. *Very exceptionally*, however, there has been a presumptive connection

---

[71] Minutes of a meeting held at the Ministry of Health, 4 November 1963, PRO MAF 282/75.

[72] R. E. J. Goodman to Dr Barnell, 18 November 1963, PRO MAF 282/75.

[73] Minutes of a meeting held at the Ministry of Health, 6 November 1963, PRO MAF 282/75.

[74] G. O. Lace to J. Hensley; G. O. Lace to J. M. Ross, 5 November 1963, PRO MAF 282/75.

[75] R. E. J. Goodman to Dr Barnell, 18 November 1963, PRO MAF 282/75.

[76] G. O. Lace to R. L. Briggs, 29 November 1963, PRO MAF 282/75.

[77] Minutes of a meeting held at the Ministry of Health, 6 November 1963, PRO MAF 282/75.

between corned beef from a particular source and recent outbreaks of typhoid in this country. The circumstances of manufacture are being investigated and as a measure of prudence the Ministry of Health has arranged for certain supplies from one source only abroad to be withdrawn from sale.[78]

It was proposed not to release the name of the firm, and, if possible, not to mention the country involved.[79] This press strategy succeeded, as may be illustrated by the number of items in *The Times* about the three corned beef-associated typhoid outbreaks during 1963. There were thirteen items which mentioned the Harlow outbreak, and eleven concerning South Shields. In the case of the Bedford outbreak, however, in spite of the withdrawal of stock that followed, only six items mentioning the outbreak appeared.[80] Public confidence in corned beef was barely dented. In the fourth quarter of 1963, consumption of corned beef slightly exceeded consumption during the same quarter of the previous year. As may be seen from Figure 2.1, corned beef consumption was much more seriously affected by the Aberdeen typhoid outbreak, and took years to recover.[81]

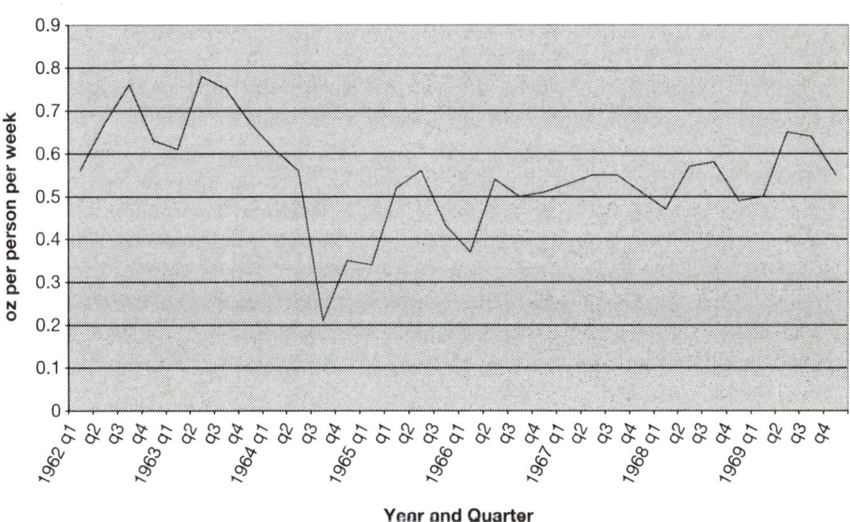

Figure 2.1 Corned beef consumption in Britain, 1962 to 1969
Source: National Food Survey

[78] T. J. B. Dawes to Mr McDowell, 11 November 1963, PRO MAF 282/75.
[79] G. O. Lace to S. S. Osborne, 12 November 1963, PRO MAF 282/75.
[80] *Official Index to the Times*, May to December 1963.
[81] Ministry of Agriculture, Fisheries and Food, *Annual report of the National Food Survey Committee*, 1965–70.

A visit to South America

Once the withdrawal of the suspect stock had been accomplished, MAFF officials turned to arranging a visit to Argentina by Leo Grace, the chief technical adviser on meat inspection, but it soon became clear that Grace would have to consider more than canning plant hygiene. After Claxton, the former veterinary attaché in Buenos Aires finally recovered from his illness and reported to MAFF, assistant secretary Lace told under-secretary Hensley in early November that 'some disquieting developments in the Argentine meat inspection position' had emerged. It now seemed that the meat inspection service presided over by the men whom Claxton had referred to as his 'colleagues' in the Argentine Ministry of Agriculture and Livestock actually left much to be desired.[82] When Lace requested approval for the trip by Grace he noted it was essential to inspect both the hygiene of meat plants and the meat inspection service.[83] Deputy secretary Humphreys-Davies commented that 'In view of the risks to public health, and a possible outcry, I am sure we shall have to do this, costly as it may be'.[84]

We have already observed that the Food Science and Plant Health division appeared to lead the concern over the stockpile, challenging more complacent views of the Food Standards, Hygiene and Slaughterhouse Policy division. During December further differences became apparent over the visit to Argentina. Food Science and Plant Health suggested that a canning expert should accompany Grace. Grace dismissed the suggestion:

> I wonder what constitutes a 'canning expert'? I make no claim to be one myself, but after a long experience of meat plants and canneries in the most important meat exporting countries I might possibly, by any reasonable standard, be considered at least knowledgeable in what constitutes good canning practice. After all, the defect in the Argentine Establishment No. 25 was discovered as a result of my prompting the Veterinary Attaché . . . one might make out an equally good case for attaching an expert bacteriologist to an advisory team. My opinion is that neither is necessary and that the suggestion is impractical.[85]

Food Standards, Hygiene and Slaughterhouse Policy division supported Grace's position. In any case, Grave's departure was planned for 13 January, and they could not afford to delay him.[86]

Grace inspected Establishment 25 and cabled London on 25 January to say he was now content for shipments to resume.[87] But he had encountered a

<hr>

[82] G. O. Lace to J. Hensley, 5 November 1963, PRO MAF 282/75.

[83] G. O. Lace to J. Hensley, 11 November 1963, PRO MAF 282/75.

[84] P. Humphreys-Davies to Mr King, 13 November 1963, PRO MAF 282/75.

[85] L. B. A. Grace to Mr Lace, 17 December 1963, PRO MAF 282/75.

[86] G. O. Lace to J. Hensley, 23 December 1963, PRO MAF 282/75.

[87] K. A. Bird to J. Hensley, 3 March 1964, PRO MAF 282/75.

situation of inefficiency overall. Many plants were running under capacity at a loss, with old and poorly maintained equipment. The morale of government officials was low. By early March Grace had obtained a 'general impression of lax meat inspection and supervision'. He had met with 'pained surprise on the part of the local people that their practices should be found to fall short', but was showing them what was expected. Plants were generally being given a month to take remedial action before a return visit from Grace or the veterinary attaché.[88]

The water in canning factories was chlorinated, except for one at Rosario, known as Establishment 1A, where the chlorination plant had broken down on 31 December 1962. Grace reported this state of affairs on 2 March 1964 by telegram, and sent a list of shipments on their way to Britain by diplomatic bag. The telegram was not received by MAFF until a week later, at the same time as the list of shipments. By this time two vessels containing Establishment 1A corned beef had arrived and their cargoes had been unloaded. In contrast to the decision of November 1963, it was decided that it would be impractical to recall the Establishment 1A stock now in circulation, but three shipments still at sea were not released on arrival. Because International Packers Ltd, the owners of Establishment 1A, disputed the facts as regards the chlorination of the cooling water, the cans were placed in bond pending Grace's return. The company were finally convinced of Grace's findings at a meeting with him on 20 April, and accepted that the stock in bond would have to be removed from the UK. However, when Bird proposed to put the decision in writing, the company's representative asked for the matter to be left 'on the present entirely informal basis'.[89] This was agreed and, once again, publicity was avoided. A month later the first cases of typhoid came to the attention of the authorities in Aberdeen, and the source was later found to be Establishment 1A corned beef.

Conclusions

In retrospect, it is easy to see that the outbreaks in Harlow, South Shields and Bedford during 1963, especially in the light of the pre-existing knowledge of the possibility of contamination of canned food from impure cooling water, might be regarded as 'unheeded warnings', in view of the Aberdeen outbreak that followed in 1964. It is noticeable, however, that knowledge of the hazards of impure cooling water was unevenly distributed, and the veterinary attaché in Buenos Aires had not been made aware of the issue. Within the Ministry of Health and MAFF the matter was initially regarded more as a theoretical

[88] K. A. Bird to J. Hensley, 3 March 1964, PRO MAF 282/75.
[89] K. A. Bird to G. O. Lace, 23 April 1964, PRO MAF 282/75; 'Corned beef and typhoid fever', 6 June 1964, PRO MAF 282/87.

rather than a practical consideration. It is also easy to suggest, with the benefit of hindsight, that had the officials been less concerned to avoid publicity, more decisive action would have been possible. The ministries' press strategy may have arisen largely from a traditional civil service culture of secrecy – a preference for taking decisions in private as far as possible – but in the case of MAFF, in particular, this was reinforced by an anxiety not to offend the Argentinians in view of other agendas.

The anxiety not to offend the Argentinians was linked with oversupply of Argentine beef in early 1963, and during the summer and autumn the Argentinians lobbied for a relaxation of the restrictions which they had previously reluctantly agreed to. This was conceded when MAFF announced in October that from that month until March 1964, Argentine beef imports would amount to between 80,000 and 89,000 tons, and a joint working party was established to agree future arrangements.[90] It emerged in early 1964, however, that Argentina would be unable to meet their commitments. Cattle prices were high in Argentina and packing stations were delaying purchases.[91] Soon officials were discussing how to encourage traders to 'scour the world' for alternative supplies, and one official even suggested taking 'calculated health risks with . . . suppliers from which imports are not at present allowed'.[92] This was a reference to animal health rather than to public health risks, but illustrates the pressures that officials faced shortly before the Aberdeen typhoid outbreak. The beef shortage eased the problem of the earlier mushrooming of the cost of the deficiency payment scheme for the support of home production, but the government soon came under attack from the public, political opposition and the press for the high retail beef prices.[93]

The process of policy formation and implementation as illustrated by the ministries' handling of the 1963 outbreaks is also worth commenting upon. First, it seems that while the Minister of Agriculture was heavily involved in the problem of regulating Argentine meat imports – due to the political and economic repercussions – there was no ministerial involvement in food safety decision making surrounding the typhoid outbreaks. As we will see in later chapters this was to change during the Aberdeen typhoid outbreak and its aftermath. Second, interaction between ministries is clearly an important feature of food safety policy making. In this case, there is no indication that the Ministry of Health acted any more vigorously in the interests of consumers in comparison with MAFF.[94] It seems to be only the fact that the outbreaks

---

[90] 'Press notice', 10 October 1963, PRO MAF 246/211.

[91] T. E. Rogers to R. M. K. Slater, 24 January 1964, PRO MAF 246/211.

[92] N. J. P. Hutchinson to Mr Franklin, 20 February 1964, PRO MAF 246/217.

[93] '*Daily Express* interview with Mr Alex Kenworthy – 21st April, 1964', PRO MAF 246/217.

[94] Unfortunately, it would appear that the relevant Ministry of Health file has not survived and this account must therefore rely largely upon the files of MAFF.

occurred in rapid succession that any action was taken in November 1963. Interactions involving these and additional government departments will be explored further in chapters 5 to 9. Third, food safety policy making also involved interaction between sections of ministries as well as between ministries. Within MAFF, we saw that such interactions involved the Food Science and Plant Health division and the Food Standards, Hygiene and Slaughterhouse Policy division. Such intra-ministry interactions formed an important feature of the process of trying to encourage improvements in Argentine meat hygiene and meat inspection, discussed in Chapter 9. Finally, Grace's response to the suggestion that a 'canning expert' might be able to take part in work for which he, a veterinarian, was formerly solely responsible, suggests that professional factors may also sometimes influence decision making. This is one of the themes of Chapter 7, which discusses the implementation of one of the recommendations of the Milne Committee.

3

The Aberdeen typhoid outbreak

Introduction

During the Aberdeen typhoid outbreak, the Director of Aberdeen university's student health service, Harold Worth, recorded in a letter to the *BMJ* details of the illnesses of two female students, the first typhoid cases. According to Worth, on Tuesday, 12 May 1964, one student visited her doctor complaining of a carbuncle on her back and was taken into residential medical accommodation at Crombie hall of residence. The following day the carbuncle was clearing, but the student developed a fever and her temperature was 103°F by the Thursday. Her flatmate sickened and, on Friday 15 May, with a temperature of 104°F, she was admitted to Crombie sick-bay. During the evening, the second student suffered diarrhoea, while the following day the first had a nosebleed. On the Saturday evening, both were transferred to the nurses' ward at Aberdeen Royal Infirmary, Foresterhill, and were there barrier-nursed.[1] An interview with Worth's colleague, Dr Campbell Murray, expanded upon the circumstances: Worth and Murray were going to a conference, and did not want to leave their patients in Crombie in their absence. Their access to hospital beds arose from their responsibility for nurses as well as students.[2]

Bacteriological investigations were carried out at Foresterhill at the laboratory of Alexander MacDonald, professor of bacteriology at Aberdeen University. Michael McEntegart, MacDonald's deputy, recalled that on 19 May he was on duty with trainee consultant J. A. Smith. Smith asked McEntegart to look at a slide of a micro-organism he had cultured and McEntegart, having experience of typhoid while in the Royal Army Medical Corps, recognised the organism as *Salmonella typhi*. McEntegart recalled that when James Brodie, Director of the Regional Hospital Board laboratory at the City Hospital was informed, 'there was a sort of gasp at the other end of the phone'. That morning, Brodie had obtained five cultures of gram negative organisms from blood samples, but assumed that they were contaminants. He phoned back later to say his assumption had been wrong. MacDonald, McEntegart and

<hr>

[1] H. Worth, 'Typhoid in Aberdeen', *BMJ*, 1964, vol. 1, p. 1706; Temperature charts, AUSHS.
[2] Campbell Murray, interview, 18 November 1999, Aberdeen, ATO/21.

58

Brodie went to the ward, and it was obvious which the typhoid patients were: they were 'flat out'. Later on 19 May, the students were transferred to the City Hospital, which was equipped for dealing with infectious diseases.[3]

The above paragraphs rely on published sources written shortly after the events, and firsthand oral evidence, but differences in detail between these and other sources have been ignored. Worth wrote to the *BMJ* to correct mistakes about the early sequence of events as related in an article by a 'Special Correspondent'.[4] However, he also gave the wrong date for the transfer of the students to the City Hospital, which is made clear by the students' temperature charts. There are also differences in the detail of the bacteriological testing between McEntegart and the report of the official enquiry into the outbreak (known as the Milne report after its chairman, Sir David Milne).[5]

Problems of conflicting evidence and identifying the precise nature and sequence of events has been noted by those investigating more recent food poisoning outbreaks.[6] Memories fade rapidly, records are incomplete, and actors quickly acquire interests in particular interpretations of events. Such difficulties are acute when the outbreak took place forty years previously: many documents have been lost and many actors are unavailable for interview. But in constructing an economical account of such an outbreak it is impossible to draw attention to every inconsistency. The only practical way to proceed is to issue warnings about the sources, and to only draw attention to important discrepancies.

Among the sources for the history of the Aberdeen typhoid outbreak are observations by SHHD officials during visits to Aberdeen, and records of their conversations with Ian A. G. MacQueen, the MOH and others. MacQueen also produced 'Rough notes' on the outbreak in mid-June 1964, and a detailed account in July. To the latter were added notes by his colleagues, and further notes were appended in August. The 'Rough notes' were written after the Milne enquiry had been announced, when it was already clear that MacQueen's performance would come under scrutiny. They were produced for a meeting of the health and welfare committee of Aberdeen Corporation, and were made available to the local press, and the secretary of the Milne Committee.[7] When MacQueen prepared the detailed account the enquiry was underway, the document forming evidence prepared in response to

---

[3] Michael McEntegart, interview, 3 March, 2000, Skipton, ATO/40.

[4] Special Correspondent, 'Typhoid in Aberdeen', *BMJ*, 1964, vol. 1, pp. 1500–2.

[5] Scottish Home and Health Department, *The Aberdeen Typhoid Outbreak*, Edinburgh, 1964 (Milne Report), pp. 9–10.

[6] For example, the precise details of how the infection responsible for the 1996 Wishaw *E. coli* 0157 was transmitted remains a mystery. T. H. Pennington, *When Food Kills, BSE, E. Coli and Disaster Science*, Oxford, 2003, p. 24.

[7] Ian MacQueen, 'Rough notes on the typhoid outbreak', ACA TH 7/6/6; 'Dr MacQueen describes victory prescription', *P&J*, 18 June 1964, p. 4a; I. N. Sutherland to J. Smith, 19 June 1964, NAS HH 61/1073.

questions put by the committee, and MacQueen's appendix answered additional questions.[8] MacQueen's accounts therefore sought to explain and defend his actions, and must be treated with caution. Their defensive character is apparent. In the 'Evidence', for example, he included 'background points' which emphasised the magnitude of the challenges he faced. He mentioned that according to the 1961 census, 19 per cent of Aberdeen's population lived at a density of more than one person per room, and 38.7 per cent of households did not have the exclusive use of a water closet. Furthermore, for a city heavily dependent on the meat, fish and tourist trades, much was at stake. He also observed that there were thirty-three staff vacancies in the health and welfare department, including fourteen health visitors and seven assistant sanitary inspectors.[9]

In this chapter, we will concentrate upon reconstructing events in Aberdeen. We will begin by continuing the account of the beginning of the outbreak and the identification of the source, and proceed to the roles played by general practitioners and the hospital and laboratory services. We will consider patient treatment and experiences, before returning to the action of the health and welfare department. Chapter 4 will consider the interactions between MacQueen, the media and the public, while Chapter 5 will cover the action at central government level, and Chapter 6 the appointment, proceedings and report of the Milne Committee.

The identification of the source

As already indicated, when the students were transferred to the City Hospital, samples were under investigation which indicated that there were other typhoid cases in the city. These included a woman admitted to the City Hospital with gastro-enteritis on 16 May, and her husband and two children admitted on 19 May. A very sick boy was also admitted on 19 May. He and his family had been under the care of a general practitioner, who on 16 May had submitted samples to the City Hospital laboratory. Four other members of his family were admitted on 20 May, together with a further patient who had been sick for two days.[10]

According to the Milne enquiry evidence prepared by Margaret Nairn, superintendent health visitor, a late-afternoon call from the nurses' ward conveyed the news of suspected typhoid to the health and welfare department on 19 May. The following morning the department learned that the students were 'quite probable' typhoid cases, and this information was conveyed to

<hr>

[8] I. A. G. MacQueen, 'Evidence submitted to Committee of Enquiry', July 1964 (main evidence) and August 1964 (further questions), EMR.
[9] MacQueen, 'Evidence', p. 7.
[10] Milne, p. 10. Day book of Dr K. L. Lipp, supplied by Mrs Lipp, entry 16 May 1964.

MacQueen. Nairn's deputy visited the students' lodgings, who found they shared toilet facilities but not meals with the landlord's family, and he left faecal specimen containers, and instructions for disinfection of the house.[11] When MacQueen telephoned the SHHD later on 20 May, he was aware of four cases in three widely separated households. The students had been in Aberdeen for longer than the incubation period, so it seemed unlikely that the disease had been contracted abroad. MacQueen was expecting further cases, had notified the neighbouring MOsH, and thought the infection was likely to be food-borne.[12]

According to the evidence of Dr A. Wilson McIntosh, senior assistant MOH, by 4 p.m. on 20 May, when MacQueen, Nairn and himself discussed the situation after the health visitors had made enquires of the two families that had been admitted to hospital, Low's cooked meat was already under suspicion. However, as yet the link was deemed 'too tenuous to justify further investigation' at the shop. McIntosh visited the hospital during the evening to obtain further information, and called at MacQueen's house at 10 p.m. to report his findings. There were three common factors: milk from the Co-op dairy, ice-cream from Holburn Ices (not common to all households), and cooked meat from a branch of the supermarket chain William Low Ltd. The latter was identified in the diets of eleven of the twelve patients. MacQueen and McIntosh concluded that in view of the frequent sampling of milk and ice-cream, Low's cooked meat was the most likely source of the infection.[13]

On Thursday 21 May, the health and welfare department focused upon Low's supermarket at 492/494 Union Street, close to the students' lodgings. This shop was the first of its kind in Aberdeen and had been open for only eight months. It was bright and clean, and popular with people from the prosperous areas of the city. Nairn and her deputy visited the shop along with Dr D. P. Brunton, another senior assistant medical officer, as McIntosh had left Aberdeen in connection with a professional commitment.[14] Brunton, who was responsible for running Aberdeen's old folks' homes and staffing welfare clinics, recalled that he was at a nursery when called by MacQueen to head-quarters at Willowbank House. He was shown a paper prepared by McIntosh indicating that Low's and corned beef were the 'common denominators'. Brunton had previously handled a small paratyphoid outbreak, and was aware of the questions to be asked and the samples to be taken. MacQueen was about to attend an important meeting, and provided a contact telephone number but preferred not to be disturbed.[15]

[11] M. Nairn, Notes submitted 23 July 1964, MacQueen 'Evidence', Appendix II, p. 38.
[12] R. M. Gordon to John Brotherston, 20 May 1964, NAS HH 58/160.
[13] A. Wilson McIntosh, 'Further appendix to evidence of the Medical Officer of Health', NAS HH 64/228.
[14] Ibid.; Nairn in MacQueen, 'Evidence', p. 39.
[15] D. P. Brunton, interview, 27 October 1999, Aberdeen, ATO/32.

After interviewing the manager, and obtaining addresses of the staff, Brunton and his colleagues interviewed each employee about recent illnesses and symptoms, and their TAB inoculation status (needed for the interpretation of Widal tests). The questions covered service in the armed forces and trips to foreign countries. Blood was taken for analysis at the City Hospital, faecal specimen jars were issued, and staff on holiday or sick leave were followed up at home. The information collected was typed and handed to MacQueen in the late afternoon. Brunton took the samples to the laboratory and spoke to Brodie, whom he knew well, since they had previously worked together.[16]

According to MacQueen's 'Rough notes', by the evening of 21 May, the 'initial investigating team' had formed a 'slight suspicion' about Low's and 'the corned beef or pressed beef sold therein', the number of cases being 'still far too few for certainty'.[17] ('Pressed beef' seems to have been used by MacQueen as an alternative for 'corned beef', referring to the same product.[18]) He emphasised that no report of the Harlow outbreak had been published – an article on Harlow did not appear in the *BMJ* until 6 June[19] – and that his department was unaware that typhoid had been associated with corned beef. The following morning he spoke with Ian Sutherland, epidemiologist at the SHHD. There were now fifteen cases, but one case was believed to have been infected upon the *S. S. Orcades* which had recently arrived in London with a case of typhoid on board.[20] Twenty-two contacts from the *Orcades* had been under surveillance in the Aberdeen area, but the possible connection with the Aberdeen outbreak was soon disregarded.[21] Sutherland noted that the only common factor among the other cases was cooked meat from a supermarket, but all save one patient obtained their milk from the same supplier, and all but one had eaten ice-cream. The dates of sickening indicated that the cause was operative for one or two days. Sutherland suggested that urine samples of the supermarket staff be examined, and MacQueen agreed.[22] Sutherland later recorded that at this time he and MacQueen thought the outbreak:

> would probably conform to the usual type of outbreak in this country and would be found to be associated with the presence in the distribution chain of some ambulant case or carrier, or perhaps a missed case. We did not think it probable that meat infected within the can was the source of this outbreak.[23]

---

[16] Ibid.; Nairn in MacQueen, 'Evidence', p. 39.

[17] MacQueen, 'Rough notes', p. 2.

[18] MacQueen, 'Evidence', p. 18.

[19] I. Ash, G. D. W. McKendrick, M. H. Robertson and H. L. Hughes, 'Outbreak of typhoid fever connected with corned beef', *BMJ*, 1964, vol. 1, pp. 1474–8.

[20] I. N. Sutherland to J. Brotherston, 22 May 1964, NAS HH 58/160.

[21] MacQueen, 'Evidence', p. 16; Nairn in MacQueen 'Evidence', p. 38.

[22] I. N. Sutherland to J. Brotherston, 22 May 1964, NAS HH 58/160.

[23] I. N. Sutherland, 'Aberdeen typhoid outbreak', 16 June 1964, NAS HH 61/11073.

All the tests on the samples collected from the shop's staff proved negative, but two workers who had been off work since 18 May were found to be suffering from typhoid and were admitted to hospital on 22 May. One worked in the cold meat department and the other in the bacon department. But MacQueen dismissed these cases as the source of infection: it was unlikely that they could have infected others who arrived at hospital before themselves. On 25 May the remaining cold meat department staff were sent home pending the results of tests, and on 24 and 28 May two more shop assistants were admitted to hospital, both of whom worked on the fruit counter. The health and welfare department's investigations revealed that four six-pound tins of corned beef were normally opened each morning for use during the day. The same slicers were used for all cold meats, and the same staff worked consistently at the cold meat counter. Cold meat samples were taken, and swabs from the counters, refrigerators and machinery – all testing negative. In view of the rapid turnover of the stock none of the meat from the suspected batches, or their packaging, remained in the shop.[24]

In his 'Evidence', MacQueen emphasised that during the early stages other possible sources were investigated, especially milk, since most of the early cases obtained milk from the Northern Co-operative Society. He even stated that for a few days, milk 'almost rivalled Low's meat department as the source of infection'. Routine test results were re-examined and further samples tested, but it became clear that the epidemiological pattern did not resemble a milk-borne outbreak (in which there is normally a preponderance of children), and patients began to mention a range of milk suppliers. As for water, recent tests showed no evidence of contamination, but the level of chlorination was raised as a precautionary measure. It was soon clear from the explosive nature of the outbreak that it was not likely to be water-borne.[25]

According to MacQueen, as further patients were admitted, by the evening of Friday 22 May his staff 'considered the corned beef hypothesis probable'. Of twenty patients, fifteen recollected eating Low's corned or pressed beef, while four remembered eating cold meat (without specification) from Low's. The following day, the PHLS identified the organism in samples taken from early cases as phage type 34. This was taken as reinforcing the 'corned beef hypothesis', since type 34 was normally found only in Spain and South America (suggesting that the view that the corned beef could not have been infected before opening had been rapidly discarded). No member of Low's staff had visited these countries, apart from the storeman, who had been to Spain, but he had no contact with the meat counter and testing revealed no suspicious results.[26]

---

[24] MacQueen, 'Evidence', pp. 9–10, 18–20, 23–4; Nairn in MacQueen, 'Evidence', p. 39.
[25] MacQueen, 'Evidence', pp. 15–16.
[26] MacQueen, 'Rough notes', p. 2; MacQueen, 'Evidence', pp. 9, 57.

MacQueen's original 'Evidence' emphasised that the involvement of a carrier was deemed 'unlikely in the extreme' as early as 22 May. It seemed improbable that a carrier would have such grossly infected hands as to contaminate corned beef without contaminating other cold meats to a similar extent.[27] Responding to a further question from the Milne Committee on this point MacQueen stated that in the preliminary investigations he:

> regarded the carrier possibility as the obvious one, and therefore instituted a careful search for a carrier. Throughout the early days, however, the difficulties of a carrier explanation became more and more apparent, until . . . I was driven in consultation with my colleagues to reject the carrier explanation.[28]

According to one interviewee, MacQueen clung to a carrier hypothesis until persuaded by colleagues that it was not viable. Bob Hughes, convenor of the Corporation's health and welfare committee, recalled that MacQueen's deputy, David Barclay, approached him on this point.[29] Since Barclay was away from Aberdeen at the start of the outbreak, not returning until 25 May,[30] this implies that following the phage typing MacQueen continued to believe that a carrier had contaminated the meat after the cans were opened. There is no documentary evidence for this, but if this version of events reached the Milne Committee, it may explain why they pressed him on this point.

As the rate of admissions accelerated, the new patients showed dietary histories following the established pattern. Of the first thirty-five cases, twenty had consumed corned or pressed beef, and six other cold meats. Five admitted no connection with Low's, while four could not be interrogated due to their clinical condition. The earliest any patient could remember eating corned or pressed beef was 8 May.[31] A health visitor recalled that many housewives were confident about the date of purchase, because it was shortly after they received their cash 'Divi' (Dividend) from the Co-op, which they used for special treats from Low's.[32] It was thought that the cases where there was no connection with Low's might be explicable in terms of unreliability of memory or conceal-ment in such cases as a cheating husband eating with a lover.[33]

According to MacQueen's 'Rough notes', on 21 May, when it seemed the outbreak might be small, he considered informing local doctors and the press. He decided to inform GPs by telephone before their evening surgeries, and to issue a press statement the following day. However, these plans were

---

[27] MacQueen, 'Evidence', pp. 24–5.
[28] Ibid., p. 56.
[29] R. Hughes, interview, 26 January 2001, Aberdeen, ATO/45.
[30] MacQueen, 'Evidence', p. 1.
[31] Ibid., pp. 3, 20–1.
[32] M. Clubb, interview, 7 June 1999, Aberdeen, ATO/12.
[33] MacQueen, 'Evidence', p. 17.

abandoned when news of the outbreak 'swept over Aberdeen on the late afternoon'.[34] On Saturday, 23 May, MacQueen arranged for a list of names and addresses of confirmed cases to be published. Anyone who had eaten food handled by a person on the list, unless already visited by a member of MacQueen's staff, was asked to consult their doctor.[35] The following day, GPs were contacted by telephone and told confidentially about the link between the outbreak and Low's supermarket, and corned beef.[36] It is the role of GPs during the outbreak that we will now consider, before returning to the activities of the health and welfare department later in the chapter.

General practitioners

During the week beginning 25 May, the number of cases increased rapidly. In total, 540 cases and suspect cases were admitted to hospital, and it was not until 20 June that MacQueen announced that the outbreak was under control. GPs performed several roles in connection with the emergency. In numerous consultations they reassured patients and contributed to their education in the rules of hygiene. They resisted demands for TAB inoculation and gave inoculations in certain cases, took blood from contacts and suspected cases, decided whether laboratory and clinical findings justified hospital admission, and made arrangements for admissions. Their 'gatekeeping' role, which is so important for the running of the NHS, continued during the outbreak, but after the first few days they received far more advice and direction than during normal times.

After the problematic start to informing GPs about the outbreak, a means of keeping them abreast of developments was established. This was the initiative of Dr Birnie, Chairman of the statutory body representing GPs, the local medical committee, who approached MacQueen. The role of the medical committee was to co-operate with the NHS Executive Council of the City of Aberdeen in administering the GP service, and it was arranged for the Clerk of the Council to circulate memoranda. The first circular, hand-delivered on 25 May, provided a definition of a contact as 'any person who has resided in the same house as a known case, or who may have taken a meal with a known case, or who has consumed food prepared or handled by a known case'. Contacts would be advised by public health staff to approach their GP who would take a blood sample using tubes and syringes available from the City Hospital, and issue containers for urine and faeces that should be despatched

---

[34] MacQueen, 'Rough notes', p. 2. There is no mention of the outbreak in *EE*, 21 May 1964, so presumably the news first broke in the electronic media.
[35] 'Plea as typhoid cases named', *EE*, 23 May 1964, p. 1a.
[36] MacQueen, 'Rough notes', p. 2.

by the contacts to the laboratory. Health visitors would also provide contacts with tubes, syringes and containers.[37]

Over the next few days, GPs were informed of various developments. On 26 May they learned that a baker employed by King's bakery was among the confirmed cases. The addresses of King's bakery and four shops were given, and four businesses and a college supplied by the firm were named. A list of eight further businesses served by King's was provided a day later.[38] Consumers of King's products were not to be treated as contacts, but GPs were asked to be on the look-out for secondary cases, which was a continuous concern of the health and welfare department.

The provision of information to GPs was enhanced on Saturday, 30 May when a 'small Special Committee representative of the main interests' was set up 'for liaison and communication', which included Birnie and another member of the medical committee.[39] According to one informant, it was Dr Denys Beddard, senior administrative medical officer for the North-Eastern Regional Hospital Board, who persuaded MacQueen of the necessity of the meetings, which were chaired by MacQueen and held at the health and welfare department at 9 a.m., immediately before MacQueen's morning press conference.[40] Besides the GPs, they involved representatives from the hospital administration, clinical staff, the regional laboratory, the university department of bacteriology, adjacent local authorities, and MacQueen's department.[41] These meetings, held daily until 20 June,[42] provided a forum in which the GPs' representatives could request information and advice. After the first meeting, GPs were sent a copy of an advice leaflet for contacts prepared by MacQueen, and, in view of the pressure the laboratory was under, they were asked to 'restrict to the absolute minimum' the submission of non-outbreak-related samples.[43]

The liaison committee allowed the procedures established by MacQueen to be scrutinised and rationalised, leading to changes in the GPs' work. Most contacts' samples had been taken too soon, when positive results could not be expected, even from those incubating typhoid, and so many tests had to be repeated. On 2 June the GPs were informed that the health and welfare

<hr>

[37] G. A. Matthew to Dear Doctor, 25 May 1964, AUSHS.

[38] G. A. Matthew, 'Circulars to Doctors Nos 50 and 51', 26, 27 May 1964, AUSHS.

[39] G. A. Matthew, 'Circular to Doctors No. 53', 31 May 1964, AUSHS; Executive Council for the City of Aberdeen, 'Report on the services for which the Executive Council are responsible for the year to 31st March 1965', NHSA GRHB D6\2\1 (1964–65).

[40] McEntegart, interview.

[41] MacQueen, 'Evidence', p. 12.

[42] 'Oral evidence taken on 23 June 1964. Dr F. D. Beddard', NAS HH 64/228. According to another document the meetings were held daily until 24 June and then every two days: E. M. W., 24 June 1964, NAS HH 61/1073.

[43] I. A. G. MacQueen, 'Prevention of the spread of typhoid instruction to contacts', May 1964; G. A. Matthew, 'Circular to Doctors No. 53', 31 May 1964, AUSHS.

department aimed to visit all contacts of a case on the day that a positive Widal was obtained. However, contacts would now receive a faecal sample container and instructions to visit their GP for blood sampling only if they had diarrhoea. If they were well, they would be visited seven and fourteen days later, when they would receive a syringe and tube for blood, and twenty-one, twenty-six and thirty-three days after the initial visit, when specimen jars for faeces and urine would be left. As time went on, other changes reduced the burden on GPs and the laboratory. From 11 June, the full contact testing procedure was no longer instituted after a borderline positive Widal result without symptoms.[44] Two weeks later, however, after the outbreak had been declared under control, GPs were warned that recent contact tracing had revealed a few asymptomatic or minimum symptom cases which could be traced to food bought at Low's. The submission of samples was encouraged in such cases in the hope of identifying carriers that might otherwise remain undetected.[45]

Notes on clinical and laboratory aspects of typhoid were circulated on 2 June, clarifying the reasons for changing the testing procedures. GPs were advised to take 'headache and high fever' as the 'cardinal features' of typhoid. In early cases diarrhoea had occurred, continuing for about two days, five to seven days after ingesting the infected material. In later cases, presumed to have arisen from lightly contaminated meats infected via the slicing machine or otherwise, '"flu"-type illness' occurred, with no diarrhoea or vomiting, seven to ten days after infection. The organism did not appear in the blood until definite symptoms developed, and was detectable in the first week of illness, but the Widal test was likely to be negative, since antibodies had yet to develop. During the second week the organism would be gone from the blood, but a positive Widal test was likely. In the third week the organism appeared in the faeces, and possibly in the urine. Patients might then excrete the organisms for weeks or months.[46] According to a circular sent to hospital staff on 8 June, GPs struck a reasonable balance between conflicting laboratory and clinical findings, the great majority of patients admitted to hospital being confirmed as typhoid cases.[47]

A further issue before the first liaison committee meeting was the possibility of using local authority clinics for taking samples to take the pressure off GPs' surgeries, especially in view of the need to re-test early contacts. By 3 June, twice-daily sessions were arranged at Holburn Street clinic, with appointments issued by the health and welfare department. The medical committee appealed for GPs to volunteer their services. It was envisaged that the clinics would

[44] G. A. Matthew, 'Circulars to Doctors Nos 54 and 59', 2, 11 June 1964, AUSHS.
[45] G. A. Matthew, 'Circular to Doctors No. 63', 25 June 1964, AUSHS.
[46] City of Aberdeen local medical committee, 'Typhoid outbreak', 2 June 1964, AUSHS.
[47] Deputy Group Medical Superintendent, Aberdeen General Hospitals, 'Typhoid committee', 8 June 1964, AUSHS.

operate for ten days, but they continued until 26 June.[48] The clinic reduced the burden of sampling, but the test results were returned to the patients' own GPs, who remained responsible for interpreting the results and arranging admissions when necessary.

TAB inoculation was discussed at liaison committee meetings and in circulars to the GPs. Demands for mass inoculation appeared in the press, but MacQueen advised that this was pointless because of the time needed for immunity to develop and the difficulties created for the interpretation of Widal tests. But it was the task of GPs to resist demands for inoculation from individual patients. On 31 May a circular advised GPs that TAB inoculation should be restricted to themselves and their staff, hospital staff, and those due to travel abroad, in view of a shortage of vaccine and the Widal test problem. The GPs, it was suggested, might emphasise that vaccination would not 'alter the course of the disease', but contrarily, two days later, a further circular stated that 'Recent inoculation with TAB *does not protect*, it merely modifies the course of the disease'. Inoculated patients usually presented with 'mild sweating and a headache, similar to mild "flu"'.[49] This confusing advice, and the fact that inoculation was available for health staff, and students on the grounds that they would shortly be dispersing to their homes,[50] hardly constituted strong arguments that GPs could use when faced with the demands of patients. The difficulty of telling whether a patient was genuinely intending to go abroad was pointed out to the committee, but GPs were urged to continue to apply the established guidelines.[51] As procedures were established for the clearance and follow-up of patients, this information was passed on to the GPs. On 1 July they were provided with guidance regarding possible relapse after discharge, and the odds of bone marrow damage from chloramphenicol.[52]

Once the emergency was over and the numbers of patients in hospital were dwindling, on 22 July a letter of appreciation of the work of the GPs from the health and welfare committee was passed on to them. This alluded to the problems which could arise between GPs and the health and welfare department:

> The Committee are very conscious of the fact that the difficulties inherent in the division of functions between the various branches of the Health Service can only be overcome by the co-operation and goodwill of all those engaged in the various

---

[48] G. A. Matthew, 'Circulars to Doctors Nos 53, 55, 59 and 63', 31 May, 3, 11, 25 June 1964, AUSHS.

[49] G. A. Matthew, 'Circular to Doctors No. 53', 31 May 1964; City of Aberdeen local medical committee, 'Typhoid outbreak', 2 June 1964, AUSHS.

[50] Secretary to the University, 'Typhoid outbreak', 1 June 1964, AUSHS.

[51] G. A. Matthew, 'Circular to Doctors No. 54', 2 June 1964, AUSHS.

[52] G. A. Matthew, 'Circular to Doctors No. 61', 17 June 1964, AUSHS; 'Circular to Doctors No. 69', 24 July 1964; City of Aberdeen local medical committee, 'Guidance notes on follow-up of patients on discharge from hospital', 1 July 1964, EMR.

branches, and they would like the general practitioners concerned to know that the manner in which they responded to the demands of the recent emergency commands the Committee's respectful and sincere appreciation.[53]

GPs had met the demands placed upon them during the emergency, but as we will see in Chapter 6, in view of the health and welfare department's clumsy start to the dissemination of information, 'co-operation and goodwill' were not the themes of GPs' evidence to the Milne Committee. Rather, complaints were made about the way the GPs heard about the outbreak from the press and the fact that contacts were advised in the press to get in touch with their GP, before any official communication about the outbreak had reached the GPs.

Hospitals

The number of cases at the City Hospital grew from twelve, when McIntosh visited during the evening of 20 May, to forty-eight by the time the *Press and Journal* of Monday, 25 May went to press.[54] Figure 3.1, based on data compiled by the SHHD for the Milne Committee, shows the numbers of confirmed and suspected cases in hospital from 26 May, when there were seventy-four confirmed and twelve suspected cases, to 30 June. The largest increase in the confirmed cases took place between Sunday, 31 May and Monday, 1 June (from 155 to 197). From 26 May to 12 June, the increase in confirmed cases averaged about nineteen per day, but from then onwards, when the total confirmed cases stood at 393, the rate of increase slowed. On 24 June there were 418 confirmed cases in hospital, after which this figure began to decline.[55] Clearly, Aberdeen's hospitals were faced with a tremendous challenge in making sufficient beds available.

According to a paper published under the editorship of William Walker, consultant physician at the City Hospital, 540 patients were admitted to hospital in Aberdeen, of whom 503 were confirmed and suspected typhoid patients, and thirty-seven rejected as non-typhoid (Table 3.1[56]). Four further confirmed cases were not admitted to hospital. Of the 507 cases, 469 were confirmed clinically or bacteriologically, but thirty-eight remained as suspects. They were from 309 households in Aberdeen and thirty-three in surrounding districts. Eight further patients contracted typhoid in Aberdeen but were

---

[53] G. A. Matthew, 'Circular to Doctors No. 68', 22 July 1964, AUSHS.

[54] 'Typhoid – 48 Cases', *P&J*, 25 May 1964, p. 1d.

[55] 'Committee of Inquiry into the Aberdeen Typhoid Outbreak Memorandum by the Scottish Home and Health Department, Appendix 1 Typhoid Outbreak – Aberdeen Hospital Services', 1 July 1964, NAS HH64/352.

[56] The data in the table are taken from W. Walker (ed.), 'The Aberdeen typhoid outbreak of 1964', *Scottish Medical Journal*, 1965, vol. 10, pp. 466–79.

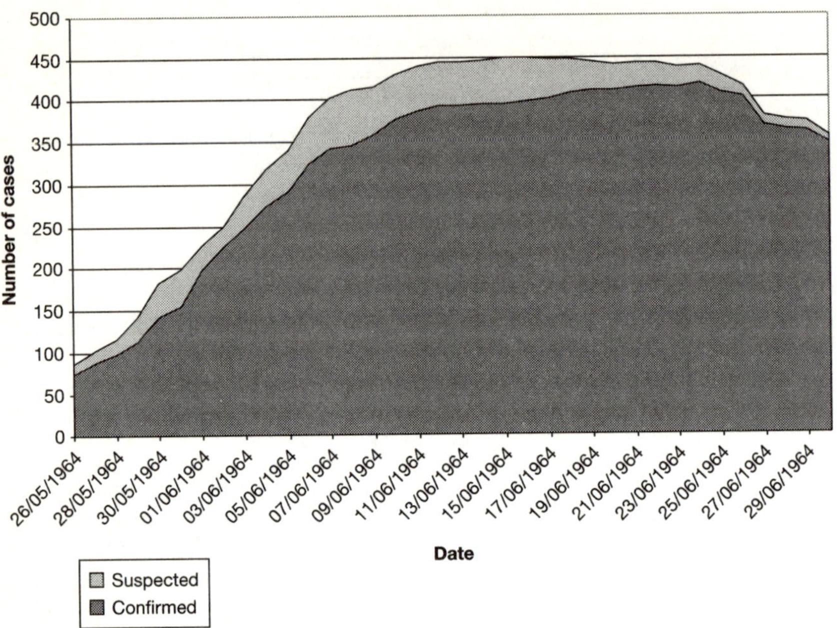

Figure 3.1 Confirmed and suspected cases of typhoid in hospital during the Aberdeen outbreak

Table 3.1 Number of patients involved in the Aberdeen typhoid outbreak

Category	Number of patients
Admitted to hospital	540
Rejected as non typhoid	37
Typhoid patients in hospital	503
Typhoid patients not admitted	4
Clinically or bacteriologically confirmed	469
Typhoid not confirmed but not excluded	38
Total number of patients	507

treated elsewhere: two in Dundee, three in Glasgow, two in Newcastle and one in Toronto.

Since 1948, the NHS hospitals in and around Aberdeen had been controlled by the North-Eastern Regional Hospital Board, under which were general and special hospital boards of management. Within the former group, the outbreak had most impact upon Woodend Hospital, about a mile west of Foresterhill. Most affected in the latter group were the City Hospital, a former municipal infectious diseases hospital, about a mile east of Foresterhill, the

Royal Aberdeen Children's Hospital at Foresterhill, Tor-na-Dee chest diseases hospital at Milltimber, six miles from Aberdeen, and Glen O' Dee convalescent hospital at Banchory, eighteen miles south-west of Aberdeen.

Besides the students, seven further patients in six wards at the Royal Infirmary were identified as typhoid victims[57] and were transferred to the City Hospital. Two came to light after the first cases were notified, but before the news was in general circulation. Dr Sandy Logie recalled that when these cases were discovered on the ward where he was a house officer, and the consultant, Alastair MacGregor, regius professor of materia medica and therapeutics, phoned MacQueen, he was 'more than somewhat surprised to be told by Dr MacQueen that he knew there was typhoid in the City. The professor was not a little upset.'[58]

As with the GPs, it took a few days for communications with hospital staff to be established, but on 25 May the general hospitals' clinical consultants were informed by the group medical superintendent that the source was 'prepared meat sold in a supermarket'. Sixty-five cases had been admitted to the City Hospital,[59] where seventy-two beds were being vacated in geriatric and general medical wards. On the advice of Alexander MacDonald, professor of bacteriology, a surgical ward at the Royal Infirmary was closed to admissions after a colostomy patient was found to be suffering from typhoid. This was probably a patient referred to by MacDonald's deputy in an interview. There was great concern because the patient had helped staff distribute meals, but no evidence of cross-infection.[60]

The immediate challenges were greatest for the special hospitals. On 27 May, the group superintendent Alex M. Duncan was authorised to recruit additional staff, purchase equipment and make other arrangements. He had already appealed for former nurses to come forward, resulting in a front-page *Evening Express* headline, 'More nurses needed as typhoid toll soars', and twenty-two responded.[61] The retired superintendent of Belvidere fever hospital at Clydeside was engaged, and the former physician in charge of the City Hospital diabetic clinic volunteered his services. Walker took up his appointment as consultant physician at the City Hospital on 1 June, a month earlier than anticipated. In total, eleven physicians cared for typhoid patients across the two hospital groups. Some junior medical staff within and beyond the

---

[57] Deputy Group Medical Superintendent, Aberdeen General Hospitals, 'To all medical staff Aberdeen General Hospitals', 30 May 1964, AUSHS.
[58] A. Logie, interview, 16 July 1999, Bowden near Melrose, ATO/21.
[59] A. M. Michie to all clinical consultants, 25 May 1964, AUSHS.
[60] J. F. Kirk, 'Typhoid outbreak in Aberdeen', 25, 26 May 1964, NAS 058/160; McEntegart, interview.
[61] Finance Committee, 27 May 1964, Board of Management, Aberdeen Special Hospitals, NHSA GRHB B2\1\1\17; 'Housewives' plea', 'More nurses needed as typhoid toll soars', *EE*, 25 May 1964, p. 1a; J. F. Kirk, 'Typhoid outbreak in Aberdeen', 27 May 1964, NAS HH 058/160.

North-Eastern Region were transferred to the typhoid wards, including two house officers and a registrar from the Western Region.[62]

As further beds in rheumatology, gynaecology and tuberculosis wards were vacated, it became clear that there was insufficient accommodation at the City Hospital. Non-typhoid patients were sent home, to Glen O'Dee Hospital, or to general medical units elsewhere. At peak, 198 beds, and all but two of ten City Hospital wards were filled with typhoid victims. Two wards were used for children and another admitted the few infant patients. For further juvenile cases, two wards at the Aberdeen Royal Hospital for Sick Children, amounting to sixty-four beds, were assigned to the outbreak, and patients were admitted from 29 May, tonsillectomies being carried out meantime at Stracathro Hospital. The number of patients at the Hospital for Sick Children peaked at forty-nine.[63]

By 29 May, Tor-na-Dee was being cleared, and the first typhoid patients were admitted there the following day. Use of the hospital was offered by the medical officer in charge, Douglas Kay, a tuberculosis specialist who had seen typhoid in India and in Fife. None of the fifty patients at the hospital were critically ill, and they were sent home or housed at Glen O'Dee. The retired superintendent from Belvidere acted as consultant for Tor-na-Dee, a registrar was lent by the Royal Infirmary and nursing staff were seconded from the Infirmary, Woodend Hospital and Ruchill, Strathclyde and Belvidere hospitals in the West of Scotland. The nursing staff included a retired fever hospital matron from Glasgow. Tor-na-Dee took 105 typhoid cases, the last admission taking place on 14 June. A total of 108 beds were available at the hospital, with families accommodated in double rooms. Normal capacity was seventy-eight beds in single rooms.[64]

Within the general hospital group an atmosphere of relative calm persisted during the first week of the outbreak. On 30 May a circular to medical staff stated that it was unnecessary to stop admissions of waiting list patients as long

[62] A. M. Duncan, Report of the Board of Management for Aberdeen Special Hospitals, 1964, NHSA GRHB B2\2\11; A. M. Duncan, 26 May 1964; J. P. Sexton, 'Board of Management for the Aberdeen Special Hospitals, Typhoid Outbreak Second Interim Report', 10 July 1964, GRHB B2\3 [20\7]; I. A. Porter and M. J. Williams, *Epidemic Diseases in Aberdeen and the History of the City Hospital*, Aberdeen, 2001, pp. 167, 177, 178.

[63] J. P. Sexton, 'Board of Management for the Aberdeen Special Hospitals, Typhoid Outbreak Second Interim Report', 10 July 1964, NHSA GRHB B2\3 [20\7]; A. M. Duncan, 'Report of the Board of Management for Aberdeen Special Hospitals', 1964, NHSA GRHB B2\2\11; Porter and Williams, *Epidemic Diseases*, pp. 175–6; Walker, 'Aberdeen Typhoid', p. 472; 'Note by Dr Macgregor', NAS HH 58/160.

[64] G. A. Matthew, 'Circular to Doctors No. 52', 29 May 1964, AUSHS; A. M. Duncan, Report of the Board of Management for Aberdeen Special Hospitals, 1964, NHSA GRHB B2\2\11; D. T. Kay, interview, 16 June 1999, Milltimber, ATO/17; J. P. Sexton, 'Board of Management for the Aberdeen Special Hospitals, Typhoid Outbreak Second Interim Report', 10 July 1964, NHSA GRHB B2\3 [20\7].

as the wards did not become too overcrowded in view of the twenty-nine-bed convalescent facility at Cults being held empty for possible use for the outbreak. Precautions had been taken similar to those instituted in the special hospitals. Staff had been immunised and visitors had been asked not to bring eatables into the hospitals. Catering officers reduced the handling of food to a minimum and avoided prepared cold meats, salads, fresh fruit and artificial cream. Cloth towels were replaced with paper.[65]

A few days later, it became clear that general hospital beds were needed. On 4 June, following a meeting of representatives of the physicians, surgeons, bacteriological department and senior nursing staff, a notice was issued to all medical staff. Beddard, senior administrative medical officer, explained that it had been decided to confine typhoid patients within the region, and to this end beds were being made available at Woodend Hospital. Eleven cases were already in an annexe at Woodend, two wards providing eighty beds would be clear by 5 or 6 June, and two additional wards would be available by 8 June. The vacancies were achieved by sending patients home or to other wards at Woodend and Aberdeen Royal Infirmary, encouraging cottage hospitals to take convalescent patients, and informing GPs that beds were now extremely scarce.[66] On 5 June, GPs received a memorandum warning of a major reduction in the beds for certain specialties, and that patients would be discharged earlier than in normal circumstances.[67] Plans were made for a ward at the Infirmary to be made available, but seem not to have been implemented. The task of persuading consultants to give up beds was delegated to James Kyle, a consultant surgeon and secretary of the medical staffs committee, a statutory body that advised the hospital board. Kyle recalled that 'from the word go' the consultants accepted that 'they had to completely alter their views about their sovereignty over their own ward'. A total of 530 beds were made available during the outbreak, consisting of 198 at the City Hospital, 108 at Tor-na-Dee, 64 at the Royal Hospital for Sick Children, and 160 at Woodend.[68]

When beds became available at Tor-na-Dee, GPs were told to make direct contact regarding admissions, but from 2 June all contact was to be with an 'Admission Centre' established in the City Hospital nurses' training department. GPs were to contact the senior house physician, Elizabeth Russell, or her deputy, providing patient details, TAB status and laboratory findings,

<hr>

[65] Deputy Group Medical Superintendent, Aberdeen General Hospitals, 'To all medical staff Aberdeen General Hospitals', 30 May 1964, AUSHS; M. C. Y. Hudson, 27 May 1964, NHSA, GRHB B2\3 [20\7].

[66] Deputy Group Medical Superintendent, Aberdeen City Hospitals, 'Typhoid outbreak', 4 June 1964, AUSHS.

[67] D. Beddard to all general practitioners in the region, 5 June 1964, AUSHS.

[68] Deputy Group Medical Superintendent, Aberdeen General Hospitals, 'Typhoid outbreak', 4 June 1964, AUSHS; J. Kyle, interview, 4 February 1999, Aberdeen, ATO/1; J. P. Sexton, 'Board of Management for the Aberdeen Special Hospitals, Typhoid Outbreak Second Interim Report', 10 July 1964, GRHB B2\3 [20\7].

if known. The Centre would tell the GP which hospital the patient would be admitted to, and notify the hospital of the details.[69]

The workloads of the regional laboratory and, to a lesser extent, the university bacteriology department, increased dramatically. By Monday, 1 June, the bacteriological examinations per day had increased twentyfold over normal times. Figure 3.2 shows the number of typhoid investigations undertaken at the City Hospital from 20 May to 31 December, excluding the small numbers of orthodox blood cultures (505), Vi agglutination tests (1253), and cultures of sewer swabs, foodstuff samples and so on (649). With these, the typhoid investigations totalled 70,304 at the City Hospital, and 2443 at the bacteriology department.[70]

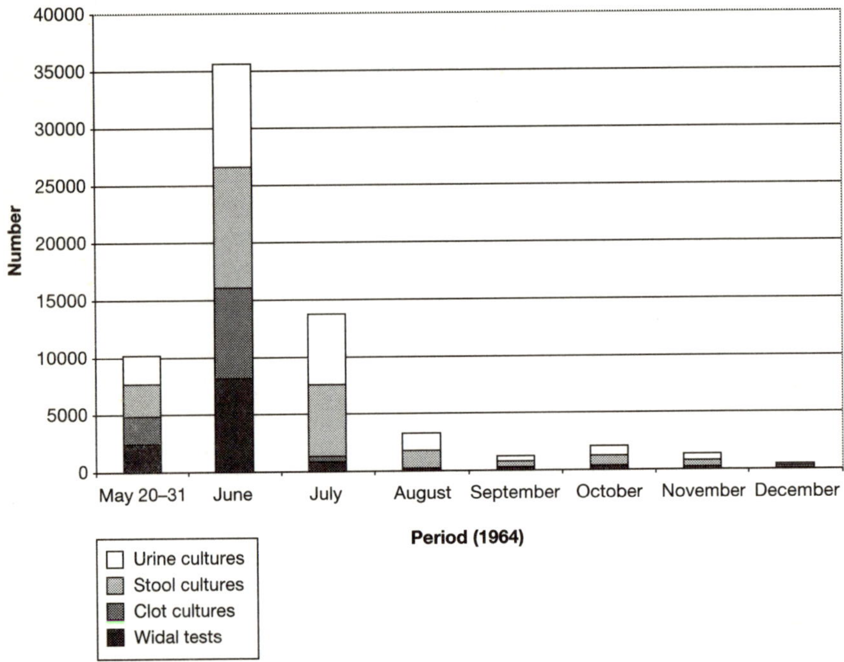

Figure 3.2 Typhoid investigations at the City Hospital laboratory, Aberdeen, May to December 1964

[69] A. M. Duncan, 'Report of the Board of Management for Aberdeen Special Hospitals, 1964', NHSA GRHB B2\2\11; G. A. Matthew, 'Circulars to Doctors Nos 53, 54, 58', 31 May, 2, 7 June 1964; North East Regional Hospital Board, 'Procedure for admission to hospital of patients with typhoid or suspected typhoid', 7 June 1964; Deputy Group Medical Superintendent, Aberdeen General Hospitals, 'Typhoid Committee', 8 June 1964, AUSHS.
[70] Walker, 'Aberdeen typhoid', p. 474.

During the height of the outbreak the regional laboratory staff worked from 6 a.m. until 10 p.m. seven days a week, and were still working until 9 p.m. on 10 July. Assistance was provided by a consultant from the Eastern Region, and technicians supplied by the agricultural college. The technicians increased from nineteen to twenty-seven, while laboratory maids increased from nine to twelve, and office staff from nine to twenty-four. Fifteen additional typists were needed to deal with the increased volume of laboratory reports.[71] The laboratory also had to contend with press interest and visits from officials and politicians. One technician recalled that the photographers 'were scared to put their cameras down or touch a chair. . . . They were very, very anxious.' They were 'desperate to get people working on microscopes' but since 'you don't do anything under microscopes with typhoid', shots of 'the lads . . . doing the stool samples' were 'the next best thing'.[72]

The increase in the public health work was not achieved without tensions between MacQueen and Brodie, Director of the City Hospital laboratory. Difficulties between the two began early and emerged later at the liaison committee meetings. Ian Sutherland at the SHHD recorded on 26 May that MacQueen 'had a minor complaint about the adequacy of laboratory services', and the following day noted that Brodie had been 'making independent investigations in the history of a number of patients'.[73] A day later he was more explicit:

> Relations between the Public Health Department and the Laboratory are no more than fair and I think Dr Brodie has some cause for his grouse that he has not been brought into full consultation. One example is that he is not sent the completely suitable specimens for blood culture and he is doing what is second best in the form of clot culture from specimens primarily submitted for serology.[74]

Brodie had been surprised when he received sewer swabs for examination, which he thought 'a pointless addition to his troubles'.

Sutherland suggested to MacQueen that he might contact Brodie by telephone to keep him in the picture. And when Sutherland visited Brodie in Aberdeen on Saturday, 30 May, he suggested that Brodie might attend the liaison committee meeting that MacQueen had called. This, thought Sutherland, might 'help to improve the relations between the M.O.H. and the laboratory men'. At the meeting, however, Sutherland witnessed 'an explosion from Dr Brodie who complained that he had received . . . about 50 specimens from Lows which had not been fully documented'. The complaint was partly

---

[71] J. P. Sexton, 'Board of Management for the Aberdeen Special Hospitals, Typhoid Outbreak Second Interim Report', 10 July 1964, GRHB B2\3 [20\7]; J. Brodie, 'City Hospital – the laboratory', NHSA GRHB B2\2\11.
[72] Fiona Milne, interview, 1 June 1999, Aberdeen, ATO/9.
[73] I. N. Sutherland to J. Smith, 26, 27 May 1964, NAS, HH 58/160.
[74] I. N. Sutherland to J. Smith, 28 May 1964, NAS, HH 58/160.

that Brodie already had sufficient work to do, as a discussion followed about the possibility of sending food samples elsewhere. But Brodie's dissatisfaction was not all with the health and welfare department, since he also complained that GPs' specimens were often badly documented. This discussion preceded discussion about the contact-testing clinic, the origins of which seem to lie partly in the discontent of the laboratory.[75] On 9 June Sir John Brotherston, the CMO of the SHHD, witnessed a further complaint by Brodie at a liaison committee meeting. He recorded:

> The main event . . . was a protest from Dr. Brodie . . . about a press announcement coming from Dr. MacQueen's morning press conference which had suggested that doubts about the diagnosis of the food handler from the shop might be due to a laboratory mistake. Dr. Brodie made the point that there was no evidence to suggest a laboratory mistake and, furthermore, this kind of press announcement might affect public confidence in the laboratory.[76]

This was a reference to a positive urine test obtained from one of Low's shelf-stackers.

To avoid confusion and duplicating work, the Admission Centre, renamed the 'Co-ordinating Centre', received all laboratory reports, and controlled the admission, clearance and discharge of patients. On discharge, the wards sent patient notes to the Centre for the abstraction of information for research, and the Centre notified GPs and the health and welfare department.[77] Russell remained in charge and was appointed a temporary locum registrar from 1 August.[78]

By the time the arrangements for providing beds were complete, the outbreak was being contained and minds turned towards the criteria for discharge of patients, and how the backlog of elective admissions could be cleared. By 17 June, when MacQueen thought that the outbreak was under control, many patients were approaching clearance, although 10 per cent to 30 per cent were expected to require additional treatment. The first discharge of a confirmed case took place on 19 June.[79]

---

[75] I. N. Sutherland to Deputy Chief Medical Officer, 3 June 1964, NAS, HH 58/160.

[76] J. Brotherston to Dr Smith, 10 June 1964, NAS HH 61/1073.

[77] Alex. M. Duncan, 'Typhoid clearance and test procedure', 12 June 1964; City Hospital, 'Documentation and procedure for clearance tests', 12 June 1964, EMR.

[78] J. P. Sexton, 'Board of Management for the Aberdeen Special Hospitals, Typhoid Outbreak Second Interim Report', 10 July 1964, GRHB B2\3 [20\7]; A. M. Duncan to V. O. Cruikshank, 12 June 1964, NHSA, B2\3 [20\7]; E. Russell, 17 June 1964, NHSA, B2\3 [20\7].

[79] Deputy Group Medical Superintendent, Aberdeen General Hospitals, 'Typhoid committee', 8 June 1964; 'Typhoid Outbreak Report at Meeting of medical staff committee, 17th June 1964', 18 June 1964, AUSHS; MacQueen, 'Evidence', p. 15; 'She's first patient out', *P&J*, 20 June 1964, p. 1a.

At a meeting of medical staff on 17 June, it was reported that two of the cleared wards at Woodend would not be needed, while the other wards and the annexe would be empty in about twenty-one days, and six to seven weeks respectively. Measures for the terminal disinfection of wards were agreed. By early July, it was envisaged that within a few weeks all cases would be concentrated at the City Hospital, but Beddard thought that it would take twelve to eighteen months to clear waiting lists.[80] It was therefore decided not to return Tor-na-Dee to normal use immediately, but to use it for surgical and gynaecological cases. Chest cases would be cared for meantime at Glen O' Dee and the City Hospital. By 21 July, a total of 230 typhoid patients had been discharged, although a few were readmitted following relapse at home.[81] Tor-na-Dee was empty of typhoid patients by 30 July, and all patients were moved out of the Sick Children's Hospital by 16 August. The last typhoid patient was discharged from the City Hospital on 22 September. Tor-na-Dee was closed for redecorating from 31 July to 27 August, but could not be used immediately for operations due to staff shortages. Stracathro Hospital and the City Hospital also contributed to the clearance of waiting lists, and Tor-na-Dee and Glen O' Dee hospitals returned to their normal uses towards the end of November.[82]

Patient treatment and experiences

One distinctive feature of the Aberdeen outbreak was the high proportion of female victims. As seen from Table 3.2,[83] women constituted almost 60 per cent of confirmed typhoid patients, and in the 15 to 29 age group there were almost twice as many women as men. These differences were explained by a difference in eating habits, as 'reducing diets' of cold meat and salads were popular among the younger women.[84]

Of the 507 patients in which typhoid was confirmed or suspected, 391 said they had eaten food from Low's, of whom 383 ate cold meat, and eight ate fruit

[80] 'Typhoid Outbreak Report at Meeting of Medical Staff Committee, 17th June 1964', 18 June 1964, AUSHS; 'Note of an extraordinary meeting of the Chief Medical Officer and senior administrative medical officers', 29 June 1964, NAS HH 64/351.

[81] Medical Services Committee, North East Regional Hospital Board, 7 July 1964; Finance Committee, North East Regional Hospital Board, 14 August 1964 NHSA GRHBA1\1\9; 'Minute of a meeting held at the North-Eastern Regional Hospital Board (Scotland) Offices on 21 July 1964 to continue discussion of Policy for Discharge and Surveillance of Patients suffering from Typhoid', EMR.

[82] Finance Committee, North East Regional Hospital Board, 14 August 1964, NHSA GRHBA1\1\9; A. M. Duncan, 'Report of the Board of Management for Aberdeen Special Hospitals', 1964, NHSA GRHB B2\2\11.

[83] E. M. Russell, 'Typhoid fever in Aberdeen: a critical analysis', MD thesis, University of Aberdeen, 1965, p. 466.

[84] Walker, 'Aberdeen typhoid', p. 467.

Table 3.2 Age and sex of confirmed patients

Age groups	Male	Female	Both
0–14	53	55	108
15–29	37	89	126
30–44	37	38	75
45–59	26	60	86
60 plus	29	45	74
All ages	182	287	469

only. Of the others, thirty-two fell ill at the same time as other family members. Russell suggested that the infection was probably transferred by handling from the contaminated food to other food and that these were not true secondary cases, infected via faecal contamination. The remaining eighty-four patients could give no indication of how they had been exposed to typhoid.[85]

In oral history interviews, patients frequently reminisced about how they felt during the acute stages. One, a teenager at the time, recalled:

> By the time the ambulance arrived I was kinda delirious . . . somebody came up the stairs and I dinna ken foo. My mother tellt me later that I was just raving. I thocht they had come from Gordon and Watson's [local undertakers] . . . I just assumed I was deid or deeing or something 'cos I really was that ill. My mother was awfy upset 'cos my final words as I was carted out the door were 'Dinna burn me I want to be buried.'[86]

But many patients were not admitted in such circumstances and were often told, when informed of a positive test result, to go to hospital by bus.[87] Another described how she felt during a relapse:

> My temperature had went right up and then for two or three days I cannot remember anything. I was actually getting specialed, the nurse and the doctors were coming in and out often and giving me injections too – I don't know if it was antibiotics or – and I was getting cold baths to take my temperature down. I was put on this powdered stuff – a drink, to try and get my temperature down . . . I actually went into a semiconscious state . . . it was probably about three days before I sort of came around . . . it must have been about another fortnight before I was able to get up.[88]

---

85 Russell, 'Typhoid fever', 1965, p. 54.
86 Sheena Blackhall, interview, 18 September 2001, Aberdeen, ATO/46.
87 Margaret Nairn, interview, 18 May 1999, Aberdeen, ATO/3.
88 Irene Morrison, interview, 26 May 1999, Aberdeen, ATO/6.

Because of the risk of damage to blood-forming tissues from chloramphenicol, doses used were at the lower end of the usual range. There was experimentation with other antibiotics, especially the recently developed ampicillin and cephaloridine. Ampicillin killed *Salmonella typhi* in the test-tube, and some success had been claimed for it as a treatment for carriers. In total, 332 adults received chloramphenicol, while fourteen received either ampicillin, or chloramphenicol followed by ampicillin, or *vice versa*. Three patients were given cephaloridine but were changed to chloramphenicol when they failed to respond. Of the children, fifty-eight received chloramphenicol alone and forty-seven ampicillin, or both drugs. The courses lasted about two weeks, but dosages varied with the consultant in charge.[89] Ampicillin was much less effective than chloramphenicol, but it was thought that higher doses might have worked better.[90]

Most patients responded quickly to treatment but one remembers being weak for a long time at Tor-na-Dee:

> High temperature, just in bed all the time, we never got up at all. Now I'm trying to think if it was two or three weeks or was it into the fourth week that we were allowed out because obviously we'd become stronger, become better obviously and the doctor said 'now if you feel fit enough you can go and have a walk around the grounds'. So me and my mum were hanging on to one another, and went down stairs . . . and we got a shock actually because we never realised how many – there was a lot of people . . . and everybody was sort of shuffling about, and everybody was getting a shock because they never realised being so ill, you thought you were the only one in hospital until you come downstairs and there was all these folk.[91]

Once patients felt well again, some found confinement frustrating. Televisions were introduced, occupational therapy was provided, and teachers volunteered to help children continue their education. Kay arranged for a police pipe band to play in the grounds of Tor-na-Dee to give a boost to a 12-year old girl, a band member, who was very sick, and one patient, broadcaster Harry Lockhart, started internal broadcasting, with requests from patients to their friends.[92]

One memory of patients and their relatives is the feeling of separation caused by the visiting regime. No visitors were allowed inside the hospitals; they had to talk with loved ones through closed windows. Gifts were handed in at the ward door and never came home from the hospital. Kay remembers standing at his office window updating visitors concerning the patients' progress. He used a tape-recorder to convey messages between patients and

[89] Russell, 'Typhoid fever', p. 99 and Table 100; W. Walker, 'Cephaloridine in typhoid', *BMJ*, 1964, vol. 2, pp. 1529–30.
[90] 'Note of meeting held on Thursday 19 November, 1964', EMR.
[91] Irene Morrison, interview, 26 May 1999, Aberdeen, ATO/6.
[92] Kay, interview.

their visitors.[93] Journalists and photographers mixed with the visitors in search of promising 'personal interest' stories, and it was outside the wards that some of the most striking images of the outbreak were produced. One, which appeared in several newspapers, showed a tearful boy looking out at his visitors. His father and grandmother were holding a slate with 'Mummy and Daddy send their love' written in chalk.[94]

The visiting regime was distressing for those unable to touch their sick children for weeks. A patient who gave birth was not allowed to hold her baby for three months.[95] One mother is still angry at the treatment of her son who was under 2 at the time of admission to the Sick Children's Hospital. His parents were told not to visit for the first few days, but they kept in touch by phone. On the tenth day they were told that his temperature had gone down and they could visit:

> We couldn't see our child, looked up and down, right along and on the corner, I can still see it yet, on the far corner on the right hand side was a little baby, he stood up and he . . . a skeletal little face . . . and I was just distressed . . . he was back to his birth weight.[96]

By the time the toddler went home he was virtually institutionalised, having spent nearly a tenth of his life in hospital.

All patients, no matter the circumstance, had to meet strict criteria for discharge. The subject came under discussion at the liaison committee on 31 May, when Beddard suggested discharging some patients before they completed the customary three consecutive negative tests, in order to ease pressure on the hospitals. Brodie opposed this and was supported by others. He argued that the average patient would be infective for three weeks after admission, and that the test of cure should start on convalescence and last for at least ten days. The bare minimum hospital stay would be a month, and five weeks more usual.[97] The issue was discussed on 2 June, when Brotherston was present. It was deemed a 'national problem' and decided that the SHHD would consult expert opinion.[98] Brotherston subsequently chaired a meeting on 9 June, which included experts from Colindale, Edinburgh, Glasgow and Dundee. A 'negative clearance test' would be one on stools and urine which was negative using direct plating and enrichment techniques. Patients would be classified as 'routine', posing no special risk of communicating the disease, 'minor risk' including housewives and those not involved in occupational food handling,

[93] Ibid.

[94] See e.g. *Observer*, 7 June 1964, p. 5d.

[95] Joyce McKain, interview, 22 June 1999, Aberdeen, ATO/20.

[96] Aileen Pettit, interview, 10 February 2000, Aberdeen, ATO/39.

[97] I. N. Sutherland to Deputy Chief Medical Officer, 3 June 1964, NAS HH 58/160.

[98] R. M. Gordon, 'Enteric epidemic Aberdeen', 3 June 1964, NAS HH 58/160.

and 'major risk', or food handlers. For all, three negative tests at four-day intervals, beginning not less than four days after the cessation of treatment, were required before discharge. Then, at seven-day intervals, routine, minor and major risk cases required three, six and nine further negative tests respectively. Patients producing a positive test during the hospital clearance phase would remain in hospital until three consecutive negative tests were obtained. Once these patients had achieved clearance in hospital, their post-hospital clearance phase would involve six, nine and twelve tests for the three risk categories.[99]

A leaflet explained to patients that although they might feel well, their continued stay in hospital was essential so that they could be 'quite rid of the infection' and 'no longer a risk' to themselves, families and friends. If any test was positive, patients would 'remain under hospital care for a little longer while steps are taken to clear up the infection', and all would provide specimens after discharge to ensure there was 'no lingering risk'. The document was signed by Beddard, MacQueen, and the MOsH of the adjoining local authorities.[100]

Many of the patients interviewed spoke of the routine of their stay in hospital awaiting clearance and how they adapted to it. Problems sometimes arose between the patients, due to the enforced incarceration and the stress of getting the three clear samples. Sheena Blackhall, who has written about her experiences, remembers being ostracised because she was late for ward rounds and could have had the patients' walks outside stopped. But two days later 'a woman left the toilet, and omitted to wash her hands – the greatest sin you could commit. Instantly communal attention switched.'[101]

Many patients felt aggrieved at being confined to hospital after Aberdeen celebrated the end of the outbreak with the Queen's visit on 27 June. There were still over 400 people in hospital who felt forgotten in the rush to demonstrate that Aberdeen was returning to normal. After speaking to MacQueen's deputy, David Barclay, Ian Sutherland told his senior colleagues:

> . . . some patients who have become aware that they have given two consecutive negative tests in hospital and who are feeling 100% fit are beginning to insist on their right to go home. So far this has not been the cause of any serious trouble but Dr Barclay is afraid that word may get round and about the extreme difficulty that there would be in holding these people in hospital against their will.[102]

Sutherland reminded Barclay of the MOH's powers to certify carriers, but admitted that 'in the past the procedure has proved ponderous and not very

[99] Minute of Meeting, 9 June 1964, NAS HH 61/1073.
[100] F. D. Beddard, J. A. Buchanan, J. Dewar, G. G. Dickie, D. Livingstone, I. A. G. MacQueen, 'To patients receiving treatment for typhoid fever', EMR.
[101] S. Blackhall, 'The Jam Jar' in S. Blackhall, *Reets*, Aberdeen, 1990, pp. 58–61.
[102] I. N. Sutherland to Deputy CMO, 29 June 1964, NAS HH61/1074.

effective'. But on the whole, the patients were well disciplined. Besides their confinement to hospital, some patients at Woodend Hospital were further inconvenienced when their belongings were damaged by steam sterilisation, but they were soon compensated by the hospital board.[103]

Besides the clearance tests, a V_i agglutination test was performed on discharge and Dr Anderson of the PHLS Central Enteric Reference Laboratory advised that the results suggested that three patients, released as doubtful cases, might be or become carriers. A further V_i test was therefore instituted for all cases three months after discharge, a comparison between the two results assisting in the identification of carriers. The blood samples were also examined for signs of damage from choramphenicol, but no long-term haematological effects were reported by Walker and his colleagues.[104]

As the outbreak progressed, minds turned to research opportunities. The meeting on 9 June recommended that a trial be carried out of the efficacy of ampicillin in the control of *S. typhi* excretion on patients failing clearance tests in hospital, and on 12 June a detailed proposal was discussed at a meeting of doctors involved in patients' care. The idea was later attributed to a suggestion by A. B. Christie in the *BMJ*, but an SHHD memorandum dated 3 June records that Robert Cruickshank, professor of bacteriology at Edinburgh University, also intended approaching Brotherston about the matter. The meeting on 12 June noted problems of 'statistics, ethics, public relations and practical procedure', but agreed that a double-blind trial should be carried out. Professor MacGregor, and E. Maurice Backett, professor of social medicine, would assist the project, and Dr Audrey Sutherland would play a co-ordinating role. Sutherland was appointed senior house officer to assist the trial, her role being liaison between the hospitals and the personnel involved. The question of obtaining legal advice was raised in case patients claimed they were kept in hospital unnecessarily, but it was agreed this was not needed. However, on the 'insistent advice' of Beddard and Backett, it was decided to tell the patients about the trial and to invite their co-operation in an explanatory leaflet, which was to make 'no specific mention of prolonged stay'.[105]

---

[103] Medical Services Committee, North East Regional Hospital Board ,7 July 1964; Finance Committee, North East Regional Hospital Board, 11 September 1964, NHSA GRHBA1\1\9.

[104] 'Appendix to Minute of a meeting of staff concerned with the care of typhoid patients, 15 June 1964, 17 June 1964', EMR; Walker, 'Aberdeen typhoid', pp. 466–79.

[105] Minute of Meeting, 9 June 1964, NAS HH 61/1073; Minute of a meeting of staff concerned with the care of typhoid patients held on 12 June 1964 at the City Hospital, Aberdeen, EMR; A. B. Christie, 'Treatment of typhoid carriers with ampicillin', *BMJ*, 1964, vol. 1, pp. 1609–11; E. M. Russell, A. Sutherland and W. Walker, 'Ampicillin for persistent typhoid excretors, including a clinical trial in convalescence', *BMJ*, 1966, vol. 2, pp. 555–7; I. N. Sutherland to Deputy Chief Medical Officer, 3 June 1964, NAS HH 58/160; Correspondence in NHSA GRHB B2\3 [20\7].

On 15 June, MacGregor, Backett and Walker circulated a memorandum announcing the trial and protocols. The antibiotic had been tried before with variable outcomes, but the size of the Aberdeen outbreak offered the prospect of definite results, with 'national and international implications'. The patients included would be those giving a positive clearance test, antibiotic sensitivity and clinical relapse being the only grounds for exclusion. Following the ten-day course of ampicillin or placebo, the patient would again go through the clearance procedure. Russell would be in charge at the City Hospital and Tor-na-Dee, while others would be responsible elsewhere.[106]

An explanatory leaflet prepared by Walker was approved. The leaflet explained to patients that they were 'still harbouring' and excreting the germ, and that while they were likely to become clear within weeks, there was no guarantee of this, and no known treatment to hasten the process. Experts had suggested there was an opportunity to find out whether a kind of penicillin would help, and perhaps prevent the germ continuing in the body indefinitely. The document continued: 'it is our duty to obtain this information in the interests of the community and the world at large, as well as your own.' Patients would take a ten-day course of capsules which might or might not contain the drug. If it became clear that the drug was working, those not receiving it would be given it at once.[107]

According to the minutes of a meeting held in November, only one qualifying patient declined to take part, twenty-four were withdrawn because of relapse and one because of penicillin rash. Eighty-nine completed the trial, forty-eight in the ampicillin group and forty-one in the placebo group. The proportion that achieved clearance was higher in the ampicillin group, although the difference was not quite significant statistically. A significant difference was obtained, however, when only patients under age 20 were considered. However, the final published results were inconclusive, although it was suggested that ampicillin might have been responsible for only five carriers arising from the outbreak.[108]

At a meeting at the health and welfare department on 24 June, decisions were made about the treatment of patients who failed to achieve clearance after the trial. They would not yet be 'chronic carriers', since many would probably still clear spontaneously. It was agreed that if these patients seemed unlikely to achieve clearance within a reasonable time they could be discharged after consultation with the MOH, who would arrange follow-up

[106] A. G. MacGregor, E. M. Backett and W. Walker, 'The problem of typhoid carriers', 15 June 1964, EMR.

[107] 'Minute of a meeting of staff concerned with the care of typhoid patients', 15 June 1964; WW/SCP, 16 June 1964, EMR.

[108] 'Note of a meeting', 19 November 1964, EMR; Russell et al., 'Ampicillin'. Slightly different figures appear in the published findings compared to those under discussion on 19 November 1964. The conclusion was much the same, however, except no mention was made of a statistically significant result with patients under age 20.

examinations. Home circumstances would be taken into account, but the MOH would seldom advise against discharge. Patients giving three positive cultures at home would be asked to return to hospital for cholecystography, pyelography and possible duodenal observation (X-ray examination of the gallbladder, kidney and small intestine). They might also be started on a longer course of ampicillin.[109]

By 25 June, the problem of relapse was worrying the physicians after two patients relapsed following three negative tests. The clearance programme may have been too tight, and since relapses had been recorded three weeks after chloramphenicol, some patients were likely to relapse after discharge, but it was impractical to suggest that patients spend another week in hospital at this stage. However, there were few relapses at home, and only seventeen readmissions. Beddard commented later that while a longer hospital stay may have avoided readmissions, early discharge 'may have paid a dividend in good will and have contributed to the small number of refusals to co-operate'.[110]

There were three deaths for which typhoid was regarded as partly responsible. One 60-year-old woman, who was very sick on admission, died from a pulmonary embolism following a relapse, six days after responding to chloramphenicol. A. M. Duncan was quoted in the press as saying that the elderly spinster 'probably would have died anyway as she was suffering from two other fairly serious illnesses'. There were two other deaths. Another 60-year-old woman was admitted in poor condition on the eighth day of her illness and collapsed twenty-four hours later, an ECG suggesting a heart attack. She died the following day. The third death was a 76-year-old man who developed congestive heart failure and broncho-pneumonia.[111]

On 21 July, the discharge and surveillance policies were reviewed at a further meeting chaired by Brotherston. By this time, sixty patients had experienced relapse, which was mostly treated with chloramphenmicol. In total, eighty-six patients relapsed, although Walker and his colleagues admitted the distinction between 'relapse' and 'post-treatment pyrexia' was somewhat arbitrary. The high relapse rate may have been the result of using relatively light initial doses of chloramphenicol. By 21 July, thirty patients were thought unlikely to obtain clearance for a considerable time. It was agreed that they would be started on a three-month course of ampicillin and discharged after three negative specimens or three months' stay in hospital. Patients producing a positive test at home would also take a three-month course of ampicillin. Samples would be taken weekly from such patients and they would go through the home clearance procedure appropriate to their risk group.[112]

[109] W. Walker, 'To physicians in charge of typhoid patients', 25 June 1964, EMR.

[110] Ibid., 'Note of a meeting',19 November 1964, EMR.

[111] 'Did germ come from 13-year-old bully?', *P&J*, 30 May 1964, p. 1c; Russell, 'Typhoid fever', pp. 85–6.

[112] Minute of a meeting', 21 July 1964; 'Note of a meeting', 19 November 1964'; W. Walker,

The 21 July meeting also settled the longer term follow-up of cleared cases. Patients would submit specimens at six months, and at one and two years after their last negative test. They would also visit the City Hospital for V_i testing and blood examination at three and six months, and probably at one and two years. But these arrangements did not satisfy everyone, since Anderson of the PHLS wanted a more stringent regime. He gathered that one family which had not completed the clearance tests was now somewhere in London, and told Brotherston:

> My fears in connection with this outbreak are obviously that persistent excretors may start new foci . . . unremitting vigilance will be necessary for some considerable time in order to restrict the sphere of activity of this organism to the original outbreak.[113]

James Howie, Anderson's boss as Director of the PHLS and a member of the Milne Committee, reinforced Anderson's concern, expressing his alarm that 'a symptomless excreter . . . had been allowed to leave Aberdeen and might actually be on holiday in London'. While 'second waves' were not a marked feature of typhoid in Britain, Howie told Brotherston that now was the time 'when it will be worth keeping a sharp lookout for them'.[114]

Sutherland checked the situation with MacQueen, who explained that several people who had given 'the odd positive result in a series of negatives' had gone on holiday, and whenever possible he had warned the appropriate MOH. MacQueen thought the danger was not great and was not prepared to accept Howie's phrase, 'allowed to leave Aberdeen'. He believed he did not possess powers against 'people who have been discharged from hospital and . . . throw up one positive result during quite a prolonged period of observation'.[115] Brotherston circulated some of Anderson's comments and made some amendments to the minutes of the meeting, but told Anderson:

> I think differently from you. . . . You clearly feel it is desirable to lay down an ideal policy. . . . In my view it is better to arrive at a policy which is near the attainable because then this can be really stringently directed.[116]

The group overseeing the discharge and surveillance policy next met in November, again including experts from around Scotland and the PHLS. It involved a wider range of people from Aberdeen, including representatives from the drainage and water departments. The meeting heard that seven

'New instructions on the management of patients recovered from typhoid', 22 July 1964, EMR.
[113] E. S. Anderson to J. H. F. Brotherston, 28 July 1964, NAS HH61/1074.
[114] J. W. Howie to J. H. F. Brotherston, 27 July 1964, NAS HH61/1074.
[115] I. N. Sutherland to Deputy Chief Medical Officer, 29 June 1964, NAS HH61/1074.
[116] J. H. F. Brotherston to E. S. Anderson, 24 August 1964, NAS HH61/1074.

patients had refused to supply samples for follow-up testing. All were cases in which the diagnosis had not been confirmed, and two had left Aberdeen. There were no powers to compel them to give samples. Five carriers had been identified, but twenty-eight people had still to complete clearance tests. The carriers were three women aged 34, 46 and 67, and two males aged 53 and 70. Three were sensitive to ampicillin, but it was thought that a further course of ampicillin might be tried with the other two. Bile function tests might also be carried out. Anderson advised that if patients were still excreting the organism in bile after a year, cholecystectomy (removal of the gall-bladder) offered a possibility of a cure.[117]

Discussion of the serological tests revealed the great complexity of their interpretation. In June 1965 a research project on the serological findings was started, funded by an SHHD grant. This eventually showed that the Widal test was of limited value in the diagnosis of typhoid. During 1965, the work of the City Hospital laboratory was still 30 per cent greater than in 1963, accounted for partly by the continuing tests on former typhoid patients. The monitoring of known and the search for unknown carriers involved sewer swab analyses, of which 1030 were conducted during the year. The swabbing work was concluded in September 1966, and by the end of 1966 the follow-up of patients was virtually ended.[118]

As for the post-discharge experience of patients, tiredness is a theme that many mention in interview. It took some as long as a year to get back to normal. At the end of September, the Governors of Robert Gordon's Technical College noted that one of their staff had been absent since 26 May with typhoid and 'was still unable to resume her duties in the College'. After discussions with the Scottish Office they decided to give her six-months' sick-leave on full pay.[119] Of the five carriers, one who became clear during 1965 recalled the visits from a health visitor to collect samples and the 'more embarrassing' drain sampling. This happened regularly at the end of her drive-way and announced her condition to everyone. This patient had experienced allergic reactions to both chloramphenicol and ampicillin, and spent three months in hospital.[120] During 1969 the four remaining carriers were treated with a new drug, septrin, a combination of a synthetic antibiotic and a

---

[117] 'Note of a meeting', 19 November 1964, EMR.

[118] A. M. Duncan, Report to the Board of Management for Aberdeen Special Hospitals, 1965, NHSA GRHB B2\2\12; A. M. Duncan, Report to the Board of Management for Aberdeen Special Hospitals, 1966, NHSA GRHB B2\2\13; J. Brodie, 'Antibodies and the Aberdeen typhoid outbreak of 1964. I The Widal reaction', *Journal of Hygiene*, 1977, vol. 79, pp. 161–80; J. Brodie, 'Antibodies and the Aberdeen typhoid outbreak of 1964. II Coombs', complement fixation and fimbrial agglutination tests', *Journal of Hygiene*, 1977, vol. 79, pp. 181–92.

[119] Minutes and Proceedings of the Governors of Robert Gordon's College, Aberdeen, 1963 to 1964, p. 166.

[120] Lorna Dewar, interview, 5 August 1999, Aberdeen, ATO/22.

sulphonamide. One was successfully cleared of *Salmonella typhi*, while the others remained carriers, probably due to gall-bladder abnormalities.[121] It was not only the carriers, however, who suffered continuing consequences from the outbreak. At the time of the outbreak some patients and their families worried that neighbours would consider them dirty, and this anxiety continued to afflict some victims. The patients interviewed believed that the outbreak had affected their lives in numerous ways. Some felt that it had influenced their career prospects or choices and a few thought that their health had been permanently damaged. One patient still feels that her fear of eating outside her own home is a result of her experience of typhoid.[122]

Having considered the experiences of GPs, the hospitals and patients, we will now return to the action taken by the health and welfare department after the identification of Low's supermarket as the source of the outbreak.

Further actions by the health and welfare department

After the source of the outbreak was traced to Low's, the shop was cleaned and remained open. Sales of cold meat were stopped on 23 May, but the cold meat department was used to serve bacon. MacQueen, and Sutherland of the SSHD, were both satisfied with the action taken,[123] but Low's were later advised to close the cold meat counter, following the intervention of Dr Betty Hobbs, Director of the food hygiene laboratory of the PHLS. Hobbs expressed concern about the situation when she visited Aberdeen on her own initiative during the weekend of 30/31 May, and on 2 June she discussed the matter with Brotherston. She referred to the Crowthorne, Pickering and Harlow outbreaks, but considered Aberdeen more complicated. Here personnel who contracted typhoid had handled food. While the evidence pointed to canned beef as the original source, Hobbs thought that infected shop assistants were responsible for further contamination. She also argued that 'once typhoid organisms get into a location it is difficult to eradicate totally except by drastic measures'.[124] As a result, Low's were persuaded to close the cold meat counter from 3 June and to suspend the use of the meat slicer for bacon, and later to close the entire shop. MacQueen welcomed Hobbs' expertise and she was seconded to the

---

[121] J. Brodie, I. A. MacQueen and D. Livingstone, 'Effect of Trimethoprim-Suphamethox-azole on typhoid and Salmonella carriers', *BMJ*, 1970, vol. 3, pp. 318–19.

[122] Interviews: Rosemary Towler, Irene Morrison, Joyce McKain, Lorna Dewar, Linsey Smith, Anne Ritchie, Sheena Blackhall, 24, 26 May, 22 June, 5, 6 August, 11 October 1999, 18 September 2001. ATO/4, 6, 20, 22, 23, 28, 46.

[123] MacQueen, 'Evidence', pp. 10, 58; I. N. Sutherland to Deputy Chief Medical Officer, 3 June 1964 (document 171), NAS HH 58/160.

[124] I. N. Sutherland to Deputy Chief Medical Officer, 3 June 1964 (document 170); R. M. Gordon, 'Enteric fever Aberdeen', 3 June 1964; J. Brotherston, 'Visit to Aberdeen – 2nd June, 1964', 3 June 1964, NAS HH 58/160.

health and welfare department, staying until 17 June, her main role being to re-examine the means of transmission by further interviews with patients.[125]

Low's personnel were kept under close surveillance. Following the initial investigations, further blood samples were taken on 25 May and 8 June. Urine and faeces samples were tested on 23 May, daily from 25 to 30 May, and every second day until 6 June, following which daily tests were conducted after the shelf-stacker's urine tested positive. The positive test reinforced Hobbs' arguments, and the supermarket, which was doing little business, closed for disinfection on 11 June. It was reopened on 22 June, the staff remaining subject to weekly tests. After admission to hospital, the shelf-stacker's infection was not confirmed. It was later presumed that the positive test was an error, perhaps a result of mixing up samples, although Brodie rejected this view.[126] Numerous other investigations were carried out. Swabs were taken from slicing and mincing machines, refrigerators and working surfaces on 25 May, and from drains the following day, all with negative results. Drain tests confirmed that there were no problems. Samples of products from Low's meat counters, unopened tins of canned meat at the shop, six tins from Low's headquarters, and corned beef purchased on 15, 16 and 18 May all tested negative.[127]

The action taken at another business may also be examined, because the proprietor, Dennis King, believed that MacQueen's department acted improperly, leading to an exchange of letters between his solicitor and Aberdeen Corporation. A 'bacteriologist' apparently visited one of King's shops on Sunday, 24 May, and intimated that a young worker from the attached bakery was a typhoid suspect, and his girlfriend was a confirmed case.[128] Brunton subsequently visited the shop on 25 May and told an assistant that the baker's sickness had been confirmed. A period of intense surveillance of King's staff followed. Two blood and four urine and faeces samples were taken per week, but no further typhoid casualties were identified. Samples of King's products and constituents were taken, as were swabs from refrigerators, machinery, surfaces, display cabinets, counters and drains, but none proved positive.[129] Brunton obtained a list of hotels and other businesses supplied by King's, and, as mentioned earlier, GPs were informed about the case, and were given details of King's branches and business customers on 26 and 27 May.[130] However, King's claimed that the health and welfare department also told their

---

[125] MacQueen, 'Evidence', pp. 1, 2.

[126] Ibid., pp. 19, 24.

[127] Ibid., pp. 16, 18–19, 23.

[128] Evidence provided by King's shop assistant, 27 May 1964, DK. Later investigations failed to identify the 'bacteriologist'. Town Clerk to Messrs Clark & Wallace (King's lawyers), 22 September 1964, DK.

[129] MacQueen, 'Evidence', p. 20; 'Appendix III – Information from Mr Parry' in MacQueen, 'Evidence', p. 43; 'Appendix IV – Swabbing particulars', in MacQueen 'Evidence', pp. 50–5.

[130] G. A. Matthew, 'Circulars to Doctors Nos 50 and 51', 26 and 27 May 1964, AUSHS.

customers to find other suppliers because they had cancelled their orders. The proprietor of a mobile shop alleged that a medical officer told him to 'get rid of' all King's goods and that he therefore burned them. According to the Corporation, however, Brunton contacted the firms simply to advise that one of King's employees was ill and that 'any cases of illness among guests and/or staff should be watched for'. It was not the Corporation's responsibility that this led to cancellations of contracts.[131]

Besides the question of what was said, King's argued that if the safety of their products was in doubt, they should have been given the opportunity of arranging alternative supplies for their customers. And if there was a real risk, the bakery should have been closed and compensation paid. As it was, the business continued at a loss, although the volume of wrapped bread sent to stores outside the city increased as customers travelled further afield to get 'typhoid-free' produce. The conflict was never resolved. King remained embittered about the cost to him of the outbreak, in his eyes due to MacQueen's actions.[132]

MacQueen's 'Evidence' gave a further example of action taken at Messrs Hardy and Marshall, a butcher's shop where one of the partners contracted typhoid. MacQueen judged the risk to be greater than at King's and the shop was given an option 'very similar to Low's meat department – seizure and destruction of the meat on sale, thorough disinfection of shop and its van, follow-up of staff as contacts, and exclusion of staff until cleared'. However, due to the difficulty of obtaining replacement staff, the well partner preferred to close.[133] The destruction of stock and closure were agreed without consulting the Corporation's legal department, the Town Clerk Depute commenting later that it was an informal decision made 'as a result of verbal discussion between the Medical Officer of Health and the proprietors of the shop'. The business claimed about £800 from the Corporation for destruction of stock, loss of profit and other items. The relevant legal provision was in the Public Health (Scotland) Act, 1897, which gave powers to close premises for cleansing and disinfection. This applied to 'houses', defined so as to include places of employment, and the articles therein, and stated that local authorities 'shall compensate' owners of articles destroyed or unnecessarily damaged. The Corporation agreed to pay £670 and the Town Clerk Depute felt they were 'well rid' of the matter for this sum.[134]

Informal methods of operation by MacQueen and his colleagues saved the Corporation money in connection with claims from other businesses. A

[131] 'Kings (Caterers Aberdeen) limited typhoid outbreak', copy of a letter from King's solicitor to Aberdeen Corporation, n.d.; Town Clerk Depute to Messrs Clark & Wallace (King's lawyers), 31 July 1964, DK.

[132] Conversation with Dennis King, January 1999.

[133] MacQueen, 'Evidence', p. 14. 'Appendix IV', in MacQueen, 'Evidence', pp. 45, 52–3.

[134] Town Clerk Depute, Aberdeen to The Town Clerk, Scarborough, ACA, 7/6/7.

request for compensation for the destruction of lettuces, for example, was rejected because there was no evidence of an order or request by the MOH, while claims for such items as loss of trade by an innkeeper were not entertained. Three claims arose from the prohibition of some milk. From 1 June only 'heat-treated' milk, or milk produced and bottled outside the city were permitted, while from 19 June all incoming milk had to be pasteurised, the restrictions remaining in force until 17 July. One of the claims was withdrawn, but the largest of the remaining two amounted to only £111 12s 5d.[135]

Besides Low's, King's, and Hardy and Marshall's, action in connection with businesses in Aberdeen was not extensive. On 6 June, a trawler whose skipper was sick was visited, the catch detained, and arrangements made for disinfecting the boat and bedding.[136] According to one informant, by this time MacQueen was determined to take drastic action in such cases, and suggested to the liaison committee that the catch might be incinerated. However, Brodie dismissed the idea, remarking that it would be different if the crew were in the habit of defecating into the hold – with which the meeting passed on to other business. The catch was released. But trawlers were required to use fresh water for cleaning, and the water used in the fish market, and the standard of hygiene at fish houses, were checked.[137]

Much of the practical action in connection with the food trade was carried out by the sanitary inspectors, who took the food samples and swabs, and followed up enquiries arising from the dietary and employment records of the latest hospital admissions. H. B. Parry, the chief sanitary inspector, and his colleagues, checked the ingredients used by ice-cream manufacturers, and the standards of hygiene of shops, restaurants, bakehouses and market stalls. They sampled meat pies of the Northern Co-operative Society and ice-cream at city-centre cafes, and were also involved in delivering an advice leaflet and giving talks to food handlers.[138]

MacQueen had previously published his views on 'teamwork' as the organising principle of local authority public health, and claimed that well-established teamwork helped in the fight against typhoid: 'most of the heads and deputy heads of the various sections . . . had worked together for some years, so that the staff really functioned as a team.' However, he admitted to difficulties with the sanitary section, as the Corporation had been considering whether it should remain in his department. Parry claimed the right to autonomy, but was opposed by MacQueen, and shortly before the outbreak

[135] 'Appendix III', in MacQueen, 'Evidence', pp. 44, 47, 49; Town Clerk Depute to D. Tudor Evans, 20 November 1964, ACA TH 7/6/6.
[136] 'Appendix IV', in MacQueen, 'Evidence', p. 54.
[137] McEntegart, interview; 'Appendix III', in MacQueen, 'Evidence', p. 45.
[138] 'Appendix IV', in MacQueen, 'Evidence', pp. 43–4, 54. For a further account of the work of the sanitary inspectors during the outbreak, see 'The role of Aberdeen's PHI's during typhoid outbreak', *Municipal Engineering*, 1965, vol. 142, pp. 1290–1.

the Corporation ruled that a unified department would continue.[139] The SHHD officials were aware of this situation. On 28 May, when Sutherland was frustrated by the difficulty of obtaining information about the corned beef involved in the outbreak, he recorded that perhaps the inspectorial staff had been 'less than 100 per cent co-operative', because of 'the poor relationship which has . . . existed between the M.O.H. and the City Sanitary Inspector'. The officials realised that Parry's department was chronically understaffed, and three sanitary inspectors were temporarily seconded to Aberdeen from other local authorities, along with two Royal Army Medical Corps personnel, and a member of the SHHD's Food and Dairy inspectorate.[140]

In contrast to his poor relationship with the sanitary inspectors, as a champion of health visiting, MacQueen was greatly admired by the health visitors, who were loyal and well motivated, and responsible for the arduous task of following up contacts. After the publication of the first list of patients, the phone lines to the health and welfare department became continuously engaged and new lines had to be installed, and the subsequent escalation in the number of patients rapidly multiplied the number of contacts to be dealt with. In Aberdeen city alone, about 4500 contacts were interviewed during the outbreak.[141]

The superintendent health visitor Miss Nairn, her deputy and assistant, and four health visitors responsible for training and health education, were normally based at the health and welfare department's headquarters at Willowbank House. About sixty health visitors were based at outlying clinics, each responsible for a nearby district, supervised by a clinic superintendent. During the outbreak, routine services were maintained by one-third of the staff and the rest were recalled to headquarters, mostly for contact tracing. Nairn initially sent her staff to visit contacts with few guidelines, as the headquarters staff had little knowledge of typhoid. However, a questionnaire was soon compiled, on the advice of a clinic superintendent who had wartime experience of the disease. As the outbreak progressed, leave was cancelled and a shift system organised. Besides their routine work, the remaining clinic staff answered inquiries about the outbreak, and engaged in hygiene education as the opportunity arose. At evenings and weekends they also helped with contact tracing. Nairn attended liaison committee meetings and, when procedures were adjusted, the clinic superintendents were called to briefings.[142]

---

[139] I. A. G. MacQueen, 'Teamwork and leadership in public health', *Public Health*, 1960, April, pp. 244–52; MacQueen, 'Evidence', p. 8.

[140] I. N. Sutherland to Deputy Chief Medical Officer, 28 May 1964, NAS HH 058/160, Appendix III, in MacQueen, 'Evidence', pp. 43–6.

[141] MacQueen, 'Evidence', p. 10; M. Nairn, 'Health visitors in the Aberdeen typhoid outbreak', *Nursing Times*, 8 January 1965, pp. 59–60.

[142] Nairn, 'Health visitors'; Nairn, interview.

Four health visitors were normally responsible for tuberculosis contact tracing and worked closely with the City Hospital and laboratory. One of them, Mabel Clubb, a tuberculosis health visitor since 1949, was assigned to checking medical records and interviewing patients from 25 May. The interviews with the first patients about their food consumption and contacts had been conducted by Dr McIntosh, but once the link with Low's cold meat was regarded as conclusive, concern shifted to possible secondary infections. The workload made it difficult for Clubb and Norma Michie, another health visitor assigned to this work, to interview all cases thoroughly, so they were later re-interrogated by other staff.[143]

Clubb and Michie became responsible for liaison between the hospitals and the health and welfare department, reporting to Barclay, the deputy MOH. Test results were communicated to Willowbank House three times a day. Clubb and Michie checked admissions records, and, when necessary, interviewed patients for information about contacts, shopping habits and foods eaten. They collected fresh specimen jars from the City Hospital and delivered them to Willowbank House for their colleagues to take on contact-tracing visits. Contacts were supposed to despatch or deliver their samples to the City Hospital, but would often hand them in at Willowbank House, frequently to 'the nearest office girl' walking along the corridor.[144]

Each day, the contact tracers called at Willowbank House for a list of visits, a pad of forms to be completed and a supply of specimen jars. They would then plan a route, travelling by bus or car. After the schools closed at the beginning of June, transport for those who did not own cars was provided by teacher-volunteers, the teachers also assisting with the paper work. Nairn recalled that health visitors were frequently assailed by reporters at Willowbank House and on one occasion a newspaper's representatives attempted to persuade them to pose for a photograph dragging a mattress down a tenement stair. Three health visitors worked with Brunton following up staff at food premises at which typhoid victims worked, and others were assigned to the special testing clinic.[145]

During interviews with contacts, and in other encounters with the public, health visitors dealt with questions about eating, toilet and food hygiene, and reassured people that the spread of typhoid could be prevented by following simple rules. Some interviews tested the health visitors' tact, as most of the patients and contacts were from the wealthier West-end and many housewives

---

[143] Clubb, interview; MacQueen, 'Evidence', p. 17. The later interviews were carried out by McIntosh, Jean Pattullo, assistant MOH, Elspeth Warwick of the SHHD, and Betty Hobbs. Like Hobbs, Warwick was seconded temporarily to the health and welfare department.

[144] Nairn, in MacQueen, 'Evidence', p. 40; Nairn, interview; Michie, interview; Clubb, interview.

[145] Nairn, in MacQueen, 'Evidence', pp. 39–40; Nairn, interview.

were anxious about having to say they had eaten corned beef because 'this wasn't the best-quality meat'. They were equally worried about questions such as whether all members of the family used the same towel. In houses where hygiene standards were judged inadequate, or where persons shared toilet facilities with confirmed cases, the inhabitants were followed up as contacts even if they had not eaten with the typhoid victim. Where whole families had been taken to hospital, arrangements were made for a member of the welfare section to obtain the key, and consent for the cleaning of the house. Disinfection was arranged by Parry and cleaning by relatives or a home help followed.[146]

Contacts were given a duplicated sheet of instructions prepared by the health visitor tutors, which was also distributed to GPs.[147] This conveyed seven 'simple and vital rules' of hygiene. Contacts were advised to wash their hands thoroughly after visiting the toilet and before preparing food. They were asked not to invite people home for meals or drinks, and not to visit the homes of others, or to eat in a restaurant. The leaflet stated that food prepared by the patient should be destroyed by burning or mixing with disinfectant and disposal down the lavatory, and that their bed should be stripped, and all linen, underwear and towels soaked in a solution of disinfectant. Crockery and cooking utensils should be treated similarly. Any contact working with food should stay away from work and collect sickness benefit until given permission to return. Finally, any child who was a direct contact of a patient in hospital should be kept off school.[148]

Health visitors also participated in the distribution of a booklet, *How to Stamp out Typhoid*, an initiative of a businessman, R. A. Williamson, Director of the firm which supplied small grocers in the area. After receiving enquiries from his customers as to how to combat the disease, Williamson contacted MacQueen, who had no suitable guidelines available. He therefore offered to provide a brochure, which was produced in consultation with the health and welfare department, and with the support of the Chamber of Commerce, the *Evening Express* providing the artwork. The result was a 45,000-copy print-run of a twelve-page booklet featuring 'Wee Alickie', the newspaper's cartoon character, a loyal supporter of Aberdeen's football team, the Dons.[149]

In October 1964, MacQueen estimated that the health visitors worked eighty hours a week on average during the first four weeks of the outbreak, fifty-six to sixty hours during the next ten weeks, and forty-six to fifty hours a week thereafter. All the overtime was unpaid. During the later phases, as

---

146 Wilma Craigmile, interview, 28 May 1999, Aberdeen, ATO/8; Nairn, interview; Nairn, in MacQueen, 'Evidence' pp. 40–1.
147 Nairn, 'Health visitors'; G. A. Matthew, 'Circular to Doctors No. 53', 31 May 1964, AUSHS.
148 I. A. G. MacQueen, 'Prevention of the spread of typhoid fever', May 1964, AUSHS.
149 R. Williamson, interview, 19 November 1999, Aberdeen, ATO/35.

contact tracing diminished, the follow-up of discharged patients became increasingly important. Clubb, with a small team of health visitors, was responsible for this. MacQueen praised the health visitors in a six-page report to the Corporation's health and welfare committee, and detailed the greater living expenses they incurred. He considered asking the committee to award an honorarium of half a month's salary, but, in a vote, the health visitors indicated they did not desire monetary acknowledgement of their overtime. MacQueen claimed, however, that they resented the lack of recognition signalled by the absence of a health visitor in the party presented to the Queen on 27 June, and asserted that several had resigned because of this. (He had been the only representative of the health and welfare department.) As a remedy, he proposed that £2000 be set aside for a health and welfare department library, in view of the 'outstanding and self-sacrificing work of the health visitors and related staff', and that a memorandum to this effect be circulated. The committee, however, favoured recognising the efforts of a wider range of personnel, and a year later it was agreed to pay twenty guineas each to ninety-seven people which included, besides health visitors, medical and sanitary staff, social workers and others.[150]

Conclusions

This chapter has provided an outline of the 1964 Aberdeen typhoid outbreak, in preparation for the various aspects of the episode which will be examined in the following three chapters. Clearly, Aberdeen's health services were severely tested by the outbreak. For several weeks, the health and welfare department, general practitioners, the hospitals and the laboratories were all involved in intense activity aimed at controlling the outbreak and identifying and treating victims. The roles of the general practitioners and hospitals, however, received little attention in the report of the Milne Committee, and the experiences of the patients received no consideration. This chapter has therefore gone some way towards recovering these relatively hidden dimensions of the outbreak.

From the perspective of 2005, the mounting of the contact-tracing and -testing operations, and especially the provision of over 500 hospital beds for the typhoid victims within the space of a few weeks, seem remarkable achievements. However, prior to our consideration of the Milne enquiry in Chapter 6, it is already clear that there were tensions between the three

[150] I. A. G. MacQueen, 'Report as to work of health visitors, etc. throughout the typhoid outbreak and as to their reluctance to accept honoraria and compensation', 19 October 1964, p. 1, ACA 7/6/6; 'Royal bon accord', *P&J*, 29 June 1964, p. 1a; 'Payment of honoraria for work in typhoid outbreak: joint report by City Chamberlain and Medical Officer of Health', 30 September 1965, ACA 7/6/6; Clubb, interview.

sectors of the health services. There appeared to be no planned system for co-ordination of the sectors: the special liaison committee seems to have been an *ad hoc* arrangement, established as a result of problems that emerged during the early days of the outbreak. There are signs of tensions between the health and welfare department and the GPs, as in the Croydon outbreak,[151] as well as between the department and the laboratory, and at least one hospital doctor. In connection with the Croydon outbreak, the need for a committee representing GPs to aid communication during outbreaks had been a matter of controversy. During the Aberdeen typhoid outbreak, the GPs' local medical committee, part of the structure of the NHS, proved useful, its administrative machinery being pressed into service on the initiative of the GPs' leaders.

As for the health and welfare department, in this chapter we have mainly considered its roles in establishing the source of the outbreak, and in taking action at the food premises most directly involved, and in connection with other food businesses. We have also considered the activities of the health visitors. However, there are other aspects of the health and welfare department's responsibilities we have yet to consider. The MOH also played a high-profile role in the media, in providing information to the public as to the latest developments, offering advice to the public and announcing control measures, and it was the MOH's media performance that received greatest critical attention in the Milne report. It is to these matters that we will now turn in Chapter 4.

---

[151] See pp. 13–14.

4

The medical officer of health, the media and the public in the Aberdeen typhoid outbreak

Introduction

This chapter expands the account of the local dimensions of the Aberdeen typhoid outbreak, and focuses upon the media role of the MOH, Ian MacQueen. It provides further insights into the actions of the health and welfare department, especially in terms of advising the public, and gives some indications of the experiences of Aberdeen's population. We will explore MacQueen's involvement with the media largely by examining the coverage that arose from his press conferences, held once or twice daily from 22 May to 19 June, but will also refer to some oral history and archival evidence. We will concentrate upon reports in Aberdeen's *P&J* and *EE*, which served as a means of interaction between MacQueen and the local population.[1] Coverage in the Sunday papers will be included, since it provoked comment from MacQueen and civic leaders on several occasions. In the Milne report, as we will see in Chapter 6, MacQueen was condemned for his alleged extravagant use of the media, which was blamed for the sensationalisation of the outbreak. At the end of this chapter we will see, however, that during the outbreak SHHD officials remained sympathetic towards MacQueen regarding the pressure he was under from the media, and largely supportive of his strategy throughout the outbreak.

The press coverage arising from MacQueen's press conferences may be considered in three overlapping phases. During the first, prior to about 29 May, the conferences were the main source of information about the outbreak. MacQueen's statements and predictions dominated the headlines, and he came under pressure from journalists, and Aberdonians via letters to the newspapers, to release more information about the source of the outbreak, and further advice about the symptoms and prevention of typhoid. Faced with an unplanned and unknown situation, his handling of the press and the public appears to be largely reactive during this phase. As he responded to criticism he began to receive more positive and supportive coverage.

---

[1] The outbreak was also extensively reported via the electronic media but little of this material has survived.

The beginning of the second phase is characterised by some of the most dramatic headlines, over the weekend of 30/31 May, generated initially from announcements made by MacQueen on 29 May. The oral history evidence suggests that it was partly MacQueen's lack of awareness of the ways of the press that led to sensationalism at this stage: journalists were able to 'feed MacQueen a line', which gave them their headlines. But MacQueen also explained to a professional colleague at the time that some precautions were announced for other than strictly medical reasons – to bring home to citizens the seriousness of the situation and the need for scrupulous hygiene.[2] During this period, journalists became more active and the sources of information within and beyond Aberdeen expanded, as did the volume of coverage. As in the first phase, MacQueen consistently attempted an optimistic interpretation of the outbreak statistics, but after his hopeful predictions were shattered he became increasingly circumspect.

During the third phase, from around the weekend of 5/6 June, there are signs that MacQueen was beginning to learn from his experiences when he mounted a careful defence of his actions on the Saturday, and the majority of the Sunday headlines were unsensational. Nevertheless, there was objectionable coverage in several newspapers which he subsequently attacked. He also used his press conferences to counter what he described as hysteria outside Aberdeen. During this phase the end of the outbreak came into sight and MacQueen's prominence in the news faded as more and more typhoid stories featured other civic leaders, officials and businessmen concerned with the return of the city to normal. Some stories continued to appear, however, in which MacQueen's profile was high, and despite the experience he had gained, his handling of certain issues continued to generate sensational stories.

Fighting and winning the public relations battle

On Friday, 22 May, *P&J* led with the headline 'Typhoid schoolboy is serious', and the news that a boy in the City Hospital was one of fifteen typhoid patients. Some details were given, including the numbers of men, women and children, and a picture of MacQueen, who had emphasised that there was 'no need for public alarm'. He had been leading a five-man team for the past thirty-six hours, and they were confident that they had identified the cause of the outbreak and located all contacts. But MacQueen refused to be drawn on the precise identity of the source, merely explaining that it was 'food that has been contaminated either by a case or a carrier as a result of faulty food hygiene'. He thought the infection had originated in the city and that, if there were to

[2] I. N. Sutherland to Deputy CMO, 3 June 1964, NAS HH 58/160.

be more cases, they would appear within three or four days.[3] *EE* devoted one-third of its front page to the outbreak, based mainly upon MacQueen's remarks at a press conference, the most prominent headline being 'Another typhoid suspect in hospital/'Prepare for rise' – MOH'. An inside-page article drew upon an interview with MacQueen. He sought to allay fears by emphasising that only people who had consumed food or drink handled by a carrier were at risk, and warned that the number of suspects was likely to increase, as doctors played safe with stomach upsets. Already 200 contacts had been interviewed and given instruction on food hygiene. MacQueen advised that immunisation was impractical because of the time needed for it to take effect. He was reasonably confident that the outbreak was under control, but could not guarantee it.[4]

The following day, *P&J* reported two more admissions, and a comment from MacQueen that this was what he had predicted and that there was no need for alarm.[5] The small item in *EE* included a list of the names and addresses of twenty-four people in hospital, which had been released by MacQueen. Further lists were printed intermittently. Anyone who had eaten food handled by someone on the list during the past eighteen days, but who had not already been contacted, was advised to 'have a word' with their family doctor. This 'additional precaution' was taken because sick and confused patients 'could not be expected to tell . . . all the people who had been in their homes'.[6] Most Sunday papers mentioned the outbreak only briefly or not at all,[7] but *Sunday Post* made front-page news of MacQueen's appeal to contacts, using the headline '400 warned of typhoid contact risk'.[8] And the *People* included the first hint of criticism. At the bottom of page 1, under the headline 'Typhoid "over" – then 7 victims', the paper reported that the latest cases had come forward after MacQueen 'said he believed the outbreak was ending'.[9]

According to *P&J* on Monday, 25 May, MacQueen's latest predictions were that there would be more cases, about 500 were at risk, and that the outbreak would 'tail off' by Wednesday. The danger of missed cases starting a second wave remained, and if this were to occur it would be clear by the end of the week. 'Wild rumours' were circulating about the source, but while stating that the food believed responsible was no longer on sale, MacQueen refused to elaborate, explaining that further laboratory results were awaited. But he 'nailed one of the rumours', stating that he believed no restaurant was

<hr>

[3] 'Typhoid schoolboy is serious', *P&J*, 22 May 1964, p. 1a.

[4] 'How it spreads', 'Another typhoid suspect in hospital', 'Typhoid – inside story', *EE*, 22 May 1964, pp. 1a, 1a, 5a.

[5] 'Now 17 Cases Confirmed', *P&J*, 23 May 1964, p. 1a.

[6] 'Plea as Typhoid Cases Named', *EE*, 23 May 1964, p. 1a.

[7] See, for example, '21 typhoid cases', *Observer*, 24 May 1964, p. 31; 'City's typhoid cases mounting', *Sunday Mail*, 24 May 1964, p. 2c.

[8] '400 warned of typhoid contact risk', *Sunday Post*, 24 May 1964, p. 1a.

[9] 'Typhoid "over" – then 7 victims', *People*, 24 May 1964, p. 1f.

involved.[10] *EE*, however, led with an item showing that discontent was growing. 'Housewives' plea' quoted a woman who phoned the newspaper, questioning MacQueen's failure to reveal the source. She had remarked: 'If we knew we had bought food from any place involved we could take precautions and consult our doctors. . . . There is too much secrecy.' MacQueen was not available for comment, but David Barclay, the deputy MOH, responded:

> We have our strong suspicions, but until we have the vital clue we cannot rush into print with a statement. We think we know what the picture is, but we cannot make a statement until we have full evidence.[11]

Barclay stated that 'the best service that can be given' was to stress 'the need for personal hygiene'.

The following day *P&J* included a response from MacQueen. He claimed there was no benefit in divulging the source because now there was 'no chance of anybody getting it from that source'. The rise in the number of cases had 'borne out what we all expected' but he warned that some people could still be incubating the infection.[12] But a letter appeared alongside MacQueen's comments under the headline 'Platitudes – says reader':

> The citizens of Aberdeen face the typhoid outbreak, not with alarm, but with grave concern; the alarm we reserve for the pussyfooting platitudes issued by the MOH about the original source of the infection.[13]

The letter pointed out that on Saturday MacQueen said that that there would be 'one or two more cases . . . and one or two false alarms' while by Monday there were sixty-nine confirmed cases. The writer then claimed that:

> if the original source of the infection had been made public at the earliest possible moment, many, if not all, of the subsequent victims could have come forward earlier, thereby reducing the risk to the public at large, and presumably speeding their own recovery.[14]

Instead, Aberdeen's citizens were 'fed a smokescreen' about the source being 'pretty definitely located' and the food responsible no longer on sale.

A second letter, 'Hygiene – for 3d!', from 'Shocked Mother', complained that the public conveniences at the beach charged 3d for using the wash-hand basin, and claimed that this would deter kiosk holders from washing their hands after using the toilet. In 'enlightened cities' the toilet paper was marked

---

[10] 'Typhoid – 48 cases', *P&J*, 25 May 1964, p. 1a.

[11] 'Housewives' plea', *EE*, 25 May 1964, p. 1a.

[12] 'The source: MOH answers critics', *P&J*, 26 May 1964, p. 1b.

[13] 'Platitudes – says reader', *P&J*, 26 May 1964, p. 1c.

[14] Ibid.

'NOW WASH YOUR HANDS', but in Aberdeen the motto was 'IF YOU WANT HYGIENE THREEPENCE EXTRA'. The letter also noted that there had been an appeal for nurses and observed:

> it is nice to know that Aberdeen has a large staff of health visitors who are all qualified nurses. . . . In the present emergency, when patients must take precedence over paper work, this reserve could be invaluable.[15]

Tuesday's *EE* displayed further pressure upon MacQueen to reveal the source. Aberdeen's hotels, food shops and restaurants were all losing business.[16] The Chamber of Commerce therefore urged MacQueen to 'kill many wild rumours regarding the cause of the outbreak'. MacQueen told a representative of the Chamber that 'it would not have been opportune for certain medical reasons to name the source before now', but agreed that the time was approaching when this information should be disclosed.[17] Another disgruntled letter appeared from a housewife who found it 'shocking to be kept in the dark'. She understood that the 'medical authorities no doubt wish to make the minimum comment in order to avoid panic', but observed that 'lack of guidance, and therefore ignorance, will cause much greater damage'. She advocated that the public be told where the typhoid cases worked, and that information be given about 'hygiene, preparation of food, safest types of food etc', and the symptoms of typhoid.[18]

According to notes of a telephone conversation between MacQueen and Ian Sutherland at the SHHD, MacQueen now felt inclined to reveal that 'tinned beef is the suspect vehicle . . . and that in all probability only one large tin was involved'. This, he thought, 'should help put the situation into better perspective'.[19] His announcement was reported in *P&J* on 27 May under the headline 'Typhoid in bully tin', outbreak news covering over two-thirds of the front page for the first time. MacQueen stated that a tin of corned beef from abroad was the source of infection, and other cold meats had become contaminated via a slicing machine, and now declared that no carrier was involved. The meat was contaminated 'where it had been made', and 'with no fault in Aberdeen and no fault in the shop'. He explained that if this information had been revealed earlier, 10,000 families who had bought cold meat at the shop would have been 'infernally worried' and 'thronging along to the department and doctors' surgeries asking for help that nobody could give'. This would have disrupted the fight against the outbreak. A conference of MacQueen's colleagues had agreed that it was 'impossible in the public interest to say anything about the source, without creating public alarm, until

[15] 'Hygiene – for 3d!', *P&J*, 26 May 1964, p. 1c.

[16] 'Typhoid total rises to 75: city hotels are losing bookings', *P&J*, 26 May 1964, p. 1a.

[17] 'MOH will name source of outbreak', *EE*, 26 May 1964, p. 1a.

[18] J. Robertson, 'Shocking to be kept in the dark', *EE*, 26 May 1964, p. 1a.

[19] I. N. Sutherland to Deputy Chief Medical Officer, 26 May 1964, NAS HH 058/160.

we reached the stage when the period of risk of the first wave was over'. There might be a few further cases but if anyone had eaten corned beef from the shop between 5 and 10 May and were now feeling all right, they had escaped. But it remained to be seen whether there would be a secondary wave caused by infectious cases before admission to hospital.[20]

In MacQueen's evidence to the Milne Committee prepared in July, he recorded that it was around 26/27 May that he calculated the number of people at risk. According to this, he surmised that the infection had spread beyond the original source and took the period of infectivity to be 7 to 23 May. The shop manager claimed that most of his 10,000 customers per week visited the cold meat counter, but, since some entered the shop more than once weekly, MacQueen took 10,000 as an estimate of the number buying cold meat over the sixteen-day period. He deduced that 10,000 families or 40,000 individuals were at risk, which he reckoned was an underestimate, since hotels, restaurants and so on were taken as families. According to MacQueen's evidence this reasoning led him to launch a publicity campaign. It was impractical to identify and monitor so many people, so he resolved to use the media to create 'scrupulous personal hygiene, avoidance of all potentially dangerous foods and – for the safety of other areas – avoidance of all needless travel'.[21]

It is noticeable that while the figure of 10,000 families agrees with that in the press at the time, MacQueen was then working with a shorter period of infectivity. Otherwise, the talk of the imminent end of the 'first wave' would not have made sense. However, the content of *P&J* on 27 May shows that this was certainly when the advice to the public changed gear. Besides the corned beef revelation, the newspaper also reported MacQueen's most comprehensive hygiene guidance to date. Detailed travel advice came later. But from the way the outbreak news unfolded, far from being a policy decision based on the calculations presented in MacQueen's Milne Committee evidence, the publicity campaign, like the timing of the corned beef announcement, appears as much a response to the criticism and demands of the public and press. He advised the public to 'avoid cream cakes, pre-cooked cold meats, lettuce and tomatoes that have not been pulled from your garden, and in fact anything that has been handled by someone and not cooked again'.[22] Food retailers were quoted as saying that they would withdraw foods blacklisted by MacQueen, and an inside column detailed precautions that MacQueen had advised. Individual towels should be used in the home, and, when eating out, people were advised to take paper towels for drying their hands after washing them before eating.[23]

[20] 'Typhoid in bully tin', *P&J*, 27 May 1964, p. 1a.
[21] I. A. G. MacQueen, 'Evidence submitted to Committee of Enquiry', July 1964 (main evidence) and August 1964 (further questions), EMR, p. 11.
[22] 'Typhoid in bully tin', *P&J*, 27 May 1964, p. 1a.
[23] 'Taking the terror out of typhoid', *P&J*, 27 May 1964, p. 10c.

MacQueen also responded to 'Shocked Mother', ignoring her remarks about charges at public conveniences (it was reported elsewhere that the cleansing committee convenor, after consultation with the Lord Provost and MacQueen, had granted free washing facilities.[24]) But he vociferously attacked her 'sneer' about the 'paper work' of health visitors. Describing the letter as 'appalling, stupid, idiotic, time-wasting', and the author as a 'cowardly, arrogant, stupid know-all', MacQueen claimed that it had caused 'indignation' in his department. His staff, especially the health visitors, had been working fifteen or sixteen hours a day, including Sunday, and were in 'danger all the time'. If a second wave was avoided, it would be because of their 'tireless' work.[25]

MacQueen's brutal attack for what seemed to another reader 'an innocuous remark that health visitors were trained nurses'[26] emphasises the extent to which MacQueen had been plunged into a situation outside his experience. As Keith Webster, junior reporter for the *Glasgow Herald*, explained, normally MacQueen (as well as George Dickie, the county MOH) 'sat with their committee chairman' when they talked to journalists. Dickie gave only a few press conferences during the outbreak, but Webster consistently spoke of both officials. The journalists, he said, very quickly got a feel for 'what are the things that rattle these men, what are the things that upset them, what are the things that animate them, that get them talking with some passion'.[27] Someone at the press conference probably realised that health visitors were one of MacQueen's passions. Webster further described the effect upon MacQueen of a pertinent question:

> Instead of lolling back in his seat . . . with his pipe in his hand, when he became animated, he'd sit up and his glasses would go on and the pipe would turn and the stem would come towards you, and sometimes it would tap the desk and sometimes it would get poked towards you.[28]

The front-page story of *EE* on 27 May showed that MacQueen's counter-attack continued during the day. He had spoken out against the 'critics of the army of "front-line" troops', declaring that during a war everything possible should be done to keep up morale. Little further was said about the source of the outbreak, but MacQueen did reveal that the corned beef was not from Europe or North America. On questioning, he also said there was 'no need to believe it was 15-year-old ex-Army meat'.[29] This remark was a reference to a

[24] 'Now, free wash-up', *P&J*, 27 May 1964, p. 1e.
[25] 'MacQueen slams woman letter writer', *P&J*, 27 May 1964, p. 1d.
[26] 'By a mother who once had typhoid', *P&J*, 28 May 1964, p. 4.
[27] K. Webster, interview, 2 June 1999, Aberdeen, ATO/10.
[28] Ibid.
[29] 'MacQueen hits out at critics as total tops 100', *EE*, 27 May 1964, p. 1a.

story originating in *Grocers' Gazette* on 16 May,[30] which had been taken up prominently by the *Daily Mail* on 22 May. This revealed that government-released corned beef, black from being too long in the tin, was on sale for 6d a pound cheaper than other brands.[31] This story appeared as part of larger items about high beef prices in other newspapers, including *EE* on 22 May, next to an item about the typhoid outbreak.[32]

Having claimed that if a further wave of cases was avoided it would be as a result of his staff's self-sacrifice, MacQueen then blamed Aberdeen's citizens, in advance, for any new wave that did materialise. On 28 May *P&J* reported him as saying that public health, hospital and laboratory workers were all performing their respective roles well, and now he wanted the general public 'to play their full part':

> If every citizen had co-operated from the start by having perfect personal hygiene . . . then they could have guaranteed there would be no second wave. . . . If every citizen started tomorrow to play their full part, then, while there might be a second wave incubating, they could guarantee there would be no third wave.[33]

But if some citizens did not bother with hygiene, MacQueen claimed, 'we could get wave after wave of typhoid'. So far, there was no evidence of a second wave, but the next few days would be 'crucial'.

In *EE* MacQueen was reported as having handed out 'Bouquets . . . and brickbats', the bouquets to businesses for their 'public-spiritedness' in stopping sales of blacklisted foods, and the brickbats to citizens who were failing to maintain a good standard of hygiene. He listed a 'six-point reminder' of the rules to be followed:

1 Remember that boiling and pasteurisation kills off germs very quickly
2 All cooked foods are best eaten soon after cooking.
3 Remember hand washing before meals and after going to the lavatory, but also remember to use clean, individual towels – and clean DISH towels.
4 The public should remember to keep their nails short.
5 People should handle food as little as possible.
6 Any person who does not feel that he or she is fit and well should not work until given official clearance. [34]

30 'Ministry corned beef scandal', *Grocers' Gazette*, 16 May 1964, p. 9.
31 'Tin-beef shock', *Daily Mail*, 22 May 1964, p. 1a. See also 'Beef', *Daily Mail*, 23 May 1964, p. 9d.
32 'Up go Aberdeen meat prices as crisis worsens', *EE*, 22 May 1964, p. 1h.
33 'Health, hospital workers – and you', *P&J*, 28 May 1964, p. 1d.
34 'Schools may have to close, warns MacQueen', *EE*, 28 May 1964, p. 1a.

The prevention of 'wave after wave', he warned, 'requires the emphatic co-operation of everybody'. But although the number of confirmed cases had risen to ninety-eight, MacQueen regarded the situation as promising, 'for it followed the pattern he had forecast – a gradual tailing-off of primary infection cases. . . . We should have a very good idea by tonight or tomorrow. And if we reach the next day without any more cases, we have every reason to feel optimistic.'[35]

The latest press conference also covered what might happen if a second wave hit the city, leading to the headline 'Schools may have to close'. As for travel, as long as strict personal hygiene was observed, MacQueen advised that holiday-makers and others leaving town could 'carry on', but that large outings, camps and picnics, especially involving mingling with people from elsewhere, should be scrapped. As for those coming into the city the hazard was slight, as long as they took normal precautions.[36] This was the first time that restriction of gatherings and movement had been advised, although cancellations of events, and trips, to and from Aberdeen, had already been reported.[37] Many more followed.

Some of the advice produced amusing incidents, especially involving children. A small boy, having urinated in the gutter, burst into tears because he did not know where to wash his hands, and a girl, watching a shop assistant clumsily trying to put rolls into a bag using tongs, enquired, 'Wouldn't it be quicker if you washed your hands?' Some adults invented their own precautions. For example, one woman reported soaking her bacon in 'Milton fluid' before cooking.[38] And when a senior civil servant visited Aberdeen, he and his colleagues found the Lord Provost's car was heavily dosed with antiseptic, with the seats covered by white sheets.[39] Aberdeen University responded to MacQueen's advice with a series of notices to students and employees. The swimming pool was closed, dances called off, and sporting fixtures and field trips involving travel beyond twelve miles from Aberdeen were cancelled.[40] A later memorandum even stated that 'There is a remote risk of infection through perspiration on examination scripts. Examiners who wish to take precaution on this score should wear cotton gloves.'[41]

---

[35] Ibid.

[36] Ibid.

[37] 'Partick's about turn', *EE*, 26 May 1964, p. 1f; 'School campers stay put', 'Bus trippers avoid City', *EE*, 27 May 1964, pp. 1a, 1f.

[38] D. L. B. King, 'Typhoid', *Scottish Master Baker*, 1965; A telephone conversation between a member of the public and D. F. Smith on 4 September 1998, following press publicity concerning the project upon which this book is based.

[39] L. P. Hamilton, interview, 11 October 1999, Edinburgh, ATO/27.

[40] University secretary, 'Typhoid outbreak', 1 June 1964, AUSHS.

[41] W. Angus, Typhoid outbreak notice No. 3, 3 June 1964, AUSHS. This notice was later changed as an addendum to Notice 4 to 'There may be a remote risk of infection through handling examination scripts. It can be obviated by adequate washing of hands.'

The main *P&J* headline on Friday 29 May, 'New typhoid wave? Touch-and-go – but MOH still hopeful' indicated that the latest figures were beginning to dash MacQueen's optimism, but he still attempted a hopeful interpretation:

> The signs are relatively favourable. If for example we had a wave beginning like the original wave I would have expected so many early cases that it would have become quite obvious by now. Either we are being very lucky and not having a second wave, or else our second wave is a small one.[42]

While preparing citizens for the worst, there were signs that MacQueen was now winning the public-relations battle. Two letters appeared under the heading, 'We're right behind you, Doc!', one of which remarked: 'In Aberdeen, I think we are well off, with a keen and clever MOH, Dr MacQueen and his able colleagues and assistants. Long may they live, and have power for their noble calling.'[43] And an item about Margaret Nairn, superintendent health visitor, described her as 'one of the gallant band of women who have been working at full pressure to try to halt the spread of typhoid'. Nairn stated that she and her colleagues were part of a team, explaining: 'We are doing no more or less than our colleagues in the City Hospital. . . . Every single nurse . . . is doing her bit.'[44] An editorial supported the proposal to close schools, but added, with a hint of criticism, that many parents wondered why this had not happened earlier.[45]

Having declared that eight or more new cases on 29 May would indicate the start of a second wave, the tension was mounting when, by the time of *EE* going to press, eleven were confirmed. MacQueen, however, was still 'not convinced' that a second wave had started. He now said that if there had been an increase of twenty cases then he would say a second wave had started. But there were further signs that he was winning the media battle. He claimed he had received many letters expressing 'appreciation of the work of all the people concerned in fighting the outbreak'.[46] In addition, an editorial acknowledged that there was a 'general need for reassurance that the health authorities are doing all in their power', and revealed that MacQueen had agreed to be 'ready and willing to answer any questions when he feels it is in the public interest to do so'.[47] Next to the editorial, under the heading 'Questions you ask' was a list of questions and MacQueen's answers, including, for example, a negative response to a query about whether there was any danger in posting

<hr>

42 'New typhoid wave?', *P&J*, 29 May 1964, p. 1a.
43 'We're right behind you, Doc!', *P&J*, 29 May 1964, p. 6b.
44 Pearl Murray, 'Gallant band', *P&J*, 29 May 1964, p. 8d.
45 'Schools warning', *P&J*, 29 May 1964, p. 6a.
46 'Fears of second wave as 11 more cases confirmed', *EE*, 29 May 1964, p. 1a.
47 'Our view gag these rumour pests!', *EE*, 29 May 1964, p. 1a.

mail.[48] Another inside-page item was a report on 'Typhoid and hygiene: a lesson to be learned',[49] a 'special investigation' which had been advertised the previous evening.[50]

The local press had realised that typhoid was good for sales. Over the next few days, as more dramatic news came from Aberdeen, national newspapers began to follow suit with their own special articles. The *EE* feature, dubbed 'An "E E" inquiry', included a picture of MacQueen, but was based on an interview with Herbert Parry, the chief sanitary inspector, and a shopping trip to city centre stores. Parry discussed deficiencies in shop hygiene, highlighting the need for tighter regulations covering street traders, the greater use of refrigerated displays, the use of tongs, and the banning of communal towels in food premises. He urged housewives not to buy from unsanitary shops, to 'force the "dirty" trader out of business or into line with the standards'. The shopping trip found dirty overalls and 'sliced meat handled with anything but clean fingers'.[51]

This effort to create additional news around the outbreak provided a mouthpiece for the health and welfare department and amplified their messages. After a difficult start, MacQueen was getting on better terms with the media and the public. The hygiene campaign had begun, but appears as much a response to criticism as a planned strategy. However, as the implications and political dimensions of the outbreak became apparent, and the news from Aberdeen became increasingly dramatic, intensifying press interest, it became clear that MacQueen still had much to learn about how to handle the media.

Sensationalism and the proliferation of typhoid news

On Saturday, 30 May, *P&J* was spoilt for choice with regard to headlines, and used 'First typhoid death' alongside 'Tor-na-Dee made ready', 'Corned-beef shocker', and 'City schools closed'. A dramatic account of the opening minutes of MacQueen's late Friday press conference was given. A few minutes after it began, an 'urgent call' revealed that twenty-nine people had been admitted to the City Hospital in the past three hours. It now seemed obvious to MacQueen that a second wave had begun. Nobody could forecast how big it would be, but it was too early for him to comment about any secondary source, or whether he would have to advise against travelling to Aberdeen.[52] Little space was given to the death of a typhoid patient, and the preparation of

---

[48] 'Questions you ask', *EE*, 29 May 1964, p. 1a.

[49] Bill Mackie and Ruby Turberville, 'A lesson to be learned', *EE*, 29 May 1964, p. 6a.

[50] 'Warning – the lesson learned', *EE*, 28 May 1964, p. 1c.

[51] Bill Mackie and Ruby Turberville, 'A lesson to be learned', *EE*, 29 May, 1964, p. 6a.

[52] 'Urgent call – and MOH knew fresh wave had begun', *P&J*, 30 May 1964, p. 1b.

Tor-na-Dee hospital, but a separate item covered the schools closure, during which MacQueen advised parents not to allow children to mix. The domestic science college would also close, but other further education institutions would remain open.[53] Two items dealt with MacQueen's claim that the corned beef starting the outbreak was ex-government stock.

An article headed 'Dr MacQueen explains: the 6lb tin that started it all' quoted MacQueen's revelation that according to a director of a canned meat manufacturer, the shop's invoices showed that some of its corned beef had been imported in 1951. MacQueen thought this 'devastating news'. A reporter asked: 'There seems no doubt now that this is some of the stuff the Government shipped on to the meat market because of the meat shortage?', but MacQueen answered carefully. All he could say was that some of the corned beef appeared to be thirteen years old and that of two brands in the shop he could not tell which was responsible for the outbreak. He declined to name the firms, but did say that he believed the meat originated in South America. He also thought that if the meat lay for years with the germs multiplying, its heavy contamination could mean the incubation period was unusually short in this outbreak. With this in mind, the outbreak could be 'into a third wave now, and what had appeared to be a peak of the first wave, had, in fact, been a second'.[54] A further item quoted Hector Hughes, Labour MP for Aberdeen North, stating that it was scandalous if the outbreak was caused by ex-Ministry corned beef, and that he would call for a 'searching inquiry'.[55]

The front page of *EE* showed a fleet of ambulances moving patients out of Tor-na-Dee. Now MacQueen's travel advice was blunt, summarised as 'Don't leave the city if you are an Aberdonian' and 'Don't come to Aberdeen unless it is absolutely necessary'.[56] According to MacQueen, 'the food hygiene of the citizens of Aberdeen had not stood up to the strain, and they already had this second major wave'. Public baths and youth clubs for the under-15s would close, while canteen facilities would be suspended at clubs for the over-15s, at community centres, and at the Arts Centre. He suggested that a football match be cancelled, dance and bingo halls shut, cinemas closed in the afternoons, and Sunday schools suspended. He added: 'One has to think of Aberdeen in the sense of being a "beleaguered city" ', from which the newspaper took its headline 'Now a beleaguered city'.[57] Shopkeepers, already suffering a 50 per cent down-turn in trade, were 'stunned', one café proprietor describing Aberdeen as a 'ghost town'. However, sales of frozen foods, spring cabbages, oranges and bananas had been brisk, and Woolworth's trade in paper towels,

[53] 'Domestic college shut, too', *P&J* , 30 May 1964, p. 1a.
[54] 'Dr MacQueen explains: The 6lb tin that started it all', *P&J*, 19 May 1964, pp.1e, 4f.
[55] George Gardiner, '"Atom" meat storm is blowing up', *P&J*, 30 May 1964, p. 1b.
[56] 'Quarter million people at risk', *EE*, 30 May 1964, p. 1.
[57] 'Now a beleaguered city', *EE*, 30 May 1964, p. 1a.

disinfectants and nailbrushes had been 'tremendous'. The three ballrooms had responded to MacQueen's advice, but some cinemas and bingo halls had yet to act.[58]

A note on a visit to Aberdeen on 30/31 May by Ian Sutherland, the SHHD's epidemiologist, indicates the thinking behind some of MacQueen's recommendations. MacQueen told Sutherland that the schools closure had been decided 'less on purely medical merits than as a somewhat drastic measure to impress all the public of the desirability of avoiding a congregation of people, especially young people'. The ballroom closures were recommended for similar reasons.[59] The former decision appears to have been welcomed, despite the inconvenience. But if these measures were meant to dramatise the typhoid risk, this was certainly achieved, leading to headlines that MacQueen was to regret. On 31 May, all the Sunday papers covered the outbreak, mostly under sensational headlines such as 'Don't come, even if it means no holiday',[60] 'Typhoid city shuts down', [61] and 'Typhoid rise: Aberdeen a siege city'.[62] The first of various 'spin-off' stories also appeared, concerning a pile of decaying corned beef on a wharf at London Docks. This was the main feature in *News of the World* but also appeared in other newspapers, and will be discussed in Chapter 5.[63]

The *People* developed its earlier critical line with a headline '"I was wrong" says typhoid city health chief'. The story included quotes from MacQueen, admitting that he should have instituted drastic measures from the start, and pointedly used the subheading 'Fever shop stays secret'. It claimed that Aberdonians felt that MacQueen should have instituted a 'standard epidemic drill', involving boiling water, mass inoculations and special hygiene instructions for children.[64] The *Observer* included more subtle criticism. Their reporter thought that the 'whole lesson' was that Aberdeen was 'an average city in its standards'. There was no set drill for a typhoid epidemic, and it was five days before schoolchildren were warned about hand washing, and public lavatory charges were abolished. There remained the question of 'whether Aberdeen was right to be secretive about the source . . . this big anonymous grocer's shop, the subject of strong rumours but no certainty'.[65] The *Sunday Times*, without naming Low's, included a picture of a counter laden with bacon,

---

[58] 'Stay away decision will kill trade', 'No dancing in the city tonight', *EE*, 30 May 1964, pp. 1a, 1f.

[59] I. N. Sutherland to Deputy CMO, 3 June 1964, NAS HH 58/160.

[60] 'Don't come, even if it means no holiday', *Sunday Post*, 31 May 1964, p. 1a.

[61] *Sunday Citizen* reporters, 'Typhoid city shuts down', *Sunday Citizen*, 31 May 1964, p. 1a.

[62] Special correspondent, 'Typhoid rise: Aberdeen a siege city', *Sunday Telegraph*, 31 May 1964, p. 1a.

[63] R. Mount, 'New bully beef scandal', *News of the World*, 31 May 1964, p. 1a.

[64] Ken Gardner, '"I was wrong" says typhoid city health chief', *People*, 31 May 1964, p. 1e.

[65] Ron Perrott, 'Typhoid seals off Aberdeen: "Don't come, don't leave"', *Observer*, 31 May 1964, p. 1b.

a weighing machine and a meat slicer, with the caption, 'Where the trail ended: the shop in Aberdeen which sold the corned beef and meat-cutter which spread the infection'. Below this, a headline 'Typhoid cases leap to 155: Aberdeen "beleaguered"'.[66]

Keith Webster gave some insight into how such headlines were generated:

> There was one occasion I recall in a news conference . . . when MacQueen, who was doubtless very good in the medical issues, but in terms of politics and in terms of public performance and information could be pretty naïve. You could feed MacQueen a line and I recall someone saying to him 'is it fair then Dr MacQueen to call this a beleaguered city, do you agree that Aberdeen is a beleaguered city?' and of course he said 'yes'

After the Sunday coverage the local press objected to the sensationalisation of the outbreak. On Monday 1 June, *P&J* led with 'In the beleaguered city but not the city of fear/(A *Sunday paper's description yesterday*)/More hopeful – but don't relax – MOH'S warning'. A 'ray of hope' had broken the 'cloud of gloom' when MacQueen said the previous evening that 'There is at least the possibility that the second wave of cases is on the decline'. Only ten patients had been admitted between Saturday and Sunday night, but he warned citizens not to relax. He now explained the first wave as arising from the infected corned beef and other meat contaminated by the meat slicer, accounting for around 100 cases up to 26 May. As for the second, he believed that one of the three typhoid victims in the shop was responsible through 'faulty hygiene', around 16 May. When questioned about the need for outside help, MacQueen said that such help was a phone call away, but that, from his forecast of likely trends, the outbreak would be under control before any new staff had 'got into the run of the thing'.[67] He gave a similar response whenever asked this question over the next few days.[68]

One story focused on the impending 'Commons storm',[69] and others were about restrictions on places of entertainment, travel and gatherings. Cinema managers were due to discuss the exclusion of unaccompanied children (which was agreed[70]). Public house licensees were also due to meet, although

[66] Stephen Fay, 'Typhoid cases leap to 155: Aberdeen "beleaguered"', *Sunday Times*, pp. 1d, 2c.

[67] 'In the beleaguered city but not the city of fear', *P&J*, 1 June 1964, p. 1a.

[68] MacQueen also addressed the issue in his notes on the outbreak produced for Aberdeen Corporation's health and welfare committee in mid-June: 'Rough notes on the typhoid outbreak', ACA TH 7/6/6. He did, in fact arrange and accept help from various personnel from outwith Aberdeen, who he listed in the July 1964 number of his department's *Health and Welfare* bulletin. I. A. G. MacQueen, 'Random reflections on the outbreak', *Health and Welfare*, 1964, No. 23, pp. 1–6, at p. 5 (NHSA).

[69] Joseph Tobin, 'Commons storm this week', *P&J*, 1 June 1964, p. 1d.

[70] 'Cinema ban on city children', *EE*, 1 June 1964, p. 1g.

MacQueen did not envisage closing the pubs, as there were limits to the public's co-operation, and it was impossible to 'turn the city into a monastery or an isolation ward'.[71] The City's ballrooms had closed, but under the headline 'Critics of the selfish dancers' the county MOH condemned Aberdonians who had travelled to a dance in Inverurie.[72] To prevent this recurring, MacQueen agreed that Aberdeen's dancehalls could reopen as long as the toilets were supervised and no food or drink was sold.[73] But in contrast with his earlier condemnation of the population for any second wave, an inside-page story was headed 'Aberdeen's commonsense earns a pat on the back/Praise for the people – from Dr MacQueen'. Citizens had 'responded magnificently to the appeal not to travel unnecessarily, to keep their children at home, to exercise good personal hygiene and avoid food that is not going to be cooked again'. Speaking on Sunday morning, MacQueen had not heard of a single case of faulty personal hygiene over the past twenty-four hours. He described unnecessary travel as 'bad citizenship' and appealed to those outside Aberdeen 'to stay away from the battlefield until the battle is over'.[74]

The front-page *EE* headlines of 1 June included 'Typhoid jump in city' and 'Now the big probe starts', the latter referring to an impending statement in Parliament. The number of cases had risen to 227, from 209 on Sunday, and there were now no optimistic remarks by MacQueen.[75] The main items that quoted him encouraged the public to complain at unhygienic shops and reiterated his views about the second wave.[76] In an item headed 'Criticism? I don't care a damn, for myself', MacQueen also responded to the *People*. He had not given an interview to the *People*, and their claims, he suggested, were a distortion of his remarks at press conferences. His main concern was retaining the confidence of Aberdonians. He denied he had made significant mistakes, and claimed that those calling for a 'standard epidemic drill' did not understand how typhoid spreads, or that inoculation would not provide immunity until July.[77]

On 2 June, *P&J*'s front page relied only secondarily upon MacQueen. The newspaper announced an increase of sixty-four cases with the headlines 'Not so bad as it looks/Fewer new cases, says Hospital Board Chief/"Second wave may be on decline" – MacQueen'. The article quoted Dr Beddard, senior administrative medical officer of the North-Eastern Regional Hospital Board before MacQueen. But they both claimed an optimistic interpretation was

---

[71] 'Pubs to close? Trade will meet this week', 'Cinemas may ban children', 'Oldmeldrum games may be off', 'Schools close until further notice', *P&J*, 1 June 1964, pp. 1e, 6d.

[72] 'Critics of the selfish dancers', *P&J*, 1 June 1964, p. 1a.

[73] 'Aberdeen dance halls reopen this weekend', *P&J*, 5 June 1964, p. 1a.

[74] 'Aberdeen's commonsense earns a pat on the back', *P&J*, 1 June 1964, p. 6b.

[75] 'Typhoid jump in city and Banffshire shock', *EE*, 1 June 1964, p. 1a.

[76] 'Boycott unclean shops – MOH', *EE*, 1 June 1964, p. 1g; 'How the second wave started', *EE*, 1 June 1964, p. 1e.

[77] 'Criticism? I don't care a damn, for myself', *EE*, 1 June 1964, p. 1a.

possible. There were only nineteen new admissions: the jump in cases was due to the confirmation of a high proportion of the previous day's suspects.[78] The newspaper contained a further account of MacQueen's reply to the *People*,[79] and supported his position in an editorial. This reiterated the view that nobody could yet assess the effectiveness of the measures taken, and that nothing could have stopped the cases which had so far appeared, because they were 'infected and incubating the disease' before typhoid was identified in the city.[80] However, 'Letters to the editor' showed that the local public relations battle was not over. A letter from 'Furious' headed 'Better to be alarmed than to be greatly infected' complained that it took several days for a full list of precautions to be issued. 'Shocked citizen' asserted that MacQueen was wasting time 'castigating the general public when vital matters have been overlooked', and a further letter demanded mass immunisation.[81] Items based mainly or solely upon MacQueen's press conferences or otherwise generated by his department were now significantly outnumbered by other items. These included the story about calls for a government enquiry, but also concerned the impact of the outbreak upon schools and Aberdonians' travel plans, readers' experiences of shop hygiene, and a rumour that Aberdeen harbour was in quarantine (it was not). In addition, quotes from Beddard, A. M. Duncan, superintendent of the City Hospital, and Dickie, the county MOH, also featured in several stories.[82]

The main *P&J* headline on 3 June, 'Another big jump in new patients/– But don't treat totals as a scoreboard – Hospital Spokesman', again introduced an article which quoted Beddard before MacQueen. Beddard thought it silly to get 'frantically worried' or 'jubilant' if the number of new cases went up or down. When asked whether they indicated the start of a third wave, he said MacQueen had the information on which such a judgement could be made. According to MacQueen, it was too early to say what would happen. He thought a new large wave unlikely, but at worst such a wave 'might be many times bigger than that which we have yet had'. Instead, there might just be a number of small family outbreaks.[83] Another official was quoted in a further

[78] 'Not so bad as it looks', 'Second wave may be on decline – MacQueen', *P&J*, 2 June 1964, pp. 1a, 1f.

[79] 'We did not make any vital errors', *P&J*, 2 June 1964, p. 7b.

[80] 'Bitter blow', *P&J*, 2 June 1964, p. 1a.

[81] Furious, 'Better to be alarmed than to be greatly infected'; 'Shocked citizen', 'Methinks the doctor doth protest too much'; Valerie Middleton, 'Money back if you wash your hands . . .', *P&J*, 2 June 1964, pp. 6c–e.

[82] For example, 'Not so bad as it looks', 'Top-level inquiry demanded – at once', 'No plans to cut summer holidays', 'Aberdeen Harbour NOT in quarantine, says port boss', 'Butcher gave me maggoty bones – Aberdeen Housewife', 'Shock for city pair bound for Jersey', *P&J*, 2 June 1964, pp. 1a, 1a, 1b, 1d, 1d, 1h; 'Why twice more women than men', *P&J*, 3 June 1964, p. 6b; 'No move to close county schools', *P&J*, 3 June 1964, p. 7a.

[83] 'Another big jump in new patients', *P&J*, 3 June 1964, p. 1a.

prominent item. Below a photograph of a lorry spraying disinfectant in Aberdeen's main street, the cleansing department's superintendent explained that his vehicles had been working late, and that the exercise would 'help bring home the importance of hygiene to the people'.[84] MacQueen featured notably, however, in a story about the previous day's parliamentary statement. Secretary of State for Scotland, Michael Noble, had said that corned beef might have caused the outbreak, but that ex-government stock was certainly not involved. MacQueen, however, stood by his previous positions. In contrast to Noble's tentative remarks, he thought there was 'no shadow of doubt . . . that the outbreak was started from corned beef'. Labour MPs were said to be suggesting that MacQueen and the government were 'at loggerheads', but this was denied by Scottish Office officials.[85]

With the headline 'Dr MacQueen – I'm displeased but not alarmed', MacQueen's views again dominated the main *EE* headline, a comment on an increase of sixteen cases since Tuesday. He still thought it 'too early to say that a third wave has appeared'.[86] Another story, 'Act now to salvage what's left of the season', based on quotes from Harry Webber, Aberdeen's publicity director, showed that some officials were already considering the post-outbreak rehabilitation of Aberdeen.[87] *P&J* reported that at a meeting of hoteliers, one speaker claimed that each post brought hundreds of pounds' worth of cancellations.[88] According to *EE*, the tourist season had been 'crippled . . . because extravagant and over-dramatised accounts have been circulated throughout Britain'. This was an allusion to coverage arising from MacQueen's press conferences, but Webber suggested that MacQueen could help the situation by making a statement that 'this was not the time for people to cancel their July and August holidays'.[89]

It would be some days before a concerted effort to rehabilitate the city developed and the implications of the numbers continued to dominate the headlines. Under the headline '30 more typhoid cases/Still some room for optimism' and 'No third wave yet – just wavelets', *P&J* of 4 June reported MacQueen's latest views. There was, he thought, no indication of a major third wave but rather 'a series of third wavelets'. But the story below soon moved on to the cost of the outbreak, and quoted the Chamber of Commerce chairman.[90] A further prominent article on the source of the corned beef revealed

---

84 'Disinfecting Union Street', *P&J*, 3 June 1964, p. 1d. For some further discussion of this incident see L. Diack, 'Myths of a beleaguered city: Aberdeen and the typhoid outbreak explored through oral history', *Oral History*, 2001, vol. 29, pp. 62–72.

85 'Storm over bully: government probe', *P&J*, 3 June 1964, p. 1b.

86 'Dr MacQueen – I'm displeased but not alarmed', *EE*, 3 June 1964, p. 1a.

87 'Act now to salvage what's left of the season', *EE*, 3 June 1964, p. 1e.

88 'Our plight is desperate, say hotel keepers', *P&J*, 3 June 1964, p. 1f.

89 'Act now to salvage what's left of the season', *EE*, 3 June 1964, p. 1e.

90 '30 more typhoid cases', *P&J*, 4 June 1964, p. 1a.

that a representative of the canned meat company who had informed MacQueen that the corned beef was ex-government stock (which MacQueen continued to suggest was a possibility) had visited Aberdeen. However, an editorial supported the view that while the source of the corned beef was interesting, for MacQueen it was a sideline:[91]

> It is surprising that as a new period of crisis draws near, Dr MacQueen should be asked to spend a couple of hours out of a busy day to answer questions. . . . Under great pressure no doubt, the Medical Officer has allowed himself to appear more as a front-room than a back-room boy. And it is the men in the back-room and the workers they supervise who will win this fight . . . Dr MacQueen has done well. He has not spared himself. He has given out all the information that the public could ask for. Now let us push the corned beef aside for the next few days.[92]

After this, MacQueen's involvement in this aspect of the story faded.

EE on 4 June led with the headline, 'The day of destiny for a stricken city', and quoted MacQueen extensively. Until the previous day, MacQueen thought, it could be reasonably said that almost all admissions had been developing typhoid before anyone knew the disease was in Aberdeen. However, from that day on:

> and certainly after today it will be possible to say that most new admissions caught the disease after we knew that typhoid existed in the city.
>
> If there is a really sizeable reduction in new cases today or tomorrow then all health workers will be able to congratulate themselves on a singular and spectacular triumph.
>
> If, on the other hand, there is no reduction . . . today and tomorrow, and even an increase . . . then dirt, carelessness, ignorance and apathy will have triumphed over all our efforts, in which case we will have to think out still more measures of attack.[93]

In justification of his press strategy, he again explained that because he had estimated that as many as 10,000 families or 40,000 people were at risk, there had been:

> a deliberate policy by the health workers to convert television, radio and the Press into unpaid health education officers and public relations officers, to spread information and advice and allay public panic.[94]

---

[91] 'The big corned beef mystery deepens', *P&J*, 4 June 1964, p. 1c.
[92] 'Let's get on with it . . .', *P&J*, 4 June 1964, p. 6a.
[93] 'The day of destiny for a stricken city', *EE*, 4 June 1964, p. 1d.
[94] Ibid.

This, perhaps, was MacQueen's response to the implied criticism from Webber. Another item, based on an interview with Mrs MacQueen, provided some good publicity. Headed 'My husband has the courage of his convictions', this remarked that they were both used to criticism and took it as part of public life. For her husband, 'The health of the city comes first: he will not allow anything to interfere with his duty to the public'. In addition, as if in defence of MacQueen's actions at the still unnamed shop where the infection originated, she revealed that she had shopped there since the outbreak started.[95]

On 5 June *P&J* broke the news that there were '33 more in hospital', and again MacQueen sought to back-track on his previous remarks. He described the latest figures as 'a little disappointing' and 'serious but not necessarily catastrophic'. He admitted that some colleagues thought he had been premature in suggesting that a crucial turning point had arrived, adding: 'Don't let's be too pessimistic yet.'[96] The newspaper also sought to present a positive gloss by devoting most of the front page to a story contributed by a correspondent from Croydon. This detailed the story of Croydon's 1937 outbreak and expressed the hope that Aberdonians would be encouraged by the fact that the victims were now 'healthy, active, people'.[97] Inside the newspaper, MacQueen's advice to Aberdonians not to go on holiday, especially to large resorts, was featured in one item, while another was based on information he had given about the contact-testing clinic, and the need to identify carriers after the outbreak.[98] A third item, 'Dr MacQueen is "dynamo"', referred to the view expressed by Mr J. A. Stodart, the Under-secretary of State for Scotland, during a visit to Aberdeen. Stodart told journalists that MacQueen had assured him that if he needed outside help he would ask, and that there was no misunderstanding between them. He accepted MacQueen's preference for his own workers who knew the area.[99] This was a reference to concern that the Aberdeen health authorities were not receiving support from outside, which had been expressed in the press, and to the Scottish Office. One Aberdonian had claimed that 'those in charge' in Aberdeen were 'trying to "bite off more than they can chew"' with detriment to the health and prosperity of the city.[100]

The front page of *EE*, dominated by two articles, illustrates the way in which the press no longer depended upon MacQueen for typhoid news. One, headed '"Postpone trades fortnight"', concerned suggestions that the town's

---

95 'My husband has courage of his convictions', *EE*, 4 June 1964, p. 1a.

96 '33 more in hospital', *P&J*, 5 June 1964, p. 1a.

97 Leslie Hadfield, 'Take heart from Croydon', *P&J*, 5 June 1964, p. 1a.

98 'Don't go to big resorts, says MOH', 'Plan to prevent recurrent city outbreaks', *P&J*, 5 June 1964, pp. 9a, 9b.

99 'Dr MacQueen is "dynamo"', *P&J*, 5 June 1964, p. 9e.

100 M. J. M. Robertson to M. Noble, 4 June 1964, NAS HH/160.

annual business holiday in July should be rescheduled. In the second, 'We think this is madness!/Our view', the newspaper argued that the Aberdeen Links golf championship should be cancelled.[101] Other items asked readers if they were showing the 'good sense' illustrated by a picture of a shop-girl serving with tongs, and featured the advice from the city engineer's department to picnickers to stay away from rivers and streams to reduce the risk of contaminating water supplies.[102] A small article, '"Reasoned optimism" says MacQueen', appeared at the bottom of the page, according to which there seemed to be no pattern in the new cases now coming forward, such as would suggest a new major source and sizeable third wave.[103] The newspaper remained supportive of MacQueen. An inside-page feature entitled 'Typhoid: have we handled the crisis the right way?' consisted largely of an item on Croydon, the 'EE Postbag', and an article headed 'Experts back our MOH', which referred to views praising MacQueen's performance expressed by Stodart when in Aberdeen, Noble in Parliament, and SHHD officials. The letters included contributions from 'Concerned', 'Puzzled' and 'Vegetarian', expressing doubts about various policies, followed by notes of explanation from the newspaper, the chief sanitary inspector and MacQueen. And a further short letter was headed 'MOH should get a big "thank you"'.[104]

On Saturday, 6 June, MacQueen's words were responsible for the main *P&J* headline 'At last – "hopeful news"'. The number of new cases had dropped to seventeen, which MacQueen hoped indicated 'the beginning of the effectiveness of all the work we have done'.[105] However, another item showed that not all citizens were observing his advice. MacQueen agreed with the *EE*'s line on the golf tournament, and declared it should be 'scrapped'. The championship secretary, however, said the event would go ahead, arguing that it was no more dangerous than a normal Saturday's golf.[106] A story headed 'Golf tournament starts despite health chief's appeal' featured prominently in Saturday's *EE*, but the newspaper led with 'Hygiene – Wee Alickie leads the way!' This was about the impending distribution of the *How to Stamp out Typhoid* brochure, mentioned in Chapter 3.[107] This initiative of a businessman was brought to fruition with the co-operation of the health and welfare department and *EE*. But as if to avoid prompting the thought that maybe the brochure had been produced too late, an item headed '"We seem to be

<hr>

[101] '"Postpone trades fortnight"', 'We think this is madness!', *EE*, 5 June 1964, pp. 1a, 1d.
[102] 'This girl shows good sense', ' Warning!/ – Keep away from rivers and streams', *EE*, 5 June 1964, pp. 1a, 1a.
[103] '"Reasoned optimism"', *EE*, 5 June 1964, p. 1d.
[104] Bill Mackie, 'Experts back our MOH'; Herbert Catto, '"E.E." man re-lives the Croydon outbreak', '. . . and now your views/E. E. postbag', *EE*, 5 June 1964, pp. 6a, 6f, 6c.
[105] 'At last–"hopeful news"', *P&J*, 6 June 1964, p. 1a.
[106] 'Warning from MOH, but Links golf tournament is on', *P&J*, 6 June 1964, p. 1h.
[107] 'Hygiene – Wee Alickie leads the way!', *EE*, 6 June 1964, p. 1a; See also p. 93.

winning" – MOH' took a much less obvious position. MacQueen thought the latest drop in the number of cases coming forward suggested that the 'war' was being won.[108]

Learning to handle the media, and the rehabilitation of Aberdeen

At his 6 June press conferences, MacQueen included a careful defence of his performance. If this was mounted with the Sunday papers in mind, he would have been pleased with the detailed factual accounts given in, for example, the *Observer*, *Sunday Express* and *Sunday Post*. Even the *News of the World*, after the sensational headline 'Typhoid total rises to 324', closely followed MacQueen's words. The reports included the welcome he gave to the SHHD's decision to send one of their medical officers, Elspeth Warwick, to help his department. He also disclosed that he was assisting attempts to limit the economic damage, by writing to intending holiday-makers assuring them that the outbreak was likely to be over by July.[109] The *Scottish Sunday Express* included a front-page item 'The bulldog snaps back at critics' which, in question-and-answer format, gave MacQueen's responses to critical questions. In conclusion, MacQueen claimed he was not bothered by criticism. Someone once told him that the essential qualities of an MOH were 'the pertinacity of a bulldog and the hide of a rhinoceros'.[110]

The *Sunday Telegraph*'s story included the comment that: 'with hotels, restaurants and even public houses practically deserted, public bitterness is building up against Dr. MacQueen. His statements about personal hygiene have given "much offence".'[111]

However, an article by Peregrene Worsthorne inside the newspaper, 'Real lesson of Aberdeen/Exaggerated fear has been a more powerful enemy than fear itself', presented a balanced view. Worsthorne thought that some citizens were responding to the outbreak with common sense, while others were gripped by irrationalism. He concluded, however, that as time passed, more and more people were 'concentrating on sensible precautions'. Hygiene had become 'a local fetish' which was 'just what admirable Dr. MacQueen – who reminds one reassuringly of Charles Hill[112] – ordered'. Worsthorne found

---

[108] '"We seem to be winning" – MOH', *EE*, 6 June 1964, p. 1c.

[109] 'New jump in typhoid cases: 379 ill', *Sunday Express*, 7 June 1964, p. 1a; 'Typhoid: we're winning the war, says M.O.H.', *Sunday Post*, 7 June 1964, pp. 1a, 2b; Roy Perrott, 'Another 22 cases of typhoid', 'Balancing the perils of panic and diseases', *Observer*, 7 June 1964, pp. 1f, 5a; 'Typhoid total rises to 324', *News of the World*, 7 June 1964, p. 1a.

[110] 'The bulldog snaps back at critics', *Scottish Sunday Express*, 7 June 1964, p. 1b.

[111] '22 more typhoid cases', *Sunday Telegraph*, 7 June 1964, p. 1a.

[112] Charles Hill was the well-known 'radio doctor' who rose to fame during the Second World War.

it fascinating to observe public morale improving as people realised that 'immunity from typhoid' lay in their own hands. He added that Aberdeen might now be 'less in the grip of typhoid fear than any other city in the realm'.[113]

The *Sunday Mail's* front-page item began with the headline 'Your health', and the following statements: 'The news from Aberdeen is heartening. But Scotland needs a startling new appraisal of health and hygiene. The typhoid outbreak has put the spotlight on other dangers lurking in our midst.'[114] This introduced 'Shock Issue!' articles over five pages, which ranged over the shortage of sanitary inspectors, the safety of canned food, poor housing, and the need to complain about unhygienic shops. Another item, 'The victims of fear' concerned the reaction of locals to an Aberdonian family staying in Law, Lanarkshire. The children were barred from the village school and the mother's money was refused at the local shop. The caption 'Victims of village gossip', below a photograph of the children, made it clear where the newspaper's sympathies lay.[115]

All the Sunday, 7 June coverage mentioned above contained little to offend MacQueen. The *People*, however, claimed that Harry Webber, the publicity director, had attacked MacQueen's 'daily bulletins' as 'too extravagant', saying that:

> the doctor's remarks have been, to put it mildly, highly colourful, misleading and unduly frightening to those outside the city . . . Dr MacQueen goes from one extreme to the other. He minimised the situation, now he exaggerates it.[116]

Webber apparently had the support of councillors and predicted that after the outbreak there would be some 'knuckles wrapped'.

The Sunday Times also contained a feature which offended MacQueen and civic leaders, spread over two inside pages.[117] According to 'Design for epidemic: the vulnerable city', behind the 'fine granite facades' in Aberdeen were the:

> classic ingredients of epidemic. There is tightly-knit community life with more than half the population living in tenements or flats. There is serious overcrowding, most families living, sleeping and eating in two or three rooms. And there is a great deal

[113] Peregrine Worsthorne, 'Real lesson of Aberdeen', *Sunday Telegraph*, 7 June 1964, p. 14c.

[114] 'Your health', *Sunday Mail*, 7 June 1954, p. 1a.

[115] 'How safe is YOUR food?', 'They call this home', 'How it all began', 'The victims of fear', *Sunday Mail*, 7 June 1954, pp. 1a, 2a, 5a, 7a.

[116] Hugh Farmer, 'Row as typhoid city toll leaps to 379', *People* (Aberdeen edition), 7 June 1964, p. 1b.

[117] 'Insight on Aberdeen', *Sunday Times*, 7 June 1964, pp. 6–7.

of Victorian plumbing, with an exceptionally large number of families sharing facilities with their neighbours.[118]

Graphics compared Aberdeen with a typical large British town, showing the proportions of homes having no separate water closet, hot water system, or fixed bath (36 per cent, 27.7 per cent and 38.2 per cent in Aberdeen against 2 per cent, 15 per cent and 18 per cent). In addition, an annotation to a map of Aberdeen's dock area, headed 'Danger spot', stated that only sixty-five out of 3200 families who lived there had their own toilet. Aberdeen was characterised by 'poor sanitation and inadequate housing – classic allies of typhoid', and few cities, it was claimed, 'could be more vulnerable to epidemic'. Photographs showing the exterior, interior, inhabitants, stair, back-green and toilet of a dockland tenement illustrated the contrast between the external appearance and slum conditions within.

Monday's *P&J* reported MacQueen's response to *The Sunday Times* under the heading '"Vulnerable city": Aberdeen seethes over smear'. MacQueen pointed out that it was the better parts of town, not the docklands, which had been most affected by the outbreak. There was overcrowding, but rehousing had been 'going ahead vigorously' and the city's infectious diseases record was remarkably good.[119] In the only surviving video footage of MacQueen's press conferences, recorded by Grampian Television, he made a further reply to *The Sunday Times*, claiming that the newspaper had distorted the facts with out-of-date figures.[120] MacQueen and Webber both commented on the *People*'s allegations. Webber assured *P&J* that there was no ill feeling, while MacQueen claimed there was not 'a shadow of disagreement' between them, and branded the *People* as 'a poisonous rag'.[121] Around this time, MacQueen reduced his contact with the press, cutting his press conferences to one a day. But he explained that this was because he had nearly reached 'cracking point' on Sunday, when he had been unable to 'speak or read coherently', despite having had only one whisky.[122]

The *P&J* leading front-page story was on the ostracism of Aberdonians, the *Sunday Mail*'s example being only one of several similar incidents. Another involved an elderly couple who were asked to leave a Greenock hotel at 1 a.m., and who, after wandering the streets, found refuge in a police cell.[123] MacQueen found this 'quite shocking' and condemned 'exaggerated fears', giving *P&J* its main headline 'We're not a leper colony!/End this hysteria

[118] 'Design for epidemic: the vulnerable city', *Sunday Times*, 7 June 1964, p. 6b.

[119] '"Vulnerable city": Aberdeen seethes over smear', *P&J*, 8 June 1964, p. 1d.

[120] Press conference at Willowbank House, Aberdeen, 9 June 1964, recorded by Grampian Television.

[121] 'No row, say city chiefs', *P&J*, 8 June 1964, p. 4c.

[122] 'MacQueen "near cracking point"', *P&J*, 8 June 1964, p. 7f.

[123] 'Night in cell for cast-out couple', *P&J*, 8 June 1964, p. 1a.

outside – MOH'. MacQueen claimed that Aberdonians were now more hygienic than citizens of any other Scottish town, and he was horrified by the 'large number of cancellations far far ahead both by people coming to the city and by outside hoteliers dealing with Aberdeen holidaymakers'.[124]

The theme of ostracism continued in Tuesday's *EE*, and the following morning's *P&J*, exemplified by the advice of Grantown Town Council, Speyside, for hoteliers to decline custom from Aberdonians, and for shopkeepers not to obtain perishable goods from Aberdeen.[125] Grantown's Town Clerk told *P&J* that 'they were only following the advice already given by Dr MacQueen in trying to reduce contact with the city to a minimum'. MacQueen countered that there was a 'vast difference between his advice to people coming to or leaving Aberdeen not to make the journey if it was not necessary, and the complete refusal of Grantown to accept people from the city'. He described Grantown's reaction as 'panic', especially in view of the recent trend in the number of cases.[126] Positive efforts of civic leaders and officials to rehabilitate Aberdeen also appeared. The front pages of the *P&J* and *EE* of Thursday, 11 June were dominated by appeals from the Lord Provost to citizens to assist in the restoration of the image of the city as clean and healthy, and to return to the city centre shops.[127]

MacQueen also continued to attack local criticism. A former RAF nurse had alleged to *P&J* that the contact-testing clinic was unhygienic because the doctors were not wearing white coats. On Monday MacQueen declared that these 'irritable, peevish criticisms' of someone who was 'either very tired or very stupid' should be 'jumped on from a very high height'. Staff 'working 14 or 15 hours a day' should not be subjected to such remarks.[128] Later in the week, however, when responding to further criticisms about the outbreak control measures, he merely claimed that he was content to 'leave it to the experts' to decide whether his decisions had been sound.[129] And local favourable opinion of MacQueen was also evident in the same edition of *P&J*, which reported that Aberdeen Trades Council had expressed full support for MacQueen's efforts.[130]

As for the latest outbreak news, on 8 June *P&J* reported the closure of a butcher's shop, named by MacQueen and pictured by the newspaper. One of the owners was a typhoid suspect and MacQueen explained that the stock

---

[124] 'We're not a leper colony!/ End this hysteria outside – MOH', *P&J*, 8 June 1964, p. 1a.
[125] 'Autumn plan for trades fortnight', 'Boycott of Aberdeen is urged', *EE*, 9 June 1964, pp. 1b, 1g.
[126] 'Aberdonians – Keep out! Says Grantown', *P&J*, 10 June 1964, p. 1a.
[127] 'Aberdeen begins the fight-back', *P&J*, 11 June 1964, p. 1a; 'Come on, housewives!', *EE*, 11 June 1964, p. 1a.
[128] 'Dr MacQueen blasts Holburn clinic hygiene complaint', *P&J*, 8 June 1964, p. 4b.
[129] 'Dr MacQueen replies . . .', *P&J*, 11 June 1964, p. 1d.
[130] 'Up 15, but "not bad"', *P&J*, 11 June 1964, p. 1a.

would be destroyed to 'play for safety'.[131] This led to further questions as to why he had not named the original shop, and he agreed to consider whether the latter might now be identified.[132] MacQueen's naming of Low's was subsequently reported unsensationally in *P&J* on 10 June,[133] and on 13 June *P&J* reported that Low's had closed voluntarily for cleaning 'largely to restore public confidence'.[134] Most Aberdonians were already aware of the shop, and, according to Keith Webster, journalists had known about Low's a day and a half after the start of the outbreak.[135]

A further *EE* item on 8 June reported that a young female employee of the shop where the outbreak started was now a suspect. MacQueen stated initially that this might be 'one of the last links in the chain',[136] but the following day said that he thought the positive test was probably an error.[137] On 9 June, *P&J* reported that he had described the ten cases admitted during the last twenty-four hours as the 'most spectacular decrease yet',[138] and two days later *EE* quoted him as describing the latest increase of four as 'down to penny numbers'. He observed, however, that now would begin 'an enormous but back breaking job of trying to tie up all the loose ends and trying to make all the arrangements to make and keep Aberdeen safe'.[139]

On 10 June, two-thirds of *EE*'s front page was taken up with typhoid news, most concerning cases in other areas, the effect of outbreak on Aberdeen's harbour, and progress with the withdrawal of suspect corned beef. The only brief quotes from MacQueen were at the bottom of the page,[140] while the following day the only reference to MacQueen was a statement that he had taken the first day off since the outbreak began.[141] On 12 June he was reported announcing the first relaxation of the outbreak control measures. Senior secondary school pupils would return to their desks, for mornings only.[142] Favourable comments by MacQueen on the trend in the number of cases continued, coupled with warnings that the population should not relax.[143]

---

[131] 'Focus on two sides of life in a typhoid hit city', *EE*, 8 June 1964, p. 1a; for further details of this episode see also p. 89.

[132] 'Why I didn't name food shop', *P&J*, 9 June 1964, p. 7h.

[133] 'Low's named', *P&J*, 10 June 1964, p. 1a.

[134] 'Brighter – but "don't let up"', *P&J*, 13 June 1964, p.1g, 'Bustle in the streets again – as Aberdeen begins to get back to normal', *P&J*, 13 June 1964, pp. 1g, 1f.

[135] Webster, interview.

[136] 'Focus on two sides of life in a typhoid hit city', *EE*, 8 June 1964, p. 1a.

[137] 'Evidence suggests 4th shopgirl "not typhoid carrier"', *P&J*, 9 June 1964, p. 7e.

[138] 'Only 10 new cases/"Most spectacular decrease yet"', *P&J*, 8 June 1964, p. 1a.

[139] 'North boats give city a wide berth', 'New cases down to penny numbers', *EE*, 10 June 1964, pp. 1a, 1d.

[140] Ibid.

[141] 'MOH takes a break', *EE*, 11 June 1964, p. 1g.

[142] 'If you relax', 'School again for seniors', *EE*, 12 June 1964, pp. 1a, 1a.

[143] 'Aberdeen gets back to normal – but "don't relax"', *EE*, 13 June 1964, p. 1d.

Most of the Sunday papers on 14 June included only small items about the outbreak, and quoted MacQueen's comment that the absence of new cases on Saturday made him feel like opening a bottle of champagne. As Keith Webster observed, MacQueen realised, as the outbreak progressed and his experience grew, that he could feed 'good lines' to the media.[144] Several Sunday papers also quoted his remarks about shop hygiene following a tour of the city. Among the items on sale he found barbecued chicken and unwrapped ice-cream, but according to the *People* he did not mean to 'castigate' shopkeepers, he merely pleaded with them not to 'throw temptation in people's way' a little longer.[145] Only the *Sunday Post* and *Sunday Mail* made typhoid their leading story, the former concentrating on the 'champagne' theme. The *Sunday Mail*, however, with the headline 'Barred because they're from Scotland', revealed that a group of students from the West of Scotland had been banned from summer jobs at the English food manufacture Bird's Eye, because of fear of typhoid.[146]

That week, there was no response by MacQueen and others to the Sunday press. Rather, *P&J* reported signs that the city was coming back to life over the weekend. The shops were busier, the trade of restaurants and public houses had picked up, and traffic was heavier.[147] During the early part of the week, the profile of MacQueen's press conference reports, which told consistently good news, continued to decline. On Monday it was reported that by the time of Aberdeen's trades' fortnight, 13–27 July, Aberdonians would be free to travel and would be welcoming visitors.[148] However, in spite of the encouraging trends, the total outbreak-related column inches in Monday's *EE* were the highest since the emergency began. The front-page news included only a small item which reported MacQueen had stated he hoped that salads and cream cakes would be back on the menu within weeks. The extensive coverage consisted of a six-page supplement on hygiene, 'The new crusade'. This included articles about sanitary regulations based upon an interview with Parry, the sanitary inspector, and health visiting, based on an interview with Joan Lamont, the principal tutor of the health visitor training school.[149]

On Tuesday, 16 June, *P&J* reported another 'quiet day on the typhoid front'[150] and the following day observed that MacQueen was now so confident

---

[144] Webster, interview.

[145] *Sunday Telegraph* reporter, 'First day without new typhoid cases', *Sunday Telegraph*, 14 June 1964, p. 3a; 'That champagne feeling', *People* (Aberdeen edition), 14 June 1964, p. 11b; 'No new typhoid – and M.O.H. "feels like champagne"', *Scottish Sunday Express*, 14 June 1964, p. 1d.

[146] 'Barred because they're from Scotland', *Sunday Mail*, 14 June 1964, p. 1c.

[147] 'A sunshine bonus', *P&J*, 15 June 1964, p. 1a.

[148] 'City trades holiday gets the O.K.', *P&J*, 15 June 1964, p. 1c.

[149] Staff writers, 'Hygiene is the watchword in constant war against unseen enemy', 'What a tragedy – after all city's good work', *EE*, 15 June 1964, pp. 7a, 8a.

[150] 'Aberdeen schools and colleges are coming back to life', *P&J*, 16 June 1964, p. 1c.

that he had decided not to postpone his holiday.[151] *EE* included details on his report to the Council's health and welfare committee,[152] which was used as the basis for a detailed *P&J* article the following day.[153] But MacQueen's press conference once again provided a leading headline on 18 June: 'At long last – it's over/The outbreak has been contained, says MOH'. He announced that while strict personal hygiene was still advisable, visitors need no longer be discouraged from travelling to Aberdeen, and Aberdonians could travel risk-free to other areas. The following week, all secondary schoolchildren would return to their desks, while primary and nursery children would return for half days.[154] *EE* announced further steps in the return to normality. The ban on children attending cinemas would be lifted on Saturday, and Aberdonians were no longer discouraged from visiting Butlin's holiday camps.[155] MacQueen was quoted as saying: 'I am all for getting back to normality and getting as quickly as we can to the stage where we can forget typhoid.' He added that:

> the ordinary person . . . is no more likely to get typhoid through coming to Aberdeen than through going to London, and considerably less likely than the person who goes on holiday to the Costa Brava.[156]

Despite these remarks, a further shock headline, 'Beach bombshell', appeared in *P&J* on 19 June, inspired by remarks by MacQueen about the risk of swimming and paddling in the sea, because of the possible presence of typhoid infection in sewage discharged into the rivers. Harry Webber was described as a 'disappointed man', who could not understand why the 'all-clear' had been given and then seemingly retracted. He had already sent letters all over the country saying that everything was back to normal and he would not issue any new statement: 'As far as I am concerned it is all clear and it is going to stay all clear.' The convenor of the links and parks committee remarked, in contrast, 'this may well be the death knell for the summer'.[157] But *EE* made it clear that the Lord Provost and Webber were pushing ahead with plans to attract visitors. Further explanation about the risk of bathing was provided by MacQueen. While patients were in hospital their excretions were disinfected before flushing, but after discharge the infectious waste of a few carriers might go into the sewers and end up in the sea. He advised that 'Until we have rounded up all possible carriers coming out of hospital I think it would be wise to stick to the paddling pool and the chlorinated swimming

---

[151] '. . . and MOH decides to take his holidays', *P&J*, 17 June 1964, p. 1f.

[152] 'MOH talks about Low's', *EE*, 17 June 1964, p. 1a.

[153] 'Dr MacQueen described victory prescription', *P&J*, 18 June 1964, p. 4a.

[154] 'At long last – it's over', *P&J*, 18 June 1964, p. 1a.

[155] 'Aberdonians told cancel your holiday bookings', *EE*, 2 June 1964, p. 1e.

[156] 'Its back to normal in a big way', *EE*, 18 June 1964, p. 1c.

[157] 'Beach bombshell', *P&J*, 19 June 1919, p. 1a.

pool'.[158] MacQueen's final headline-catching statements did little to dent the drive for the rehabilitation of Aberdeen. On Saturday, 20 June *P&J* was dominated by the news that the first typhoid patient had been discharged from hospital, a 23-year-old woman, who was given a bouquet and sash by staff and patients proclaiming her 'Typhoid Queen 1964'.[159] The Sunday press was subdued.

Monday's *EE* led with an account of a special Council meeting, called by ten councillors for debate about the establishment of a relief fund and other matters. The Council's treasurer, however, condemned the meeting's sponsor as a publicity seeker, and a motion calling for the fund was decisively rejected. As for the other matters, the treasurer argued that it would be wrong for the Council to consider 'the alleged action or behaviour of a head of department, when he would not have an opportunity to reply to any criticism made'.[160] With this, the possibility of a local municipal 'inquest' into MacQueen's actions was rejected. That evening MacQueen, who had been listening to the debate, went on holiday.[161] The still-frequent typhoid-related headlines became increasingly dominated by the actions of the Lord Provost, Webber, and the Chamber of Commerce in furthering the rehabilitation of the city, as well as the Queen's flying visit on 27 June.[162]

It was estimated that Aberdeen had lost £7 to 10m as a result of the outbreak and, to limit the damage, the Corporation spent an extra £15,000 on attracting tourists. The Lord Provost wrote to 25,000 people who had cancelled their holidays, explaining that the city was now safe. By the middle of July, Aberdeen was back on course as a tourist centre and the hoteliers were doing good business.[163] R. A. Williamson, on whose initiative *How to Stamp Out Typhoid* had been produced, with his brother, the President of the Chamber of Commerce, were instrumental in setting up the Bon Accord festival, a further effort to rehabilitate Aberdeen. From 25 July to 8 August Aberdeen celebrated with special events including an ox roasting at the beach, a procession, and a further visit by the Queen. While Robbie Shepherd's 'Northern Lights' variety show was cancelled due to fears about its financial viability,[164] capacity audiences totalling a record 150,000 people attended Andy Stewart's show at His Majesty's Theatre.[165] It is Andy Stewart who is given the credit for

158 'We'll be glad to see you', 'Why it's safe to do this . . . but not this', *EE*, 19 June 1964, pp. 1a, 1a.
159 'She's the first patient out', *P&J*, 20 June 1964, p. 1a.
160 'Noon call for Council', *P&J*, 29 June 1964, p. 1a; 'Bid for compensation fund is rejected', *EE*, 22 June 1964, p. 1a.
161 'Aberdeen relief fund rejected', *P&J*, 23 June 1964, p. 1e.
162 'Royal Bon-Accord!', *P&J*, 29 June 1964, p. 1a.
163 Magnus Magnusson, 'Aberdeen, Britain's gayest spot', *Scotsman*, 29 July 1964, p. 6.
164 Robbie Shepherd, interview, 29 October 2001, Aberdeen, ΛTO/46.
165 AULSCA, MS 3628, interview with Andy Stewart in *A City Under Siege*, a BBC radio

the most famous joke associated with the typhoid outbreak – that only in Aberdeen could people get 500 slices from one can of corned beef.

Professional and political sympathy

In MacQueen's evidence to the Milne Committee, he presented his dealings with the media as a decisive strategy, designed to create 'perfect food hygiene' in Aberdeen, and claimed that this strategy was responsible for his ability to sound the 'all clear' after only one month. There is no doubt that MacQueen's media campaign was conditioned by his existing interest in the potential of the media for mass health education. As we saw in Chapter 1, he had used a small food poisoning incident in 1961 as an opportunity to generate press publicity about food hygiene.[166] However, the account in this chapter of MacQueen's press coverage during the typhoid outbreak shows that the timing and content of the information and advice that he released were conditioned as much by his interactions with the press and the population as the outbreak unfolded, as by any preconceived strategy.

At the time of the outbreak, MacQueen's handling of the press was accepted uncritically by the journal of the Society of Medical Officers of Health, which reported on 5 June 1964:

> Dr MacQueen has been holding daily press conferences during most of the course of the epidemic with the result that this has probably been the best 'covered' outbreak of its kind. With an infection so difficult to bring under control, it is fortunate that Aberdeen's population has been so accustomed to accepting guidance on health matters, and there must be a firm hope that strict personal hygiene will bring the outbreak to an end.[167]

The article alluded to MacQueen's enthusiasm for health education, expressed the solidarity of rank-and-file public health professionals, and even contained a hint of envy at the opportunity for re-creating an historic role of the MOH, which had faded with the retreat of infectious diseases. Archival evidence also suggests that Ian Sutherland, the senior medical officer who had most day-to-day contact with MacQueen, remained sympathetic regarding MacQueen's media relations throughout the outbreak, and appreciated the pressures he faced.

programme broadcast on 13 April 1984. This programme continued the theme of the beleaguered city twenty years after the outbreak.

[166] See p. 37; see also L. Diack and D. F. Smith, 'Professional strategies of Medical Officers of Health in the post war period (1): 'Innovative traditionalism': the case of Dr Ian MacQueen, MOH for Aberdeen 1952–1974', *Journal of Public Health Medicine*, 2002, vol. 24, pp. 123–9.

[167] 'Epidemiological notes. Typhoid in Aberdeen', *Medical Officer*, 1964, vol. 111, p. 335.

On 22 May, when there were fifteen known cases of typhoid, after a telephone conversation with MacQueen, Sutherland prepared a memorandum for the Chief Medical Officer, Sir John Brotherston. According to Sutherland, the outbreak was already receiving considerable publicity and MacQueen was under 'bombardment . . . by news agencies'. Sutherland added, 'he will cope with that', but intimated that while MacQueen had avoided naming the shop under investigation, he doubted whether his defences could 'stand very long against the methods of the Press'.[168] From Sutherland's point of view MacQueen's situation was unenviable: when he was in Aberdeen on 30/31 May, he deliberately avoided the press conferences.[169]

MacQueen's handling of the press created some difficulties for Sutherland and his colleagues, and he recorded on 16 June that MacQueen had acquired 'a habit of telling the Press Conferences of recent developments which he had not yet communicated to this Department', which had 'led to some awkward moments'.[170] The most problematic episode was when MacQueen announced that the corned beef responsible for the outbreak might have passed through the hands of the Ministry of Agriculture, Fisheries and Food.[171] As we will see in Chapter 5, this seriously alarmed the government, but when Mr Stodart, the Under-secretary of State for Scotland, quizzed John Smith, the deputy chief medical officer about MacQueen's press conferences, Smith was supportive of MacQueen, explaining that:

> the Medical Officer of Health was not responsible to the Secretary of State for Scotland and . . . it was probably easier for him to handle the press through the medium of press conference than to have continual questions asked by different sections of the press throughout the 24 hours.[172]

A few days later, a minute from Stodart to the Secretary of State, commenting on MacQueen's performance on television, made excuses for his shortcomings:

> It is unfortunate that MacQueen has done his televising in the evening when he has clearly been tired. He was much more spry on the morning of the day I was there. . . . Consequently a lot of people I have met have been very sceptical of my remarks about his ability. He has made a poorish impression in television, but I think this has been the reason.[173]

Stodart's positive remarks about McQueen, mentioned above, therefore do not appear to have been expressed solely for the sake of public relations. There

---

[168] I. N. Sutherland to CMO, 22 May 1964, NAS HH 58/160.
[169] I. N. Sutherland to Deputy CMO, 3 June 1964, NAS HH 58/160.
[170] I. N. Sutherland, 'Aberdeen typhoid outbreak', 16 June 1964, NAS HH 61/11073.
[171] I. N. Sutherland to Mr Stodart, 29 May 1964, NAS HH 58/160.
[172] J. Smith to CMO, 3 June 1964, NAS HH 58/160.
[173] L. P. Hamilton to Mr Baird, 8 June 1964. NAS HH 58/160.

was genuine empathy in the Scottish Office about the pressures MacQueen
was under. Soon afterwards, Brotherston reported that Elspeth Warwick, the
SHHD medical officer seconded to MacQueen's staff, had helped MacQueen,
who was obviously tired, 'to decide to reduce his press conference to one a
day.[174]

Sutherland, when preparing a review of the outbreak, placed no blame upon
MacQueen for the nature of the reporting. He observed that the outbreak was
'grossly overplayed' by the press, 'particularly outwith Scotland', causing much
additional work for his colleagues in Edinburgh and staff in Aberdeen. Spurious
travel bans and other measures had 'caused as much disorganisation and
misrepresentation as, say, a localised outbreak of smallpox'. He continued:

> For that I think some blame must be laid at the door of global media, including
> particularly television and the Press. They were ready to seize the opportunities
> given them by a Medical Officer of Health who was acutely Health-Education
> conscious and to apply outside Aberdeen measures which it was his effort, and
> indeed his duty, to try and apply within the City. [175]

On the same day, Sutherland recorded, after a conversation with MacQueen,
that MacQueen was intending to make a statement which would 'lead to
the restarting of visitors including holiday makers', and also wanted to reverse
the advice to bakers about the production of such items as cream cakes. But
Sutherland hoped that MacQueen would not 'take precipitate and/or unilateral action'. He thought that a telephone conversation between MacQueen
and Brotherston might be useful and intimated that 'I have a feeling that if
the subject is simply left with him he may once again make a public statement
which *might* cause difficulty here'.[176] Thus while Sutherland was sympathetic,
he was also wary of MacQueen's handling of the press. We will see in Chapter
6 that during the deliberations of the Milne Committee, opinion regarding
MacQueen's supposed press strategy and its impact moved against him. Civil
servants in London, in particular, were highly delighted when his dealings with
the press were explicitly and strongly criticised in the Milne report.

[174] J. Brotherston to Dr Smith, 10 June 1964, NAS HH 61/11073.
[175] I. N. Sutherland, 'Aberdeen typhoid outbreak', 16 June 1964, NAS HH 61/11073.
[176] I. N. Sutherland to Deputy CMO, 16 June 1964, NAS HH 61/1073.

5

Ministers, officials and the Aberdeen typhoid outbreak

Introduction

In Chapter 3 we referred to some of the interactions between officials of the SHHD and personnel in Aberdeen. In this chapter we will initially consider some further activities of SSHD officials, particularly their efforts to understand the epidemiology of the outbreak. We will also consider their involvement, with other civil servants and their ministers, in dealing with additional aspects of the outbreak, including the identification of the origin of the corned beef, and subsequent action.

We will see that once the probable source of the outbreak was admitted, much work was done on formulating and presenting explanations for past and current decisions. This was with a view to questions in Parliament and from the press, and with an eye to the impending committee of enquiry which was announced at the beginning of June. As the interest of the press and politicians intensified, ministers became increasingly involved in decision making. A co-ordinating group of ministers was formed on the instructions of the Cabinet to oversee the handling of the outbreak, and to take decisions about sensitive issues. Selwyn Lloyd, Lord Privy Seal, and William Deedes, Minister without Portfolio, played central roles. Michael Noble, Secretary of State for Scotland, was initially the main spokesman, but this role, and that of the Scottish Office generally, later became less prominent. Past decisions that had made the outbreak possible had not involved the Scottish Office, but rather the Ministry of Health and the MAFF, which were, in practice, responsible for the Imported Food Regulations.

After the initial action, the key questions were not directly concerned with Aberdeen. Attention shifted to the withdrawal of canned meat produced under similar conditions to the corned beef involved in the outbreak. Ministers and officials wavered between precautionary action and avoiding action, but by the end of June, canned meat produced at two plants, in addition to the one associated with the Aberdeen outbreak, had been withdrawn. A stop was placed on releases of an even wider range of canned meat in the government stockpile. However, the eventual fate of the suspect stock, like many questions thrown up by the outbreak, would have to await the deliberations and report of the official committee of enquiry, which will be discussed in Chapter 6.

Interpretation of the epidemiological evidence

As indicated in Chapter 4, MacQueen's use of the media was heavily criticised in the Milne report. Part of the committee's case was that MacQueen over-estimated the risk of secondary infections and that there was therefore no need for the intense publicity campaign that he orchestrated. It was also upon this basis that the committee criticised the closures of schools, cinemas and dance-halls, and the travel restrictions. MacQueen's warnings of 'waves' of infection led to newspaper headlines using this terminology, and at least one local joke: 'Why's Dr MacQueen sitting alone at the beach? He's waiting for the next wave to come in.'[1] We will see, however, that MacQueen was by no means alone in these concerns. Assumptions and worries about existing and further waves of secondary infections are apparent in the thinking of SHHD officials, and informed some official circulars. Furthermore, MacQueen arrived at the interpretation of the outbreak accepted by the Milne Committee – as consisting almost entirely of a single wave of infection – earlier than Ian Sutherland, SHHD's epidemiologist.

Sutherland had been MacQueen's immediate superior when MacQueen worked at SHHD from 1947 to 1952, and from the beginning of the outbreak he was in touch with MacQueen, passing regular reports to John Smith, deputy CMO. On 25 May, Sutherland told Smith that MacQueen believed that 'the worst of the first wave has now been revealed', but that 'the size of the secondary wave cannot at present be estimated'. Sutherland added: 'My personal feeling is that the numbers will soon start to stabilise,'[2] and reported the following day that MacQueen was 'hopeful that the first wave may have reached, and even passed, its peak.'[3] That day, Smith sent the first official SHHD communication about the outbreak to MOsH. It intimated that seventy-five cases had been identified, that the evidence pointed towards food from one shop, the organism was of phage type 34, and that there were very few cases outside Aberdeen. But two-thirds of the document concerned typhoid among a group of schoolchildren who had visited the Costa Brava, Spain. This had already been the subject of a letter from the CMO of the Ministry of Health to MOsH in England and Wales.[4]

On 27 May, having heard about the King's bakery employee who apparently 'persisted in going to work although he was ill', Sutherland commented that 'The secondary wave could be quite heavy', but concluded his long memo-randum with the remark: 'It may be that the secondary wave will not be very

---

[1] Hilda Robb, interview, 25 May 1999, Aberdeen, ATO/5.

[2] I. N. Sutherland to Deputy CMO, 25 May 1964, NAS HH 58/160.

[3] I. N. Sutherland to Deputy CMO, 26 May 1964, NAS HH 058/160.

[4] J. Smith to Medical Officers of Health in Scotland, and others, 26 May 1964; G. E. Godber to Medical Officers of Health in England and Wales, 25 May 1964, NAS HH 58/160.

large.'[5] The following day, he prepared a note for transmission by the Ministry of Health to the WHO. This intimated tentatively that 'one possibility' was 'that corned beef imported into the United Kingdom had contained the original infection' and stated that, to date, 'all cases appear to be primary'.[6] The following day, Sutherland again noted, when reporting on a survey by MacQueen of the last twenty cases, that they were still all primary infections, 'essentially part of a quite widely distributed group with a point of origin of infection in the period 5th to 10th May'.[7] At this time in Aberdeen, however, the possibility of secondary infections was being seriously entertained. A memorandum to GPs remarked that the latest figures might indicate 'the start of a second wave',[8] and a circular to medical staff of Aberdeen general hospitals stated: 'It would appear that the second wave is now with us.'[9]

Over the next few days, Sutherland and R. M. Gordon, one of SHHD's medical officers, and John Brotherston, the CMO, visited Aberdeen. The idea of several waves of infection was now becoming entrenched. On 30 May, Sutherland attended a meeting at the health and welfare department, and observed that Aberdeen's public health doctors were in no doubt that the infection stemmed from Low's and that the most likely source was corned beef, this applying particularly to 'the first wave of cases'. During discussion about the 'form of the wave', Sutherland saw a graph which 'conveyed quite definitely the impression of a normal frequency curve with mean age [sic] of onset at 15th May'. But he noted that another curve, including a larger number of cases, 'showed some bimodality and to me appeared to have the qualities of two super-imposed curves of which the first would be that which I have already mentioned and the second another curve with peak 7 to 10 days later'.[10] Earlier, following a discussion with Dr Brodie, the consultant bacteriologist, and David Barclay, MacQueen's deputy, Sutherland noted that there was evidence of an abnormally short incubation period. One family bought cold meat on 9 May and sickened on 13 May.[11] After his visit to Aberdeen he recorded that Barclay rejected the textbook two-week incubation period for the current outbreak, suggesting that seven or eight days was more accurate. With this in mind, he interpreted the data as indicating two periods of infectivity concentrated on 9 to 10 May and 15 May, the latter leading to a large wave of cases.[12]

---

[5] I. N. Sutherland to Deputy CMO, 27 May 1964, NAS HH 58/160.

[6] I. N. Sutherland to Deputy CMO, 28 May 1964; Stephen to Roffey, 29 May 1964, NAS HH 58/160.

[7] I. N. Sutherland to Deputy CMO, 29 May 1964, NAS HH 58/160.

[8] G. A. Matthew, 'Circular to Doctors No. 52', 29 May 1964, AUSHS.

[9] Deputy Group Medical Superintendent Aberdeen General Hospitals, 'To all medical staff Aberdeen general hospitals', 30 May 1964, AUSHS.

[10] I. N. Sutherland to Deputy CMO, 3 June 1964, NAS HH 58/160.

[11] I. N. Sutherland to Deputy CMO, 27 May 1964, NAS HH 58/160.

[12] I. N. Sutherland to Deputy CMO, 3 June 1964, NAS HH 58/160.

The implication was that one or more of the three shop assistants who contracted typhoid may have been responsible for the 'second wave', and this notion appeared in a letter from Brotherston to MOsH on 1 June. According to this it was probable that 'the cases admitted up to about 28th May were primarily from the meat or by contamination of the meat slicer and the period of incubation was fairly short'. The period of infectivity was also short and was 'most probably on 7 May'. The cases among the shop assistants had created 'another short period from which infection has been possible from the same shop'. Cases admitted after 28 May were 'likely to have been secondary', and the possibility of further cases developing among contacts was 'still considerable'.[13] These views were in accord with those of Betty Hobbs of the PHLS.[14]

Opinion in favour of consecutive sources of infection within Low's became more entrenched over the next few days. Gordon, who was still in Aberdeen, recorded on 3 June:

> Nothing that I have seen or heard today shakes my confidence in the fact that the main epidemic stems from Low's food store. Originally the source of infection was the infected meat but later the infected person who worked in the shop until 23 May.[15]

He also wrote that 'No doubt some of the more recent cases, although this has not been proved conclusively, are secondary cases some of which are the result of infection by way of bakery products from the case in a baker'.[16] Such anxieties about foci of secondary infections beyond Low's were a frequent feature of SHHD officials' notes. On 1 June, Gordon noted the 'disconcerting news' that a food handler from Albyn school, with 400 to 500 pupils, was among the typhoid cases,[17] and he later mentioned 'possible sources of secondary infection' involving staff at a nursery, the students' union, Woodend Hospital and the Palace Restaurant.[18]

According to Sutherland's record of his discussions during a second visit to Aberdeen on 4 to 5 June, it now seemed that a few patients had been taken ill as early as 6 May, suggesting an initial period of infectivity as early as 1 May. But Sutherland still thought that there were two waves of infection, and that a worker who entered hospital on 23 May was the 'most likely source of origin of the big wave of cases in late May and early June'.[19] On 11 June he learned

[13] J. Brotherston to Medical Officers of Health in Scotland, and others, 1 June 1964, NAS HH 58/160.

[14] See pp. 87–8.

[15] R. M. Gordon, 'Enteric epidemic Aberdeen – 1964', 3 June 1964, NAS HH 58/160.

[16] Ibid.

[17] R. M. Gordon, 'Enteric fever Aberdeen – 1964', 1 June 1964, NAS HH 58/160.

[18] R. M. Gordon, 'Enteric fever Aberdeen – 1964', 3 June 1964, NAS HH 58/160.

[19] I. N. Sutherland to Deputy CMO, 8 June 1964, NAS HH 58/160.

from Barclay that while some of the latest fifteen cases showed a history of consumption of Low's cold meat, among others there was 'a bit of variety'. Two had bought cold meat from the butcher's shop that had been closed.[20] In addition, on 13 June, after speaking to MacQueen, Sutherland noted that one new worrying case was a nurse at Woodend Hospital. She had not nursed typhoid patients, but had eaten at the Palace Restaurant. MacQueen hoped that 'this did not mean a large group of cases secondary to a restaurant infection'.[21] However, none of these anxious notes were followed by further documentation regarding relevant confirmed cases. Sutherland reviewed the outbreak and reiterated his views in a seven-page document on 16 June. This included a graph plotting the date of onset of illness of ninety-four cases which he regarded as 'most likely to show the outline of the first wave', and the subsequent curve which he described as 'much flatter'. The variation in the latter, Sutherland regarded as 'chance fluctuations'. Barclay, however, still interpreted the data as representing several 'consecutive waves', based on his theory of short incubation periods.

Sutherland thought that the explanation of the 'second wave' as caused by a shop worker was necessary to account for the size of the outbreak, which was much greater than other outbreaks of 'probably similar origins'. He thought that MacQueen's theory, namely that the outbreak was explainable by the contamination of other cold meat from an infected tin via the 'hands of the workers and the apparatus and equipment of the counter', could not account for such a large number of cases.[22] MacQueen's theory in his Milne Committee evidence, prepared in late July, accorded with that attributed to him by Sutherland. However, he also incorporated the possibility that some cases admitted in early June may have arisen by contamination of food by an infectious shop worker, and added that the King's bakery worker may have also been responsible for some cases. MacQueen also thought that persons admitted after 11 June were contacts infected as secondaries, and people who had kept infected food for days before eating it. MacQueen also mentioned, and rejected, the views of Barclay.[23]

There is, in this account of the development of the views of SHHD officials on the epidemiology of the outbreak, much evidence that the possibilities of secondary and subsequent 'waves' of infection were taken very seriously and informed official thinking. There was some disagreement over matters of detail, but on general points there was a high degree of consensus between MacQueen and his colleagues in Aberdeen and Edinburgh. The archival evidence also suggests that SHHD officials appreciated the pressures MacQueen was under

---

[20] I. N. Sutherland to Deputy CMO, 11 June 1964, NAS HH 58/160.

[21] I. N. Sutherland to CMO, 13 May 1964, NAS HH 58/160.

[22] I. N. Sutherland, 'Aberdeen typhoid Outbreak', 16 June 1964, NAS HH 61/1073.

[23] I. A. G. MacQueen, 'Evidence submitted to Committee of Enquiry', July 1964 (main evidence) and August 1964 (further questions), EMR, pp. 25–6.

during the outbreak, due to the long hours of work and media spotlight.[24] There is no indication of any serious breakdown in relations between the local and central health authorities, and MacQueen, in his notes prepared in mid-June, referred to 'existing good relationships' between his department and SHHD as one of the advantages of his position.[25] We will see in Chapter 6, however, not only that MacQueen was condemned for overestimating the infectivity of typhoid, but also that difficulties in the relationship between MacQueen and SHHD became another of the problems identified by the Milne Committee.

The identification and withdrawal of the suspect corned beef

Once the source of infection was identified as imported canned meat, tracing the source of the meat became a priority. Initial enquiries of the retailer, suppliers and manufacturers were handled locally, with monitoring from the SHHD. On 25 May, Sutherland was unable to contact MacQueen but spoke to Barclay and Brodie in Aberdeen, and Dr Anderson at the PHLS in Colindale. His notes indicate that in most respects the theories that were eventually accepted as explaining the contamination of the corned beef, and the size of the outbreak, were already well formed in some minds. In view of the phage type, it seemed that the infection had been imported, and according to Barclay, Fray Bentos canned meat had been in use at the shop.[26] Sutherland also reported that Anderson thought it possible for the organism to enter tins during cooling, and suggested that other meats could be infected in the shop. Specimens of corned beef were being examined by the PHLS and by manufacturers, but this amounted to a 'search for a rare event'.[27] Sutherland's report was sent to G. O. Lace, the assistant secretary in charge of MAFF's Food Standards, Hygiene and Slaughterhouse Policy division. Lace did not propose to circulate the information that corned beef was responsible for the outbreak beyond his division and a few other individuals, 'until we are either forced to by events, or it can be confirmed'.[28]

On 27 May the initiative remained with personnel in Aberdeen, although they were busy with other matters. Brodie was examining samples of canned meat from the shop in Aberdeen and Low's depot in Dundee, and told Sutherland that there were two possible makes involved: 'Helmet' brand corned beef, produced in Argentina, and 'Fray Bentos' pressed beef, produced

---

²⁴ See e.g. R. M. Gordon, 'Enteric epidemic Aberdeen – 1964', 1 June 1964, NAS HH 58/160; J. Brotherston, 9 June 1964, NAS HH 61/1073.
²⁵ Ian MacQueen, 'Rough notes on the typhoid outbreak', ACA TH 7/6/6, p. 1.
²⁶ I. N. Sutherland to Deputy CMO, 25 May 1964, NAS HH 58/160.
²⁷ I. N. Sutherland to Deputy CMO, 25 May 1964, NAS HH 58/160.
²⁸ G. O. Lace to A. M. Stephen, 26 May 1964, NAS HH 64/350.

in Paraguay.[29] But Alex. M. Stephen, an SHHD Principal Secretary whose duties included the administration of food hygiene regulations,[30] had been informed by MAFF that the Paraguayan meat plant had always used chlorinated water. Further enquiries were underway about the 'Helmet' corned beef, produced by International Packers Ltd. Sutherland also began to comment on possible action. He advised that 'a ban on any particular batch' would have to be carried out as 'a national exercise', but thought that there was not yet 'sufficient evidence pointing towards excessive danger in any particular batch'.[31]

MAFF quickly became aware of the possible relevance of events surrounding the discovery by Leo Grace, the chief technical adviser on meat inspection, that Argentine Establishment 1A had been using unchlorinated cooling water. At the end of May, Grace was in Washington, USA, and had his notes on his South American trip with him, so he was asked by cable to check the chlorination position of Argentine Establishments 1, 3 and 12. From the information so far available, these seemed to be the possible origins of the Helmet corned beef. The cable added reassuringly, 'Production at Establishment 1A not likely'.[32]

On Thursday, 28 May, Sutherland recorded that 'certain identifying letters and figures' had been obtained from a firm that supplied Low's, and that MAFF advised that these indicated that the corned beef may have been produced at Argentine 12.[33] The difficulty of identifying the establishment with certainty arose from the unfamiliar form of the codes transmitted to London.[34] Sutherland thought it unlikely that further information could be obtained by inspecting discarded tins at the supermarket, but further examination of records might help. He added that the poor relationship between MacQueen and Aberdeen's chief sanitary inspector, Mr Parry, might be contributing to the difficulty of obtaining information, and suggested that a member of SHHD's food and dairy inspectorate make enquiries.[35]

It occurred to MAFF officials to ask whether the Aberdeen corned beef might be ex-government stock, but Ken Bird, chief executive officer of the Food Standards, Hygiene and Slaughterhouse Policy division, was sure it was not. This information was included in a note prepared for the Minister's weekend bag, for delivery on the Saturday morning.[36] The document, prepared

---

[29] I. N. Sutherland to Deputy CMO, 27 May 1964, NAS HH 58/160; J. L. Miller to D. Barclay, 25 May 1964, NAS HH 64/228.

[30] Alex. Stephen, interview, 17 September 1999, Melrose, ATO/8.

[31] I. N. Sutherland to Deputy CMO, 27 May 1964, NAS HH 58/160.

[32] Bird to Grace, 27 May 1964, PRO MAF 282/87.

[33] I. N. Sutherland to Deputy CMO, 28 May 1964, NAS HH 58/160.

[34] K. A. Bird to A. M. Stephen, 28 May 1964, PRO MAF 282/87.

[35] I. N. Sutherland to Deputy CMO, 28 May 1964, NAS HH 58/160. See also pp. 90–1.

[36] 'Note by the Private Office', 18 June 1964, PRO MAF 282/87.

before MacQueen's allegations about the involvement of the stockpile, noted that the possible connection had already been suggested in the press. In any case, if imported canned meat was confirmed as the source of the outbreak, MAFF and the Ministry of Health would be responsible for following up the implications. SHHD hoped to complete their investigations by Monday, 1 June, when the three ministries could discuss the necessary action. The memorandum mentioned that Grace had identified problems at South American canning plants and stated that appropriate action had been taken, 'including the keeping out from this country of supplies from one plant then in transit'. The fact that part of these supplies were allowed into circulation was not admitted.[37] Lace thought that the grounds for attributing the outbreak to corned beef had not yet been provided 'in a completely convincing manner'. They appeared less convincing than at Harlow, where, in any case, the evidence was circumstantial. On the other hand, it was important not to appear inactive. Lace's division had been attempting to 'avert premature accusations against individual firms or products'. Mr Fernandez of the Argentine Meat Board, as well as Stephen in Scotland, were in agreement with this line, and the Ministry of Health did not question MAFF's actions.[38]

During the Friday evening, the Minister heard on the wireless MacQueen's allegations that the corned beef involved in the outbreak may have passed through the Ministry's hands. Lace, after extensive conversations with colleagues, explained the situation to the Minister by telephone at 9.30 the following morning, and later intimated that the officials would meet on Sunday to prepare a report. Meanwhile, it was learned that Hector Hughes, Labour MP for Aberdeen North, was submitting a parliamentary question about the outbreak.[39] As we saw in Chapter 4, the publicity during the weekend of 30/31 May was intense. There were numerous quotations in the press from Labour MPs, indicating that ministers would face many questions when parliament reconvened after the Whitsun break the following Tuesday.[40] William Ross, the Labour Party's Scottish spokesman, wrote to the speaker of the House of Commons requesting a private notice question to ask Michael Noble, Secretary of State for Scotland, to give a statement on the outbreak.[41]

MacQueen's allegation that ex-government stock might be involved took SHHD by surprise as much as MAFF.[42] Sutherland was recalled to Edinburgh from Aberdeen, and on the Sunday met with senior SSHD officials at the home of John Smith, in preparation for a meeting in London the following

---

[37] Slaughterhouse Policy division, 'Note for the Minister', PRO MAF 282/87.

[38] G. O. Lace to Mr Humphreys-Davies, 29 May 1964, PRO MAF 282/87.

[39] 'Note by the Private Office', 18 June 1964, PRO MAF 282/87.

[40] See e.g. 'Recall the old stock, MPs urge', *Observer*, 31 May 1964, p. 1c.

[41] W. Ross to Mr Speaker, 31 May 1964, NAS HH 64/351.

[42] To Mr Stodart, 29 May 1964 [*Note*: this memorandum was certainly misdated. From references to certain events in the text, it was clearly written on 30 May 1964], NAS HH 58/160.

day, which Sutherland was to attend, along with Stephen.[43] Meanwhile, the London-based officials produced a memorandum that was concerned largely with the establishment of a committee of enquiry as part of a strategy for the political handling of the affair. The memorandum briefly reviewed the evidence against corned beef and commented only on MacQueen's statements on this point:

> If the bacillus which caused the outbreak was in any of the cold meat when it came into the shop, then there is a possibility that it came in the corned beef. In fairness to Dr MacQueen . . . he has never, except under severe Press pressure, put it higher than this. His reported words are 'There is a distinct possibility of corned beef having been the source of the infection.'[44]

The memorandum seemed concerned to weaken the link between the outbreak and corned beef and suggested that as several cold meats had been on sale,

> there seemed to be no special reason for incriminating corned beef rather than cold ham etc. Any meat could have been contaminated by someone with recent connections with Spain or South America. . . . There is thus no evidence directly connecting corned beef with the outbreak. We have not so far been informed whether any other foods have been investigated. But it is unlikely that the cause will ever now be established beyond doubt.[45]

There is no indication of a desire to condemn MacQueen for his handling of the press and the comments he had made. The reference to the question of whether ex-ministry stocks were involved merely stated: 'Contrary to suggestions in the Press, there is no evidence that ex-ministry stocks were on sale in the shop.'

By the time the officials met, a further corned beef story had appeared in the media. *News of the World*, with the headline 'New bully beef scandal', made its front-page story a pile of 'rusty, battered cans of stinking corned beef' on a wharf at London's Wapping docks. The cans were from Argentina, having been imported via Houston, Texas and Rotterdam. On arrival, there were many blown cans among the 2000 cases, each containing six cans. The cases were sorted under the supervision of the MOH for Stepney, and the sound ones were distributed, with 250 being delivered to Kincardineshire near Aberdeen. The rest still lay on the wharf. The wharf director wondered

---

[43] John Smith, interview, 4 June 1999, Edinburgh, ATO/11. Besides Sutherland and Smith, the meeting was attended by Brotherston and Gordon, and the purpose was partly to brief Gordon in preparation for his visit to Aberdeen the following day.

[44] 'Typhoid outbreak in Aberdeen memorandum by officials', 31 May 1964, PRO MAF 282/87.

[45] Ibid.

whether some slightly blown tins had slipped through and ended up in Aberdeen, and telephoned MacQueen. MacQueen thought that even if there was no connection with the outbreak, the Wapping corned beef was a potential danger.[46] Other newspapers, including the *Sunday Times*, also mentioned the story.[47]

The officials' memorandum advised that there was no evidence to link the tins at Wapping with the Aberdeen shop, and that MAFF had never dealt with 'Andes brand' corned beef. Corned beef was generally 'perfectly wholesome' and had 'very rarely been associated with any outbreak of disease', and there was no reason to advise people not to eat it. Nevertheless, since the Aberdeen outbreak was already the largest in Britain since 1937, it was 'at least possible that further investigations ought to be made' into the cause. In any case, there was 'a great deal of public disquiet' which ministers would 'wish to allay'. The officials therefore suggested that the Secretary of State for Scotland should establish an expert enquiry which it was hoped would 'confirm the provisional findings . . . regarding the reliability of canned corned meat in general and of Ministry stocks in particular'.[48] As one Ministry of Health official later put it, the enquiry was originally created to 'whitewash MAFF's stockpile'.[49]

On the Monday, in preparation for the ministers' meeting, Sir John Winnifrith, Secretary of MAFF, sent an urgent teleprint to R. E. C. Johnson, Secretary of SHHD. He referred to a report in the *Guardian* which quoted MacQueen saying, 'The contaminated tin originated in Paraguay, part of the stock imported by the government 13 years ago and released on the market recently to ease the meat shortage'.[50] He asked Johnson to find out whether MacQueen had made the statement and, if so, on what evidence it was based.[51] The *Guardian*'s editorial also illustrates the pressures ministers were under. Referring to two suspected typhoid cases on a submarine, the editorial asserted that the 'possibility of a purely local infection' was becoming remote. It was therefore 'even more important for the public to be able to identify tins from the same batch' as that responsible for the Aberdeen outbreak. That service families in Malta had been asked to return tins with certain markings suggested this could be done. The editorial concluded: 'In matters of this sort the instinctive official attitude is to assume that publicity leads to panic. The opposite is the truth.'[52] The reference to Malta arose from reports that appeared on 30 May. The *Glasgow Herald*, citing the Associated Press news agency, stated that Maltese officials were searching for corned beef bearing special

[46] R. Mount, 'New bully beef scandal', *News of the World*, 31 May 1964, p. 1a.

[47] 'M o H on two lessons from epidemic', *Sunday Times*, 31 May 1964, p. 3c.

[48] 'Typhoid outbreak in Aberdeen', 31 May 1964, PRO MAF 282/87.

[49] J. M. Ross to Mr Davidson, 12 August 1964, PRO MH 148/198.

[50] 'Aberdeen may be on top of epidemic', *Guardian*, 1 June 1964, p. 1a.

[51] J. Winnifrith to R. E. C. Johnson, 1 June 1964, NAS HH58/160.

[52] 'Where are all the other tins?', *Guardian*, 1 June 1964, p. 9a.

codes, following advice to British forces to ban the issue of certain brands of corned beef.[53] According to the *Daily Telegraph*, naval catering officers were examining corned beef before it was eaten,[54] while *P&J* claimed that medical officers were checking corned beef supplies to servicemen and their families all over the world.[55]

Besides the pressure exerted by the press, ministers, including the Prime Minister, began to receive indignant letters from the public. One citizen of Aberdeen declared:

> In the total lack of supervision in the import of preserved beef into the country and the excessive age of the products which can be issued for public consumption your government stands convicted in the eyes of every intelligent citizen in Aberdeen, and I hope in the whole country, so please do not get out the whitewash buckets tomorrow, but get up like a man and confess your Government's negligence, and take steps to see that this grave trouble . . . will not be repeated elsewhere.[56]

It was against this background that ministers and officials deliberated on the action to be taken.

In response to Winnifrith's teleprint, SHHD contacted MacQueen, and prepared and transmitted a reply. MacQueen claimed that he had only said that of two brands of corned beef in the shop, one had come from Paraguay and was part of a consignment bought in 1951, based on information obtained from Messrs Liebig.[57] However, by the time of the ministers' meeting, the only aspect of the origins of the corned beef that seemed clear to officials was that MacQueen's information was erroneous. Winnifrith stated that the wholesalers had confirmed that all consignments sent to the shop were comparatively new.[58] However, in Edinburgh, after a telephone conversation with MacQueen, Johnson recorded that there was a danger that MacQueen 'might be persuaded in discussion with the Press' to throw doubt upon the conclusion of the London meeting.[59]

Besides Noble, and the Ministers of Agriculture, and Health, and their senior officials, the London meeting included the Minister of Defence for the Royal Navy, and the Minister without Portfolio, William Deedes. They agreed that an enquiry should be instituted along the lines recommended by the officials, Noble arguing that it should not be put in train until the pressure upon the staff in Aberdeen had eased. The meeting agreed that Noble would

---

[53] 'Second wave of typhoid', *Glasgow Herald*, 30 May 1964, p. 1a.

[54] 'Navy check on tinned meat', *Daily Telegraph*, 30 May 1964, p. 1b.

[55] George Gardiner, 'Atom meat storm is blowing up', *P&J*, 30 May 1964, p. 1b.

[56] A. W. Carnie to A. Douglas-Home, 1 June 1964, PRO MAF 282/88.

[57] Statement, 1 June 1964, NAS HH 64/381.

[58] Ministry of Agriculture, Fisheries and Food, 'Note of meeting on the Aberdeen typhoid outbreak and corned beef supplies', 1 June 1964, PRO MAF 246/239.

[59] R. E. C. Johnson, 1 June 1964, NAS HH 64/381.

announce the enquiry during a statement on 2 June, which would also exonerate ex-government stocks as far as possible, and would indicate that the Aberdeen authorities had acted swiftly and had all the help they needed. The enquiry would be limited to 'the immediate causes of the outbreak', to avoid it considering such questions as 'relations between central and local Government or the Government's general methods of supervising the import of meat and meat products'.[60]

A discussion followed about corned beef supplies to the armed forces. It emerged that on 27 May, the Admiralty had called in stocks of Argentine 1A corned beef in view of Grace's adverse findings, having heard about the issue from the army, which had taken similar action.[61] This created an awkward situation, because the public still had access to supplies that the Army and Navy deemed too risky. It was agreed that medical advice should be sought and if the withdrawal of these stocks could not be justified the Army and Navy orders would be rescinded. Otherwise, the manufacturers concerned would 'be invited to co-operate in a voluntary withdrawal of supplies'. Deedes advised that until a decision was taken on the basis of medical advice, as little as possible should be said about the Army and Navy actions. The final issue discussed was the corned beef at Wapping. It was agreed that a statement be issued that these supplies had been condemned and were awaiting destruction, and that none had been on sale at the shop in Aberdeen.[62] After the meeting, officials prepared a draft of Noble's statement and sent it to the Prime Minister's office for approval.[63]

While the ministers and officials were meeting, SHHD and MAFF were pursuing investigations in Aberdeen and Dundee. M. E. M. Anderson, SHHD's chief food and dairy officer, inspected the supermarket records with Mr Parry, the sanitary inspector, and then went to Low's stores in Dundee to verify the identity of the corned beef sent to Aberdeen. At Dundee, investigations were underway by Mr Maclean of Perfect, Lambert & Co Ltd, the firm employed by MAFF to manage the stockpile. The information obtained at Low's Dundee office and from the manager of the supermarket was roughly consistent with MacQueen's statements, but was more specific and sufficient for the conclusion that stockpile corned beef was certainly not involved. The Fray Bentos product was in 4lb tins labelled 'pressed beef', which had never been bought for the stockpile. The Helmet 6lb corned beef tins were all of recent manufacture, and no Helmet corned beef had been released from the stockpile since 1962, all of which had a different label. Maclean found that among the Helmet

---

[60] Ministry of Agriculture, Fisheries and Food, 'Note of meeting on the Aberdeen typhoid outbreak and corned beef supplies', 1 June 1964, PRO MAF 246/239.

[61] Ibid. The admiralty had also consulted MAFF's armed services supplies officer on 26 May. J. A. Mullington to K. A. Bird, 27 May 1964, PRO MAF 282/88.

[62] Ministry of Agriculture, Fisheries and Food, 'Note of meeting on the Aberdeen typhoid outbreak and corned beef supplies', 1 June 1964, PRO MAF 246/239.

[63] A. M. Thomson to M. H. M. Reid, 1 June 1964, PRO PREM 11/5073.

corned beef in Dundee was some from Argentine Establishment 1A. This information was conveyed to London on the evening of 1 June, and the following morning Maclean advised that out of 216 tins of Helmet corned beef sent to Aberdeen between 13 April and 4 May, all or most were from Establishment 1A.[64]

Seven ministers and sixteen officials reconvened during the morning of 2 June at MAFF's offices. This meeting was chaired by Selwyn Lloyd, the Lord Privy Seal, who reported afterwards to the Prime Minister. This became the first of a series of meetings chaired by Lloyd. He was asked at a Cabinet meeting on 4 June to continue to 'keep an eye on' the outbreak, and to convene a co-ordinating group of ministers for the purpose.[65] The Minister of Agriculture, Christopher Soames, began the 2 June meeting by explaining the circumstances of the decision to stop consignments of Establishment 1A corned beef in transit while leaving stocks in Britain in circulation. He remarked that the Ministry of Health had agreed with the course of action taken. Later, however, principal medical officer John Ross claimed that his Ministry had only been consulted about the consignments in transit. Winnifrith conveyed the latest information from Dundee. Sir George Godber, CMO of the Ministry of Health, then advised that MOsH should be notified that no further corned beef from 6lb tins manufactured at Establishment 1A between 1 January 1963 and mid-March 1964 should be sold to the public, pending further enquiries. This did not apply to smaller tins as there was no evidence that they had been associated with typhoid. And Godber did not think that all canned meat manufactured using unchlorinated cooling water should necessarily be withheld, such as stockpile corned beef which had been part of large consignments, much of which had been consumed without ill-effect.

The Minister for the Navy revealed that all three services had withdrawn corned beef, not only from the Argentine Establishments 25 (implicated in the 1963 outbreaks) and 1A, but also from Uruguay 5, owned by the British Vestey group. In the latter case, Grace found that chlorination had been introduced only recently, and that the water analyses were unreliable. Grace explained by telephone from the USA that he had taken no further action in this case because he knew that no consignments were on the high seas. In view of the need to respond to questions about the 1963 outbreaks and the mission to South America, it was agreed to recall Grace to London as soon as possible.

The meeting accepted Godber's recommendation regarding Establishment 1A, and also agreed that Uruguay 5 supplies produced since 1 January 1963

---

[64] Parry evidence p. 44; 'Evidence to show that the tinned meat in the shop in Aberdeen did not come from the M.A.F.F. stockpile'; J. M. Black to Mr Parselle, 2 June 1964; W. Maclean to Ministry of Agriculture, Fisheries and Food, 4 June 1964, PRO MAF 246/239; M. E. M. Anderson to A. M. Stephen, 2 June 1964, NAS HH 64/228.
[65] S. Lloyd to Secretary of State for Defence, 10 June 1964, NAS HH 64/350.

should be withheld, even though, before that date, there had been no chlorination at that plant. The decision would be defended on the weak grounds
that 'such evidence as there has been linking corned beef with typhoid applied
only to supplies produced recently'.[66] In preparation for announcing the
decisions, representatives of the firms were called to a meeting before Noble
made his statement, in the hope that this would encourage their co-operation.
Peter Humphreys-Davies, the MAFF Deputy Secretary, also telephoned the
Treasury warning that the announcement might 'put the Exchequer at risk of
about £2 million'. The official who followed up the call, however, recorded
that the withdrawal would probably be temporary and compensation issues
were unlikely to arise.[67] Later, Humphreys-Davies recorded that at the meeting
with the trade, Godber gave a 'masterly exposition . . . of the reasoning behind
the Government decision', who 'sorrowfully accepted it'. The representatives
were assured that the ministries would use their best endeavours to 'see that
the deservedly high reputations' of the firms 'did not suffer from the shortcomings, now rectified, of two particular plants'. No questions were raised
about compensation.[68] The Treasury's view was that compensation could not
be justified for 'normal insurable trade risks'. The food could not be condemned
as unfit and there were no powers to insist on it being removed from the
market. The operation depended on goodwill, and as the firms withdrew their
stock voluntarily, they had no viable claim against the Crown.[69]

When Noble made his statement, he remarked that 'the cause of this
outbreak has not been finally established', but announced that ex-government
corned beef was certainly not involved. However, cans produced by an
establishment that had not been using chlorinated water had been present in
the shop, and this stock was to be withdrawn from circulation. Furthermore,
as a precautionary measure, stock from another plant that had not been using
chlorinated water would be withdrawn. Because of the remaining uncer-
tainties, Noble continued, the government had decided to hold an enquiry
under an independent chairman, to 'discover the cause of the outbreak'.[70]

Noble faced a series of questions, among the speakers being William Ross
and George Brown, the Labour Party's deputy leader. They pressed Noble as
to why it had taken twelve days to decide on the withdrawal exercise, to which
Noble responded that this time was needed to trace the source of the infection.
Ross also attempted to keep the 'ex-government stock' issue alive, observing
that, as Johnson had feared, MacQueen had repeated his assertions, only half

[66] 'Note of a meeting held on Tuesday, 2nd June, 1964', PRO MAF 282/87.

[67] G. O. Lace to Mr Bird, 3 June 1964, PRO MAF 282/87; I. P. Bancroft to Mr Bretherton,
2 June 1964, PRO T 227/1655.

[68] P. Humphreys-Davies to R. F. Bretherton, 2 June 1964, PRO MAF 282/87.

[69] D. R. Collison to The Treasury Solicitor, 4 June 1964; C. F. Brooke to D. R. Collison,
9 June 1964, PRO T 227/1655; P. Humphreys-Davies to Secretary, 10 June 1964, PRO
MAF 246/250.

[70] PD(C), vol. 695, cols 925–7 (2 June 1964).

an hour before Noble gave his statement. Noble assured Ross, however, that there was no evidence of the involvement of ex-government stock. Hector Hughes and others asked questions about the scope and membership of the enquiry, the need for advice on personal hygiene, and travel and other restrictions.[71] During the afternoon of 2 June, Godber and Smith of the Ministry of Health and SHHD respectively sent letters to MOsH. They gave details of the 1963 outbreaks, explained the theory of how contaminated cooling water could enter cans, and mentioned the problem at Establishment 1A. The MOsH were asked to check stores and feeding establishments for 6lb tins marked 'Industria Argentina Estab. 1A' processed between 1 January 1963 and 9 March 1964, and to advise withdrawal. Withdrawal of 'Uruguay Estab. 5' produced during the same period was also advised as an 'additional precautionary measure' because of a chlorination problem.[72]

The co-operation of the trade achieved on 2 June proved less complete than initially assumed. At a meeting with Ministry of Health officials the following morning, they accused the government of selecting 1 January 1963 arbitrarily in relation to Uruguay 5, to protect massive stockpile stocks of canned beef produced using unchlorinated water. In addition, they would not agree to a plan to publicise the code numbers of the suspect cans until they were sent upstairs for a meeting with the Minister.[73] Further letters were then sent to MOsH setting out the codes by which the suspect cans could be identified.[74] The same information was given to the press. The press statement also including an account of the meeting between the Minister and the trade representatives, who were said to remain 'quite unconvinced' that corned beef was responsible for the outbreak. Nevertheless, 'without prejudice to the views expressed', they were co-operating. The Minister agreed that the cause of the outbreak had not been finally established but observed that 'one could certainly not rule out' the possibility that the organism had been in the corned beef.[75] During the afternoon, MAFF officials attempted to assess the likely impact on meat prices, which had become a sensitive political issue over recent weeks. However, since corned beef imports amounted to only 50 thousand tons compared to total supplies of meat and offal amounting to 2.6 million tons, they advised that 'consumer resistance' to corned beef would have only a marginal effect.[76]

---

[71] Ibid., cols 927–32.

[72] G. E. Godber to Medical Officers of Health in England and Wales, 2 June 1964, PRO MH 148/356; J. Smith to Medical Officers of Health and Senior Administrative Medical Officers, 2 June 1964, NAS HH 58/160.

[73] G. O. Lace, 'Corned beef', 3 June 1964, PRO MAF 282/87.

[74] G. E. Godber, 3 June 1964, PRO MH 148/356; J. Smith to Medical Officers of Health and Senior Administrative Medical Officers, 3 June 1964, NAS HH 58/160.

[75] Ministry of Health, 'Corned beef: official statement', 3 June 1964, PRO MH 148/354.

[76] C. J. Brown to Mr Kirk, 5 June 1964, PRO MAF 246/239.

Limiting the damage: taking further action and defending past decisions

Having launched the withdrawal of Argentine 1A and Uruguay 5 corned beef, the precautionary withdrawal of further suspect stock became necessary over the next few weeks. The decision making shifted to London, but the SHHD continued to deal with issues connected with Aberdeen. SHHD officials monitored the hospital situation, and prepared daily lists of the number of cases and suspect cases in and outside the city.[77] Brotherston also issued a letter on 8 June encouraging MOsH to use the outbreak as an opportunity to reinforce 'normal teaching on all aspects of safe food handling'. He urged them to direct their advice to all food handlers, and reminded them of the HMSO publication *Clean Catering*, and other publicity material.[78] SHHD also prepared memoranda in response to enquiries from foreign health administrations,[79] and for the WHO and Council of Europe.[80] They also communicated with six embassies in connection with the contacts of a woman who became infected in Aberdeen but who helped to prepare sandwiches for the delegates attending an international conference in Edinburgh.[81]

From before the end of May, SHHD officials answered numerous queries about whether various events should go ahead or be cancelled. These included, for example, the Forestry Commissioners' visit to Aboyne, a conference at the Torry Research Station in Aberdeen, and the Highland Show in Edinburgh, all at the end of June, and a Scout jamboree in Blair Atholl starting on 18 July.[82] They advised postponement of the first two events, but the Highland Show was thought to pose no risk so long as caterers from Aberdeen were excluded, and the jamboree could go ahead as long as scouts from Aberdeen did not take part.[83] Following discussion with the Scottish Tourist Board, James Stodart, Under-secretary of State, also became involved in considering opportunities for ministers to provide reassurance to the public.[84]

---

[77] There are numerous papers concerning these activities in NAS HH 58/160 and NAS HH 61/1073.

[78] J. Brotherston to Medical Officers of Health and Senior Administrative Medical Officers, 8 June 1964, NAS HH 58/160.

[79] Ministry of Health to Scottish Office, 1 June 1964; Scottish Home and Health Department to Han Bolin, Stockholm, 2 June 1964, NAS HH 58/160; D. P. Kennedy to J. Brotherston, 10 June 1964, NAS HH 61/1073.

[80] Howitt to Roffey, 10 June 1964; Maclehose to Roffey, 19 June 1964, NAS HH 61/1073.

[81] Letters from I. N. Sutherland to the Canadian, French, Norwegian, Belgian, American and Finnish embassies, 16 June 1964, NAS HH 61/1073.

[82] M. Roberston to McCabe, 3 June 1964; A. T. F. Ogilve to McCabe, 4 June 1964, NAS HH 58/160; Hogarth to McCabe, 10 June 1964; J. Smith to McCabe 10 June 1964; B. D. Fairgrieve to J. Brotherston, 8 June 1964, NAS HH 61/1073.

[83] Hogarth to McCabe, 10 June 1964; J. Smith to McCabe, 10 June 1964; I. N. Sutherland to CMO, 10 June 1964; J. Brotherston to B. D. Fairgrieve, 11 June 1964, NAS HH 61/1073.

[84] R. E. C. Johnson to Mr Hogarth, 11 June 1964, NAS HH 64/350.

Besides dealing with the withdrawal of corned beef, the London-based ministers and officials, especially at MAFF, also prepared defences of their past decisions. On 2 June, besides the questions following Noble's statement, a written question from the Labour health spokesman Kenneth Robinson to the Minister of Health, Anthony Barber, sought information about previous corned beef-associated outbreaks.[85] This was the first of 102 questions to ministers, related directly or indirectly to the outbreak, answered at question time or in writing between 2 June and 1 July. Of these, forty-three, twenty-four and eighteen, were addressed to Noble, Barber, and Christopher Soames, Minister of Agriculture, respectively. Five were addressed to the Prime Minister, and five to other ministers.[86] The early questions covered supplies of chloramphenicol and TAB vaccine, use of the media by the Scottish Office, arrangements for the turnover of the corned beef stockpile, travel restrictions and hygiene precautions, and the committee of enquiry.[87] Questions concerning the stockpile were most numerous (seventeen), while the enquiry, compensation, past outbreaks and imported food safety were the next most popular subjects. Questions about the provision of free toilet facilities were also stimulated by the outbreak, both within and outside of Parliament.[88] Twenty-nine MPs asked questions, twenty of whom belonged to the Labour Party. Fourteen represented English, and fifteen represented Scottish constituencies, among these being two of Aberdeen's local MPs, Patrick Wolridge Gordon, Conservative member for East Aberdeenshire, and Hector Hughes, Labour representative for Aberdeen North. Hughes was the most prolific questioner, asking thirty-six questions. Twenty-one MPs asked one or two questions. Hughes asked seven of the fifteen questions concerning the enquiry and nine of the ten concerning compensation.[89]

The question of compensation for Aberdeen's businesses had also been raised privately by Lady Tweedsmuir, Conservative MP for South Aberdeen, and Under-secretary for Health at the Scottish Office. On 5 June she wrote to the Prime Minister, mentioning an estimated £7m business losses. She claimed that the 'whole of Aberdeen' was asking about compensation, and suggested that there was a strong case in view of the compensation paid for floods and such disasters. She further advised: 'The handling and public presentation of this problem is of supreme importance, as opinion naturally is very sensitive.' But across the top of the letter was written: 'The Secretary of State for Scotland has spoken to Lady Tweedsmuir about this unorthodox approach by a member of H.M.G. [Her Majesty's Government] and I understand that Lady T will ask

[85] *PD(C)*, vol. 695, cols *149–50* (2 June 1964).
[86] Ibid., vols 695–7.
[87] Ibid., vol. 695, cols *170, 175* (3 June 1964), *205–6* (4 June 1964), *217–18* (5 June 1964).
[88] 'Shock campaign urged by hygiene official/Aberdeen as a warning', *Daily Telegraph*, 15 June 1964, p. 19a.
[89] *PD(C)*, 1964, vols 695–7.

to withdraw the letter.'[90] On 8 June, however, several newspapers reported her visit to Aberdeen under headlines such as 'Lady Tweedsmuir asks for compensation'.[91] After this, she was contrite, apologising to the Prime Minister,[92] but a few days later she wrote to the Chancellor urging 'some form of financial contribution' for those who had suffered during the outbreak.[93]

It was left to Hughes to pursue the issue publicly, but he received little encouragement from ministers.[94] On 17 June Noble admitted that he had received letters about the plight of the tourist industry, but stated that he had no powers to provide compensation.[95] The same day the Chief Secretary to the Treasury chaired a meeting attended by Noble, Deedes, junior ministers from MAFF and the Ministry of Health, and officials. Noble thought that demands for compensation could harden if problems in 'the arrangements for import and distribution of meat' were to become widely known – an allusion to the circumstances in which the Argentine 1A corned beef had entered circulation. The Chief Secretary, however, stated that there was no precedent for compensation for loss of profit except for farmland damaged by flooding, and payments to hotel keepers or other businesses would be a 'very dangerous breach' in established principles. In Croydon, damages were awarded against the local authority, which was proved negligent, but the question of whether negligence arose in the Aberdeen outbreak was not yet clear. The Ministry of Health's view was that the responsibility for fitness of food rested upon traders. Inspectors could not have 'complete oversight' and it would be 'dangerous' if the government accepted responsibility. MAFF's spokesman stated that the certificate provided by the country of origin should mean that the British hygiene requirements were met, but admitted that the regulations made no specific reference to cooling water. It was concluded that government statements should avoid raising hopes of compensation, and that the matter would have to await the report of the enquiry.[96] This line was transmitted to the Prime Minister,[97] and was consistently adhered to, although he had earlier been sympathetic towards calls for compensation.[98] Some of Aberdeen's business owners were very disappointed when Noble told Hughes that he did not intend to acquire powers to compensate them, but others accepted the

---

[90] Lady Tweedsmuir to Prime Minister, 5 June 1964, PRO PREM 11/5073.

[91] 'Lady Tweedsmuir asks for compensation', *Glasgow Herald*, 8 June 1964, p. 1a. See also: 'Hoteliers should get compensation, says Lady Tweedsmuir', *P&J*, 8 June 1964, p. 4d, and 'Typhoid jabs for Services', *Daily Telegraph*, 8 June 1964, p. 1a.

[92] Priscilla to Alex, 9 June 1964, PRO PREM 11/5073.

[93] Lady Tweedsmuir to Reginald Maudling, 16 June 1964, PRO T 227/1655.

[94] *PD(C)*, vol. 696, cols *130–1, 133–4, 148–9* (15 June 1964).

[95] *PD(C)*, vol. 696, cols *176–7* (17 June 1964).

[96] 'Note of a meeting held at the Treasury on 17th June 1964', PRO T 227/1656.

[97] T. A. B. C. to Prime Minister, 19 June 1964, PRO PREM 11/5073.

[98] Alec Douglas-Hume to Lady Tweedsmuir, 11 June 1964; M. Reid to W. Baird, 12 June 1964, PRO PREM 11/5073. *PD(C)*, vol. 697, col. *227* (23 June 1964).

position.[99] The Prime Minister at least fulfilled a promise to Noble to emphasise, in answer to a parliamentary question, that holiday cancellations were
unnecessary.[100]

Many responses to questions about, for example, the numbers of previous
outbreaks and victims were straightforward and prepared solely by officials.
Other questions, and the information released during parliamentary statements, were discussed at meetings between ministers and officials, and drew
upon successive draft narratives of actions taken during and since 1963. The
explanation of why some Establishment IA stock had been left in circulation
was particularly difficult.

The formulation of a line on the March 1964 decisions began after
the apparent discrepancies in the comments made at the meeting of ministers
and officials on 2 June. Through a conversation with Godber, Winnifrith
established that when Bird had consulted Ross by telephone, the discussion
had concentrated upon the fate of the stock in transit rather than that in
circulation. But Godber admitted that Bird had raised the latter question, and
Ross, who was under the impression that the volume of produce involved was
small, gave the opinion that no action was necessary. Winnifrith hoped this
would provide some comfort for Bird, and expressed surprise that Ross did not
enquire as to the amount of corned beef involved.[101] This point was not dwelt
upon, however, on 4 June, when Soames and his deputies and officials discussed
the sequence of events since 1963. However, there was another way of shifting
responsibility for the decision to leave Establishment 1A stock in circulation
on to the Ministry of Health. It was pointed out that in 1963 they had insisted
that withdrawal of Establishment 25 stock need only apply to post-30 May
1962 production. This was the earliest date of production associated with
the typhoid outbreaks in England, and coincided with an outbreak near the
meat plant. The decision was taken even though, as MAFF had emphasised,
chlorinated water had never been used at Establishment 25. This established
a principle of only calling in stock produced at the time of outbreaks in the
vicinity of meat plants using unsatisfactory water, making action against
Establishment 1A stock more difficult to justify. But having reached this point,
the Minister summed up with forward-looking conclusions: the next step
would be to draw up criteria to be used in future to judge whether canned meat
could be imported.[102]

MAFF officials swiftly prepared a draft statement addressing the question
'Why was earlier action not taken against the products of the two plants which

---

[99] *PD(C)*, vol. 697, cols 68–9 (24 June 1964); G. Gardner, 'Compensation blow to hotels',
P&J, 25 June 1964, p. 1a.
[100] M. Reid to W. Baird, 12 June 1964, PRO PREM 11/5073; *PD(C)*, vol. 697, cols *227–8*
(23 June 1964).
[101] A. J. D. Winnifrith to Mr Hensley, 3 June 1964, PRO MAF 282/87.
[102] M. D. M. Franklin, 4 June 1964, PRO MAF 282/87.

were failing to chlorinate?', providing an answer along the lines agreed at the 4 June meeting – that there was no evidence of typhoid outbreaks in the vicinity of the plants. The subsequent decision to withdraw stock was presented as precautionary and temporary, 'pending the results of the enquiry'.[103] The statement was discussed and approved at the first meeting of the co-ordinating group of ministers chaired by Selwyn Lloyd, which met in Lloyd's rooms at the House of Commons during the evening. Noble, Soames and Barber were present, along with Deedes, and an Under-secretary of State for Defence.[104] The statement was not to be issued, but would be used by staff when faced with questions from the press.[105] The question it addressed was the one that most worried ministers. Even after the statement was approved, Soames expressed doubts about what 'no record of any typhoid outbreaks' meant, and checked with Grace that this claim could be sustained.[106] To ensure a co-ordinated approach and prepare for possible difficulties over the following weekend, it was decided that Deedes would call together the public relations officers of MAFF, the Ministry of Health and the Scottish Office, and that guidance would be issued to the press officers. Noble's assistant private secretary would act as a central point of contact between ministers and would be informed of their movements. These arrangements were designed to pre-empt the kind of problems of the previous weekend, when ministers had been taken by surprise by several new stories.

Besides considering the arrangements for the Milne Committee, the ministers decided that Noble would make a further statement, when an opportunity would be taken to correct an earlier error.[107] He had said on 2 June that the shop in Aberdeen had been open for eight weeks rather than eight months, the error arising from a report by Maclean of Perfect, Lambert & Co. This had been the cause of disquiet, in case the claim that ex-government stock had never been in the shop could not be sustained.[108] The meeting also discussed the widespread demands for TAB inoculation, and it was agreed that Godber and Brotherston would issue a joint press statement on the matter, which was also circulated to MOsH.[109] Noble and Barber were also asked to

---

[103] 'Draft press statement', 4 June 1964, PRO MAF 282/87.

[104] 'Note of conclusions reached at a meeting of Ministers on 4th June', PRO PREM 11/5073.

[105] M. D. M. Franklin to Mr Hensley, 4 June 1964, PRO MAF 282/87.

[106] Ibid.

[107] 'Note of conclusions reached at a meeting of Ministers on 4th June', PRO PREM 11/5073.

[108] A. J. D. Winnifrith to R. E. C. Johnson, 4 June 1964; R. E. C. Johnson to Mr Hogarth, 5 June 1964, PRO HH 64/350.

[109] Note of conclusions reached at a meeting of ministers on 4 June, PRO PREM 11/5073; G. E. Godber to Medical Officers of Health in England and Wales, 8 June 1964, NAS HH 61/1073; J. Brotherston to Medical Officers of Health and Senior Administrative Medical Officers, 8 June 1964, NAS HH 58/160.

consult with their experts on the question of when and in what circumstances it might be necessary to isolate Aberdeen, and Noble was asked to investigate what action would be needed to make this possible. After consulting lawyers, officials advised that it would be difficult to justify the use of existing powers to create a *cordon sanitaire*, and it would be preferable 'to take specific powers' by 'putting through legislation very quickly'. However, they warned that this would be possible only 'if the extent of the emergency were such as to make such extreme action acceptable to public opinion'.[110] Within a few days it was obvious that such action would not be necessary.

The investigation of past events continued, and by 5 June, MAFF officials had prepared a list of dates and actions pertaining to Argentine Establishment 25.[111] Lace then constructed a seven-page draft narrative that also covered the decision making regarding Argentine 1A and Uruguay 5. This sought to vindicate MAFF by emphasising that it acted consistently upon Ministry of Health guidance. The only exception was that during 1963 MAFF put a stop on all stockpile corned beef produced using unchlorinated cooling water, although the Ministry of Health advised that action was necessary only against material also subject to withdrawal from commercial distribution.[112] A second draft explicitly claimed that MAFF's action in connection with Establishment 25 had been 'entirely correct'.[113] These documents clarified how the armed services came to take early action against Argentine 1A corned beef. On 13 March the War Office requested MAFF's advice on tenders for supplies from three plants, including Argentine 1A. In the light of the information given by MAFF, the War Office decided not to place orders with 1A, and then, in view of the Aberdeen outbreak, recalled existing stocks of 1A canned meat. The withdrawal order also applied to Uruguay 5 produce[114] (the problems with which the War Office learned from Grace on 29 April[115]). It was because the Navy's action was made public[116] that it became necessary to remove both types of corned beef from general circulation, even though only 1A produce was implicated in Aberdeen.[117]

Precautions taken by the armed forces were the subject of discussion on 8 June at another meeting chaired by Soames attended by eight politicians and fourteen officials. In this case, the matter of contention was the decision to give TAB booster inoculations to service personnel, which had been

---

110 J. Hogarth, 5 June 1964, NAS HH 58/160.
111 'Events relating to Establishment 25', 5 June 1964, PRO MAF 282/87.
112 'Corned beef and typhoid fever' (document 79), PRO MAF 282/87.
113 'Corned beef and typhoid fever' (document 108A), PRO MAF 282/87.
114 Ibid.
115 'Corned beef and typhoid fever' (document 133), PRO MAF 282/87.
116 'Withdrawal of corned beef by the Ministry of Defence', 8 June 1964; Margaret Pearson to Mr Bird, 8 June 1964, PRO MAF 282/86.
117 'Corned beef and typhoid fever' (document 108A), PRO MAF 282/87.

publicised in the *Daily Telegraph*.[118] The forces' representative explained that the normal routine was to give inoculations every three years, but that this had been reduced to one year, as was usual when there was a risk of typhoid. Godber stated that he would have advised against this, because it was at variance with the statement that he and Brotherston had issued. The inconsistency, it was decided, would have to be answered, if necessary, in terms of different circumstances applying to service personnel.[119] Lloyd subsequently sent a sharp note to the Secretary of State for Defence, which was circulated to the other ministers. He stressed the importance of the action taken by the civilian authorities and the services being in step, and asked him to refrain from taking any action without consultation.[120]

How the decision was made to leave Establishment 1A stock in circulation was again discussed. It was important for ministers to finalise an agreed version of events, because the essential facts of what happened following Graces's findings were now in the public domain. A front-page *Sunday Times* article used the headline 'Ministry knew of corned beef risk'.[121] Barber explained that Ross had assumed that Grace would have told him had there been evidence of typhoid in the vicinity of Establishment 1A. Since no such information was forthcoming, Ross felt there was no need to withdraw stocks in circulation. Summing up, Barber proposed that the government should repeat that it was not certain corned beef was the source of the outbreak, and even if it was, it was not certain the fault lay in unchlorinated water. Grace, who had returned from America, and Godber, supported this position, and Grace explained that the decision to stop shipments *en route* 'represented a means . . . of putting pressure on supplying countries to improve their hygiene standards'.[122]

A conversation between Noble and Soames indicates the difficulties ministers experienced in formulating a convincing and politically acceptable version of events, and also the role Deedes attempted to play in this connection. Soames suggested to Noble that, if pressed as to why produce of the suspect plants was left in circulation, they could say that 'the experts on whom the Government relies to take these decisions did not consider that the situation warranted it'. However, Noble told Soames that Barber had discussed the matter with Deedes, who felt that they should avoid giving any impression that the government was 'shielding behind "some hapless official"'.[123] Nevertheless, when under pressure in the House of Commons, Noble seemed to find it impossible to avoid adopting this line. In a statement on 8 June he initially outlined the numbers of typhoid patients, the precautions to avoid spread,

<hr>

[118] 'Typhoid jabs for Services', *Daily Telegraph*, 8 June 1964, p. 1a.

[119] 'Note of a meeting held at 11.30 am on 8th June, 1964', PRO MAF 282/87.

[120] S. Lloyd to Secretary of State for Defence', 10 June 1964, NAS HH 64/350.

[121] Stephen Fry, 'Ministry knew of corned beef risk', *Sunday Times*, 7 June 1964, p. 1f.

[122] 'Note of a meeting held at 11.30 am on 8th June, 1964', PRO MAF 282/87.

[123] A.M.T., 'Note for the record', 8 June 1964, NAS HH 64/350.

help given to MacQueen, and policy on inoculation. He also revealed the membership and terms of reference of the official enquiry. In response to a question from George Brown, which asserted that Noble or Barber were advised months ago to withdraw the corned beef responsible for the outbreak, Noble then explained further about the decisions of March 1964. He remarked that 'The withdrawal of vast quantities of food did not seem wise at the time' and, after further questioning, that 'In our view, and in the view of our medical advisers, the risk was not sufficient to justify a withdrawal of the meat already in the country'. As members rose to ask further questions, the speaker called the house to order, remarking 'We cannot debate this matter without a Question before the House', and, to a call of 'Very unsatisfactory', he moved on to other business.[124]

The same day, ministers gave twenty-three written answers to questions stimulated by the outbreak, the highest number answered on a single day. Ten were addressed to Barber, five to Noble, and seven to Soames.[125] Six of the latter were concerned with the stockpile. There was, by this time, no attempt to repeat the allegation that ex-government corned beef was involved in the outbreak, although, after Noble's 2 June statement, the *Scottish Daily Mail* had attempted to keep the interest alive with the headline: 'Noble: No hard evidence on beef/MacQueen: I stick to my guns.'[126] But interest in the stockpile had been aroused and in response to probing, Soames gave details of the origin, monitoring and disposal of the corned beef, but refused to reveal the quantity in storage and its location, or details regarding other foods, citing reasons of national security.[127]

Noble was certain that there would be further questions about the action taken in March and with a view to improving his response, sought from officials information on the quantity of corned beef imported since the war so that he could emphasise what a tiny proportion had been contaminated.[128] He was advised not to quote precise figures, however, but simply to refer to the few cases of typhoid associated with corned beef in comparison with the millions of tons eaten over many years.[129] But by this time the task of explaining why some 1A corned beef had been left in circulation had fallen to Barber. Noble's role as spokesman was fading, as was the involvement of the Scottish Office in decision making. The main decisions were now about whether or not to withdraw further stocks of canned meat, matters which were largely the concern of MAFF and the Ministry of Health, due to their roles in connection

---

[124] *PD(C)*, vol. 696, cols *43–9* (8 June 1964).

[125] Ibid., vol. 696, cols *15–20, 35–6* (8 June 1964).

[126] J. Haines and I. Ramsay, 'Noble: No hard evidence on beef/MacQueen: I stick to my guns', *Scottish Daily Mail*, 3 June 1964, p. 1a.

[127] *PD(C)*, vol. 696, cols *21–3* (8 June 1964).

[128] W. Baird to M. D. M. Franklin, 9 June 1964, NAS HH 64/350.

[129] M. D. M. Franklin to W. Baird, 11 June 1964, NAS HH 64/350.

with the Imported Foods Regulations. Stodart approved of the Scottish Office withdrawing from the limelight, recording on 11 June that as far as he could see the Scottish Office's 'sole responsibility has been in dealing with the epidemic' and that the 'other Ministers should have been carrying the can about import releases etc'.[130]

The explanation and justification of the action taken in March was again the subject of a ministers' meeting on 9 June, which asked the officials to prepare a text for approval at a further meeting the following day.[131] The latter meeting, which was not attended by any Scottish Office representative, approved the document, which Barber would use in his speech during a debate on the hospital service on 11 June. But there was further urgent business, because the meeting learned that J. Sainsbury Ltd, the grocer, had withdrawn Establishment 1A canned tongue on the advice of their experts. It had not been realised that this product was in circulation, and Barber was asked to see the importers with a view to arranging its withdrawal. It was also revealed that the MOH for Hull had discovered human intestinal organisms within a 12oz can, but Godber assured the ministers that there had been no evidence of typhoid infection arising from small cans. In any case, there was no risk of large-scale spread arising, as was the case with the large cans used for slicing meat on shop counters.[132]

The ministers were annoyed that it had not been known earlier that Establishment 1A had been canning meat other than corned beef during their 'unchlorinated' period, since there had been several opportunities for the importers to tell officials or ministers about the matter. Barber met representatives of the firms on 11 June,[133] and later that day it was announced that canned tongue from Argentine 1A and Uruguay 5 would be withdrawn. Godber and Brotherston conveyed the advice to MOsH.[134] Barber mentioned the matter during his contribution to the debate on the hospital service. Barber's statement focused initially on the decisions made in March. His explanation was more detailed than that given by Noble, and he emphasised that he and the other ministers had not been aware of the issue until recently. He explained that the decision had been made on the advice of a principal medical officer, who had taken the view that 'as there was no pointer to any illness arising from the product of this plant and no evidence of any typhoid outbreak in the area in which the plant operated . . . it would not be reasonable to arrange for the withdrawal of such stocks of corned beef from the plant as he knew to be in circulation'. Ministers had not been made aware of these

<hr>

130 J. A. Stodart, Minute, 11 June 1964, NAS HH 64/351.
131 'Note of conclusions reached at a meeting of Ministers on 9th June', NAS HH 64/350.
132 'Note on conclusions reached at a meeting held on June 10th 1964', NAS HH 64/350.
133 Mrs Hauff to Mr Hogarth, 11 June 1964, NAS HH 64/381.
134 G. E. Godber to Medical Officers of Health, 11 June 1964; J. Brotherston to Medical Officers of Health, 11 June 1964, NAS HH 61/1073.

matters until 1 June, and it was not known until that evening that some of the stock in question had been at the Aberdeen shop. Barber also mentioned the decision to withdraw the canned tongue 'for the time being' and, in response to an enquiry as to what this meant, explained that there was no question of condemning the stock, which he thought would be the 'height of folly'. Rather, it would be put into storage until the Milne Committee reported. He acknowledged that the decision of the principal medical officer had been an error, but reiterated that at that time no ill-effects had been associated with the corned beef concerned. Furthermore, cans admitted germs via defects only rarely, and the chance of only disease-causing and no spoilage organisms entering a can was very remote. Had Barber known about the matter he admitted that he would have endorsed the decision, and his CMO was of the same view, but further shipments were denied entry because the enquiries of the MAFF veterinary officer in Argentina had shown the official certificate to be 'inaccurate'. When pressed by William Ross to admit that his department had taken a calculated risk, Barber urged that it was important to 'keep a sense of proportion', adding:

> It is quite impossible to take steps to ensure that 100 per cent. canned food or indeed any other food is not contaminated. . . . Of course, it would be possible to go to inordinate lengths, but the consequence would be that there would be virtually nothing left to eat . . . I am advised that, in fact, canned food in general is less liable to infection than fresh food.[135]

Ross complained that Barber had made 'what is virtually a Government statement at a time when he cannot be properly questioned . . . and without the usual courtesy of a copy of that statement to the other Front Bench'. In response, Barber explained that he merely wished to correct the assumption made by George Brown on 8 June, namely that ministers had been advised in March to withdraw the Establishment 1A stock in circulation. A friendly question invited Barber to agree with the point that prior to 1955 all canned corned beef had been prepared using non-chlorinated water with 'virtually no outbreaks of typhoid on a serious scale'. Assenting to this point, Barber moved on.

MAFF officials continued working on their narrative of action taken since 1963,[136] and Winnifrith sent a much-refined version to Soames on 12 June. He thought it was now suitable to 'go round Whitehall'. He commented that MAFF was '100 per cent covered in what was done to protect the public health of this country by the action taken by Dr Ross'. He admitted, however, that

---

[135] *PD(C)*, vol. 696, cols 755–7 (11 June 1964).
[136] G. O. Lace to Secretary, 9 June 1964; P. Humphreys-Davies to Secretary, 10 June 1964; to J. A. Hauff, 11 June 1964; M. D. M. Franklin to Mr Cann, 11 June 1964, PRO MAF 282/87.

MAFF's action to enforce acceptable standards of hygiene in South American meat plants was 'less impressive' but added that 'Mr Grace's instructions to Mr Claxton [the veterinary attaché in Buenos Aires during 1963] do constitute action to enforce our hygiene standards'.[137]

A further problem

As soon as Soames and his officials settled their stories about the 1963 outbreaks, Argentine 1A and Uruguay 5, they had to turn to unpicking the events surrounding the 'Wapping Dock incident'. Following the reports on 31 May about the dockside pile of rotting Andes-brand corned beef, the veterinary officer of Edinburgh Corporation examined a can of the same brand. In February 1964 he had received a complaint about some odd-tasting Andes corned beef, but bacteriological tests proved negative. However, when the inspector heard about the Wapping incident on television, he obtained further samples from local warehouses for testing.[138] Edinburgh University's bacteriology department reported on 11 June that one of the samples produced a pure culture of the food poisoning organism *Salmonella typhimurium*.[139] This was reported to the SHHD,[140] and the English ministries, and on 12 July Winnifrith informed Soames about the situation. Winnifrith intimated that it also seemed that the official certificate which secured the entry of the Wapping consignment had not been valid, but assured the minister that this was a matter for the port health authority.[141] It was a problem concerning the precise format of the stamp on the cartons containing the cans.[142] An additional complication was that Establishment 1819, from where the cans originated, was not known to MAFF and had not been inspected. Grace had asked the Argentine authorities whether any meat plants, apart from those on his list, were exporting to Britain, but had not been informed about Establishment 1819. It might be, Winnifrith told Soames, that 1819 produce had never been imported directly to Britain, the Wapping consignment having arrived via America. MAFF officials were looking further into the situation.[143]

---

137 A. J. D. Winnifrith to Minister, 12 June 1964, PRO MAF 282/87.

138 J. Norval, 'Corned Beef – Industria Argentina Est. 1819', PRO MH 148/198.

139 J. L. Gilloran to J. H. F. Brotherston, 12 June 1964, PRO MH 148/198.

140 I. N. Sutherland to Mr Stephen, 12 June 1964, NAS HH 61/1073.

141 A. J. D. Winnifrith to Minister, 12 June 1964, PRO MAF 282/87.

142 M. D. M. Franklin, 'Establishment 1819', 17 June 1964, PRO MAF 282/87. As time went on less was made of this problem. A document in February 1966 advised that while the 'certification marks on some of the cartons . . . were not in the approved form', those on the cans were correct and that it was these which 'counted for the purpose of admission into this country'. 'Note for Mr Hensley – Briefing meeting for Minister 16th February 1966', PRO MAF 282/114.

143 A. J. D. Winnifrith to Minister, 12 June 1964, PRO MAF 282/87.

Following the press reports, Ministry of Health officials had carried out an investigation on 1 June. One of their medical officers, Dr Martin, visited the Stepney MOH and learnt that 204 of 2000 cartons, each containing six 6lb tins of corned beef, were condemned in August 1963, but had not been removed for destruction due to labour problems. Some were destroyed in February 1964, but the remainder were not dealt with until after Martin's visit. On 5 June, MAFF asked the Ministry of Health what action, if any, was needed in connection with the 1819 corned beef in circulation, and pointed out the problems with the official certificate. It was not until 12 June, however, after the discovery in Edinburgh, that further consideration was given to these matters.[144]

On 15 June, a meeting took place at the Ministry of Health, attended by Lace of MAFF and a representative of Canbury and Co, the company that had imported the Establishment 1819 Andes corned beef. It emerged that 8000 cases had arrived in four shipments between 21 June and 23 September 1963 (and later a further shipment was identified).[145] The Canbury representative explained that his firm did not normally import canned meat from the USA and was unaware that the certificate was 'phoney'. Besides the material condemned on entry, complaints had been received that the meat was 'sour' and 1000 cases were withdrawn from Edinburgh and Glasgow, although there were no adverse bacteriological findings. The meeting resolved to withdraw the meat, but Canbury did not know its whereabouts, having sold it to Produce Distributor Ltd, who had sold it to two other firms.[146] Since there was little prospect of the material being retrieved through the trade, on 15 June Godber and Brotherston sent a further memorandum to MOsH advising the withdrawal of Establishment 1819 Andes corned beef. The cans were easily identified because they were cylindrical, instead of the usual loaf shape.[147] The veterinary authorities in South America were also warned that Britain would no longer accept canned meat from any establishments that had not been visited and approved by a British inspector.[148]

MOsH immediately began to report the discovery of Establishment 1819 corned beef marketed under other brand names. Some cans were square rather than round, and some were 4lb rather than 6lb cans.[149] Since Ministry of Health officials felt that it was the plant that was primarily under suspicion, they advised, in response to enquiries, that all 1819 corned beef should

[144] 'Corned beef from Argentina Establishment 1819 Diary of Events', PRO MH 148/198.
[145] Ibid.
[146] G. O. Lace to K. Bird, 15 June 1964; Meeting with Canbury & Co, 15 June 1964, J. A. Hauff to Mr Pater, 15 June 1964, PRO MAF 282/87.
[147] J. M. Ross, 'Distribution of "Andes" brand corned beef', 15 June 1964, PRO MH 148/200; G. E. Godber to Medical Officers of Health, 15 June 1964, PRO MH 148/198.
[148] M. D. M. Franklin to Mr Humphreys-Davies, 17 June 1964, PRO MH 148/198.
[149] J. E. P. to CMO, 17 June 1964, PRO MH 148/198.

be held.[150] However, a ministers' meeting at the Lord Privy Seal's office on 16 June, at which MAFF but not Ministry of Health officials were on hand, decreed otherwise. They thought that prior to receiving a report from Argentina about hygiene at the plant, complete withdrawal of 1819 produce might be an 'excessive precaution'.[151] This created an awkward situation for the Ministry of Health. Pending further information, they now advised those enquiring about non-Andes 1819 corned beef to 'put it on one side for the time being'.[152] The Scottish Office was not represented at the meeting but when Stodart saw the minute he was uneasy, recording that 'these *repeated* [emphasis in original] discoveries are creating a very serious situation politically. They give the impression that we are not in control.'[153] By the following day, the scale of the problem had been realised: besides the material arriving via the USA, at least 20,000 cases of Establishment 1819 corned beef had entered Britain direct from Argentina.[154]

In the evening of 17 June, the Minister of Agriculture met senior officials to discuss how to follow up the notice given to the South American veterinary authorities. They decided to inform port health authorities of the situation and to publish a list of approved establishments.[155] On 19 June, the veterinary attaché, who had now visited Establishment 1819, reported that it was efficient in most respects, but that its chlorination techniques were inadequate, and the slaughterhouses at which the meat originated were below standard. A report on these developments also raised questions about whether there was other suspect meat in the stockpile or in commercial circulation, and what should be done about it. Enquiries suggested that one or more plants in Australia had been using unchlorinated cooling water and the situation in New Zealand was under investigation. In view of this a stop had been put on releases of stockpile corned beef from Australia and New Zealand, as well as South America.[156]

On 21 June, an exceptionally well-informed article about Establishment 1819 appeared in the *Sunday Times*. The author, Anthony Cowdy, was aware, for example, of the veterinary attaché's findings, and the newspaper had investigated the fate of produce offloaded at London docks via importers, haulage contractors, wholesalers and shops. The article suggested that the 1819

---

[150] J. M. Ross to Mr Pater, 17 June 1964, PRO MH 148/198; I. N. S. to Deputy CMO, 17 June 1964, NAS 61/1073.

[151] 'Note of a meeting held on 16th June, 1964', PRO MH 148/198.

[152] G. O. Lace to Secretary, 17 June 1964, PRO MAF 282/87.

[153] Hamilton to Baird, 18 June 1964, NAS HH 64/380.

[154] M. D. M. Franklin, 'Establishment 1819', 17 June 1964, PRO MAF 282/87.

[155] M. D. M. Franklin to Mr Humphreys-Davies, 17 June 1964, 'Corned beef supplies from Establishment 1819', 17 June 1964, NAS HH 64/350.

[156] 'Memorandum by the Minister of Agriculture, Fisheries and Food', PRO MH 148/198.

produce might have been traced more rapidly in this way, rather than by relying on the efforts of MOsH in checking on numerous wholesale stores and retail premises.[157] On the following day, ministers agreed that all 1819 canned meat should be withdrawn.[158] Letters to this effect were sent out to MOsH, and a list of recognised South American establishments was issued, barring any further consignments from Establishment 1819 and other plants not on the list.[159] By the end of June 1964, under the supervision of MOsH, stocks of canned meat from Argentine establishments 1A and 1819, and Uruguay 5, had been withdrawn from commercial circulation. On the advice of the CMO, however, no action was taken against the Australian canned meat produced using unchlorinated cooling water in commercial circulation.[160]

Emergency food safety policy making and the management of political risk

As we have seen, at every stage of the events described in the previous three sections of this chapter, actual or potential press publicity and political risk played an important role in prompting or delaying decisions. While politicians had not been involved in decision making prior to early June, senior minister Selwyn Lloyd, the Lord Privy Seal, subsequently played an important role in the political management of the outbreak and its consequences. The meetings over which he presided facilitated decision making and the formulation of agreed lines of explanation and action. In the emergency situation, they overcame problems of interdepartmental and inter-professional tensions, which, as we will see in Chapter 7, seriously complicated action in normal times. However, the political steer provided by Deedes was also influential. Deedes became involved before Lloyd, and attended not only Lloyd's meetings but also, for example, the meeting at the Treasury to discuss compensation. He also met with Noble, John Smith and members of the Scottish Office's information office on 15 June to discuss possible ways of limiting the damage to the Scottish tourist industry.[161] Besides the question to the Prime Minister on 23 June mentioned above, this meeting gave rise to other suggestions. These included the Queen's visit to Aberdeen on 27 June, publicity surrounding the

---

[157] Anthony Cowdy, 'Minister bars more corned beef', *Sunday Times*, 21 June 1964, pp. 1, 3.

[158] 'Note of a meeting held at the Lord Privy Seal's Room on Monday 22nd June', 23 June 1964, NAS HH 64/350.

[159] 'Corned beef from Argentina Establishment 1819 diary of events', PRO MH 148/198.

[160] The resolution of the problem of New Zealand and Australian stockpile corned beef is discussed on pp. 222–3.

[161] J. Smith to J. Brotherston, 16 June 1964, NAS HH 61/1073; W. F. Deedes, *'Dear Bill' W. F. Deedes Reports*, London, 1997, pp. 197–8.

Milne Committee's first meeting in the city, and Sir Billy Butlin's announcement that Aberdonians were again welcome at his holiday camps.[162]

Deedes' role in handling the outbreak was part of the broad responsibilities he had acquired for political management in Sir Alec Douglas-Home's government. Home had succeeded Harold Macmillan as Prime Minister in October 1963 amid a Conservative Party crisis, which included the adultery scandal involving John Profumo. With an election impending within months, the political stakes were high in June 1964. Deedes' memoirs confirm the role he played. He records that, on Sunday, 7 June, he received a phone call at home from Lloyd to say that the Prime Minister had been on to him, worried by the *Sunday Times* 'Ministry knew of corned beef risk' story. During the afternoon, he had further long telephone conversations with the MAFF press office, Soames and Selwyn Lloyd.[163]

Apart from the day-to-day decision making in response to events, the announcement of the official enquiry was the key component of the strategies of officials and ministers, to quieten the uproar of early June. And, at least temporarily, the announcement of the committee helped to lay several issues to rest, including that of compensation. After the meeting at the Treasury on 17 June, officials of each ministry prepared papers dealing with different aspects of the question, and took advice from solicitors. By 20 July the Treasury had prepared a document summarising the legal position, which advised that any claim by victims against the shop, supplier, importer or manufacturer would be unlikely to succeed. In addition, it would probably be impractical to bring action in foreign courts against the manufacturer, or the foreign government responsible for ensuring the validity of official certificates. Persons such as hotel keepers who suffered indirectly were considered 'too far removed from the proximate cause to have any chance of success'. As for the possibility of victims suing the government, local authority or port health authority, 'the *onus* would be on the pursuer to show such gross negligence or neglect of duty that the possibility of direct action . . . seems too remote to merit consideration'. The official who compiled the document noted that by mid-July public and parliamentary interest in the issue had died down, although it might revive once the official enquiry had reported. He envisaged that the document would be circulated to the participants in the 17 June meeting, but a senior colleague commented that since compensation seemed 'a dead issue for the time being' he was 'inclined not to risk reviving it' by circulating the document. Another agreed that it was best to 'sit' on the matter.[164] In this way, the issue rested. We will see in Chapter 7, however, that after the Milne Committee reported,

---

[162] W. M. B. to Secretary of State, 15 June 1964, NAS HH 64/351.

[163] Deedes, *Bill*, pp. 194–6.

[164] C. H. W. Hodges to Mr Harding, 20 July 1964, and annotations dated 21 and 23 July 1964, PRO T 227/1656.

difficulties in the disposal of certain commercial suspect stocks eventually led to bitter exchanges about compensation between the government and a section of the trade. It is to the formation, proceedings, and report of the Milne Committee that we will now turn.

6

The Milne Committee of Enquiry

Introduction

The analysis of an enquiry such as that on the Aberdeen typhoid outbreak, which looked into a wide variety of issues and evidence, is daunting. Ideally, we might aim initially for a comprehensive understanding of how the findings were arrived at, but this approach is compromised by the incompleteness of the records, the impossibility of interviewing some actors, and the size of the task. Over four months, the committee took oral evidence during fourteen days, and received evidence from 104 witnesses, as detailed in Table 6.1.[1] The report is wide-ranging. Seventy-six pages long, it is organised into three parts, thirty-nine chapters, 246 paragraphs and two appendices. An introduction lists fifteen findings, fourteen recommendations and one observation. It is impractical to analyse the production of the report in full detail. However, it is feasible to attempt to understand how the general shape of the report, and some findings and recommendations, came about.

Some idea of the 'shape' of the report may be gained from the Appendix (pp. 310–11), which reproduces the findings and recommendations. Only two findings (xii and xiii) attach explicit praise or criticism to any individual, and both are concerned with MacQueen. According to one, it was due to the 'speed and efficiency' of MacQueen and his staff and their 'close surveillance of all contacts and of sufferers' that the disease was not more widespread. The other was critical: there was a need for 'health education in personal hygiene', but MacQueen's methods were 'not wholly justified'. Censure of MacQueen's media strategy was developed in the penultimate chapter, 'The medical officer of health and the press'.[2]

The committee approved of MacQueen acting as spokesman for the health and welfare department, but argued that the measures instituted, apart from encouraging hand-washing, were unimportant in limiting the outbreak. They declared that 'the extensive and sensational publicity campaign . . . was . . . of

---

[1] Scottish Home and Health Department, *The Aberdeen Typhoid Outbreak*, Edinburgh, 1964 (Milne report), pp. 72–4, and correspondence with witnesses in NAS HH 64/378 and NAS HH 64/380.
[2] Milne, pp. 68–70.

Table 6.1 Evidence to the Milne Committee

Sector of witness	Type of evidence written/ oral	Number of oral witnesses	Venue for oral evidence	Date oral evidence given
Food retailing, manufacturing and management				
Wm Low and Co	W/O	6	Edinburgh	6/7
Robert Lawson and Sons (Dyce) Ltd	W/O	4	Aberdeen	29/7
Armour and Co Ltd (International Packers Ltd)	W/O	12	London	8/9
Liebig's Extract of Meat Co Ltd	W/O	8	London	10/9
Corporation of Argentine Meat Producers (CAP) Ltd	W/O	8	London	28/9
James Barnes Pty Ltd	W			
A. J. Mills & Co Ltd	W			
Perfect, Lambert & Co	W/O	2	London	22/7
Central government				
Scottish Home and Health Department	W/O	6	Edinburgh London	7–8/7 9/9
Ministry of Agriculture, Fisheries and Food	W/O	8	London	22/7
Ministry of Health	W/O	4	London	23/7, 9/9
Local health authorities				
Aberdeen Corporation	W/O	14	Aberdeen	29/7, 14/9
North-Eastern Regional Hospital Board	W/O	4	Aberdeen	23/6, 15/9
Medical officers of health from:				
Bedford, Harlow, Pickering, Bedfordshire	W/O	4	London Edinburgh	29/6, 7/7, 14/7
Microbiologists and other expert witnesses:				
Public Health Laboratory Service	W/O	4	London	14/7, 22/7
7 Members of staff of the Fruit and Vegetable Canning and Quick Freezing Research Association, Metal Box Company, University of Strathclyde, Edinburgh University, Glasgow University, Edinburgh Corporation, World Health Organisation	W/O	5	London Edinburgh	29/6, 8/7, 14/7

continued

Table 6.1 continued

Sector of witness	Type of evidence written/ oral	Number of oral witnesses	Venue for oral evidence	Date oral evidence given
A Fellow of the Royal Institute of Chemistry	W			
Miscellaneous written and oral evidence				
3 residents of Aberdeen and Stonehaven	W			
Aberdeen Branch of the Scottish Housewives' Association	W			
A general practitioner from Aberdeen	O	1	Aberdeen	15/9
An Aberdeen businessman	W/O	1	Aberdeen	15/9
Anglers' Co-operative Association	W			
Department of Natural Philosophy, Glasgow University	W			
Government of Paraguay	W			

little help in containing the spread of the disease'. The closures of schools and other premises had repercussions beyond Aberdeen, even internationally, giving the outbreak 'the status of a national disaster'. The committee thought that press statements rather than conferences should have been employed.[3] MOsH, the report continued, should 'have strict regard to the possible effect' of anything they said to the press. If 'conscientious attention' were given to this precept, 'the temptation to make statements, the possible effect of which may be harmful far beyond the area affected by the outbreak, should be more easily resisted'. The implication was that MacQueen had unwisely spoken too freely.

Chapters covering action at the shop, and liaison between the health and welfare department and other sections of the health service, included additional criticisms. The report hinted that MacQueen should have closed the shop immediately for cleaning and implied that consultation with the regional bacteriologist (Dr Brodie) would have improved his judgement. Later comments suggested that the initial inappropriate contact sampling procedures

[3] This issue had previously been discussed in Ministry of Health and Scottish Home and Health Department, *Memorandum on the Control of Outbreaks of Smallpox*, London, HMSO, 1964, pp. 12–13.

could have been avoided, had liaison between MacQueen and Brodie began earlier.[4]

MacQueen's dealings with the hospital authorities were also criticised. According to the evidence of Dr Beddard, the senior administrative medical officer of the North-Eastern Regional Hospital Board, making beds available would have been easier 'had it been possible for him to discuss the trend of the outbreak in the early days . . . with Dr. MacQueen'. As for the notification of GPs about the outbreak, the report repeated MacQueen's explanation that he had prepared a letter when the news broke in the press, but commented that it would have been better for his relationships with the GPs if they had not learned of the outbreak from the media.[5]

In contrast with the criticisms of MacQueen, criticisms of the London ministries, the Scottish Office, the manufacturer of the canned meat, and the shop, were less visible and carefully qualified. It is how this overall 'shape' or balance of the report was arrived at which we consider in this chapter. We will begin with an account of the appointment of the committee, the formulation of the terms of reference, and the committee's procedures. We will then consider the evidence provided by the ministries, the actors involved in Aberdeen and the commercial firms, and the publication and reception of the report. In conclusion, we will reflect upon the shaping of the report, and will finally briefly cover the implementation of the recommendations, other than those discussed in chapters 7 to 9.

Terms of reference, membership and procedure

We saw in Chapter 5 that after MacQueen declared that ex-stockpile corned beef might have caused the outbreak, the London-based officials met and produced a memorandum proposing a committee of enquiry. The officials intended that this would defuse controversy, their main concern being confirmation that MacQueen was mistaken.[6] A meeting of ministers and officials on 1 June agreed to the appointment of a committee by the Secretary of State for Scotland, Michael Noble.[7] Noble did not want the enquiry to begin until the pressure had eased in Aberdeen, but it was politically desirable to announce the committee quickly.[8] Peter Humphreys Davies, Deputy Secretary at MAFF,

---

[4] Milne pp. 56–8, 62.

[5] Ibid., pp. 61–2.

[6] See pp. 135–6.

[7] 'Typhoid outbreak in Aberdeen memorandum by officials', 31 May 1964, PRO MAF 282/87.

[8] Ministry of Agriculture, Fisheries and Food, 'Note of meeting on the Aberdeen typhoid outbreak and corned beef supplies', 1 June 1964, PRO MAF 246/239.

minuted that the enquiry would look at 'the causes and handling of the Aberdeen epidemic and see what went wrong, and whether there were any gaps in the investigation', adding that it would not 'range over the whole field of food supply, Government stockpile, and so on'.[9] MAFF was wary of opening the management of the stockpile to public scrutiny. The *Scottish Daily Express* had claimed that the stockpile cost the taxpayer £25 million a year,[10] and suggestions were made elsewhere that MAFF had taken advantage of high prices to market surplus stock that was 'perilously near the end of its period of fitness for human consumption'.[11] To exclude such matters, the terms of reference would be 'drawn tightly'.[12]

On 2 June, a further meeting agreed that the inquiry should be restricted to 'the narrow issue of the causes' of the outbreak and what the policy implications would be for the government.[13] Proposals for the terms of reference and membership were left to officials. Alex. M. Stephen, a long-serving Principal Secretary in the SHHD who had worked on food and drugs and hospital administration, and who had already been involved in the typhoid outbreak, was appointed secretary.[14] In line with concerns about controlling the scope of the enquiry, an initial suggestion of appointing a senior Scottish lawyer as chairman was dropped in favour of former civil servant Sir David Milne, who was named on 4 June. Milne had joined the Scottish Office in 1921, and from 1942 had been Permanent Under-secretary of State for Scotland until his retirement in 1959.[15]

Noble's private secretary notified him about the progress with formulating the terms of reference on 4 June. R. E. C. Johnson, Secretary of the SHHD, and Sir John Winnifrith, Permanent Secretary at MAFF, preferred 'To investigate the cause of the primary infection in the recent outbreak of typhoid fever in Aberdeen and the means by which it was disseminated, and to report'. This was supposed to indicate a restricted remit. However, Sir Bruce Fraser, Permanent Secretary at the Ministry of Health, favoured an enquiry into 'the whole conduct of the epidemic'.[16]

Fraser told his minister that the Winnifrith/Johnson proposal would confine the enquiry to scientific aspects, while his option, 'To investigate

---

[9] P. Humphreys-Davies to Mr Franklin, 1 June 1964, NAS HH 64/379.

[10] George Gardiner, 'Atom meat storm is blowing up', *Scottish Daily Express*, 30 May 1964, p. 1b.

[11] Public health correspondent, 'Typhoid and corned beef: the inspection problem', *Municipal Journal*, 5 June 1964, p. 1789.

[12] P. Humphreys-Davies to Mr Franklin, 1 June 1964, NAS HH 64/379.

[13] 'Note of a meeting held on Tuesday, 2nd June, 1964', PRO MAF 282/87.

[14] Alex. Stephen, interview, 17 June 1999, Melrose, ATO/18; R. E. C. Johnson to A. M. Stephen, 3 June 1964, NAS HH 64/379.

[15] P. Humphreys-Davies to Mr Franklin, 1 June 1964, NAS HH 64/379; PD(C), vol. 695, col. 206 (4 June 1964); *Who Was Who 1971–1980*, (London, 1981), p. 546.

[16] Secretary of State, 4 June 1964, NAS HH 64/379.

the circumstances of the recent outbreak of typhoid fever in Aberdeen, and to report',[17] would:

> enable the Committee to probe also into the way the outbreak was handled by the Public Health Services and the Departments concerned, and *might* enable them to range also into the general methods (i.e. not confined to Aberdeen) adopted by the Government and Local Authorities to safeguard public health against infected imports.[18]

Fraser argued that it would be difficult to 'get away with an enquiry so narrow that the actual handling of the Aberdeen outbreak was outwith its scope'. The matter was 'quasi political' and would have to be decided by ministers, but he favoured a broad remit, adding that 'behind the scenes' the committee could be persuaded to avoid sensitive areas.[19]

The divergence probably arose from different perceptions within each ministry about the extent to which it was desirable to investigate matters that were their own responsibility. Fraser was happy for the committee to scrutinise issues that were primarily the concerns of MAFF and the Scottish Office, or the local authority. But the Winnifrith/Johnson version was accepted, by a meeting of ministers, which agreed that the priority was to report on the cause of the outbreak. The findings would determine whether there was any need for a wider enquiry.[20]

As for the membership beyond the chairman, medical experts were discussed by Sir John Brotherston, CMO of the SHHD and Sir George Godber, CMO of the Ministry of Health.[21] They agreed that two medical members were desirable, 'one with experience in field work and one with extensive bacteriological experience, especially of pathological organisms in foods'. They identified Professor Andrew B. Semple, MOH for Liverpool, and James W. Howie, director of the PHLS.[22]

Stephen's recollections suggest that there was a little more to the selection process. He recalled that Christopher Soames, Minister of Agriculture, Fisheries and Food, indicated that since the outbreak was in Scotland and the chairman was Scottish, it was important to have English members to 'appear impartial'. The SHHD did not like this idea, but to avoid unpleasantness they sought Scottish experts working in England.[23] Howie was an Aberdonian and graduate of Aberdeen University, who had worked at the Rowett Research

---

[17] B. D. Fraser to Minister, 4 June 1964, PRO MH 148/357.

[18] Ibid.

[19] Ibid.

[20] Note of conclusions reached at a meeting of ministers on 4 June, PRO PREM 11/5073.

[21] R. E. C. Johnson to A. M. Stephen, 3 June 1964, NAS HH 64/379.

[22] J. Winnifrith to R. E. C. Johnson, 3 June 1964, NAS HH 64/369; A. M. Stephen to J. A. Hauff, 4 June 1964, NAS HH 64/379.

[23] Stephen, interview.

Institute near Aberdeen.[24] Semple came from Glasgow, where he trained. In interview, Semple suggested that he had been selected because of his interest and experience in food hygiene. He had established his reputation by prosecuting a prominent Liverpudlian café proprietor, and later organised food hygiene courses for café staff and the public.[25]

During the early discussion it was agreed that it was desirable to appoint a female, to 'inspire the housewives' confidence'.[26] SHHD officials favoured Gabriel Pike because she was English, perhaps in the light of their achievement in appointing Scottish experts.[27] Pike was a member of MAFF's Food Standards Committee, and Chairman of the Women's Institute in England and Wales. The ministers had also agreed that a trade representative should be appointed, and MAFF nominated Algernon M. Borthwick, Chairman of the meat importing business, Thomas Borthwick and Sons Ltd, which was only marginally involved in canned meat.[28] However, according to Stephen, Pike and Borthwick made little contribution. He recalled Pike as the 'obligatory woman' who was merely 'decorative', and that Borthwick 'used to fall asleep'.[29]

The membership was approved at a meeting of ministers and officials on 8 June,[30] and was announced, with the terms of reference, during Noble's statement to the House of Commons. Hector Hughes, Labour MP for Aberdeen North, declared that Noble had made a 'terrible mistake' in appointing an ex-civil servant as chair and argued that a High Court judge would have been more appropriate. He also wanted Noble to widen the scope of the enquiry.[31] The latter point was also addressed by another Labour MP who wanted the enquiry to cover possible reforms in public health organisation and policy, but Noble thought this unnecessary.[32] Hughes also asked the Minister of Health whether, since the outbreak was a 'national danger', he would appoint another committee with wider terms of reference, but received a one-word answer: 'No.'[33]

Some newspapers were critical. The *Guardian* declared that 'having taken refuge in a committee of inquiry to allay anxiety . . . the Government has now appointed the wrong people'. Milne might 'find himself inquiring into the conduct of his old department', and, while Semple, Howie and Borthwick were no doubt 'independent-minded', this was a case of 'the Establishment

---

[24] *Who's Who, 1982*, London, 1983, p. 1190.

[25] Ibid., pp. 1989–1990; Andrew Semple, interview, 1 October 2000, Liverpool, ATO/44.

[26] J. Macpherson to C. H. W. Hodges, 3 June 1964, PRO T 227/1655.

[27] Ibid.

[28] J. A. W. McDonald, 'Note for the record', 5 June 1964; M. Noble to D. Milne, 5 June 1964, NAS HH 64/379.

[29] Stephen, interview.

[30] 'Note of a meeting held at 11.30 a.m. on 8th June, 1964', PRO MAF 282/87.

[31] *PD(C)*, vol. 696, col. *47* (8 June 1964).

[32] Ibid., col. *35*.

[33] Ibid., col. *104* (11 June 1964).

being asked to inquire into the affairs of the Establishment'. As for the terms of reference, these would not cover the questions that the public wanted answered. After Noble's attempts to explain why suspect stock had been left in circulation, it needed to be asked whether 'the Ministry was wise to keep its fingers crossed?' The committee, however, was 'not qualified either in its constitution nor in its terms of reference to answer that question'.[34]

Critical questions continued. On 17 June, William Hamilton, Labour MP for West Fife, asked Noble to set up an independent committee to consider 'both the causes of the outbreak and the manner it has been handled'. Noble declined to widen the remit because it was 'of greatest importance that we should get quick answers to the main problem'. But when Willie Ross, the Labour Party's Scottish spokesman, asked for assurances that the committee would investigate the 'import, distribution, control and early withdrawal of suspect corned beef', Noble replied that it was likely that the enquiry would cover all this.[35] In answer to another question he indicated that the enquiry could include 'an examination of the dispersal and disposal of foodstuffs in dock and warehouse'.[36] It seems, then, that whatever the initial intentions, it was soon realised that to satisfy critics it would be necessary to allow the committee to interpret its terms of reference broadly.

Reports of the inaugural meeting, on 18 June at the Royal Commonwealth Society's rooms in London, based upon a press statement and comments by Stephen, confirmed that the committee's work would extend beyond the identification of the cause of the outbreak. The committee would also draw attention to any deficiencies in legislation that came to their attention.[37] Prior to the meeting, Stephen had already produced lists of witnesses and an outline of the questions to be addressed to them,[38] and on 22 June he set about inviting them to prepare evidence and to appear before the committee. MOsH and others who had been involved in the 1963 outbreaks, and microbiologists from various institutions, were called to meetings in London.[39] The MOH for Pickering, along with further microbiologists and a veterinary officer, were invited to give evidence in Edinburgh.[40] Stephen's next set of invitations was to the trade. These included the meat-packing companies, the owners of the shop, and the surveyors used by MAFF for the management of the stockpile. A further round of letters was sent to government departments.[41]

---

[34] 'The Aberdeen typhoid inquiry', *Guardian*, 9 June 1964, p. 10a.

[35] *PD(C)*, vol. 696, cols *1274–5* (17 June 1964).

[36] Ibid., cols *175–6*.

[37] 'Inquiry may visit Aberdeen next week', *Guardian*, 19 June 1964, p. 3a.

[38] A. M. Stephen to D. Milne, 15 June 1964, NAS HH 101/377.

[39] A. M. Stephen to D. J. H. Payne, I. Ash, A. R. Darlow, C. L. Sharp, A. L. H. Tomlinson and E. S. Anderson, 22 June 1964, NAS HH 64/380.

[40] A. M. Stephen to W. R. M. Couper, R. Cruickshank and J. Meyrath, 22 June 1964, NAS HH 64/380.

[41] Liebig's Extract of Meat Co Ltd, International Packers (London), Ltd, Perfect, Lambert

After a preliminary meeting in Aberdeen on 23 June, between 29 June and 29 July the committee spent four days in London, two in Edinburgh and one in Aberdeen taking evidence. Prior to the session in London on 29 June, Howie prepared a list of 'questions of a non-technical nature' for other members of the committee to put to the witnesses.[42] After the meeting, Stephen produced summaries of the evidence, and before subsequent meetings prepared notes to provide a line of questioning.[43]

Semple was on holiday from 23 June until 17 July and missed a number of meetings, but on his return Stephen briefed him and presented him with papers.[44] Semple made up for lost time by making extra visits to Aberdeen, with Stephen, in late July and August.[45] The full committee did not meet in August but took evidence in September over a further six days: four in London and two in Aberdeen. Although in practice the committee interpreted their remit broadly, they made no systematic attempt to gather information from patients and citizens affected by the outbreak. Few of the personnel involved in dealing with the outbreak in Aberdeen beyond the health and welfare department gave evidence. The report was assembled by Stephen.[46] A draft of the chapters on the cause of the original infection was ready by 23 September for discussion on 28 September, and a further drafting meeting took place on 6 October.[47] By the end of October, complete drafts of the report had been sent to government departments for comment.

The ministries and the Milne Committee

The committee met some officials at the inaugural meeting, as Stephen arranged for MAFF representatives to outline the importation and distribution of corned beef. However, they were careful not to anticipate their official evidence, attending on the understanding that they would not discuss 'the sequence of events or justification of anything done or not done'.[48] When

& Co Ltd, William Low & Company, 24 June 1964; A. M. Stephen to J. Winnifrith, B. Fraser and J. N. T. Spreckley, 25 June 1964, NAS HH 64/380.

[42] A. M. Stephen to J. W. Howie, 25 June 1964, NAS HH 64/378.

[43] A. M. Stephen to J. W. Howie, 2 July 1964, NAS HH 64/378.

[44] A. M. Stephen to A. B. Semple; A. M. Stephen to D. Milne, 17 July 1964, NAS HH 64/378.

[45] Town Clerk Depute to I. A. G. MacQueen, 6 August 1964, ACA TH 7/6/7; A. M. Stephen to A. B. Semple, 5, 7 and 12 August 1964, NAS HH 64/378; Semple, interview.

[46] Stephen, interview.

[47] A. M. Stephen to members of the Milne Committee, 23 September 1964, NAS HH 64/378.

[48] A. M. Stephen to J. A. Hauff, 9 June 1964, M. A. J. Pearson to A. M. Stephen, 17 June 1964, PRO MH 148/354; A. M. Stephen to Mr Tame, 9 June 1964, NAS HH 64/378;

Stephen wrote to the departments inviting them to prepare evidence and to send witnesses, he included lists of questions. Those to SHHD covered when the department learned about the outbreak and when MacQueen informed them that it was reaching epidemic proportions. There were also detailed questions about the assistance given to MacQueen and the laboratory service.[49] Both the Ministry of Health and MAFF were asked about the 1963 outbreaks, Grace's report of March 1964, the association of Aberdeen with Establishment 1A produce, and the Wapping incident. MAFF's questions also covered official certification and expected water treatment methods, the proportion of the stockpile produced using unchlorinated water, and stockpile monitoring and turnover policies. In addition, the Ministry of Health were asked what assistance they normally provided during epidemics.[50]

By 1 July, in preparation for their appearance before the committee, SHHD had produced an eight-page memorandum plus appendices. This included sections on action in Aberdeen and nationally, and action in relation to suspect canned meat, laboratory services, and 'clearance and rundown'. The section on Aberdeen gave the impression of a straightforward factual account. No explicit negative comments were offered on MacQueen's performance, including his handling of the press. There was no mention of his warnings about successive waves of infection, or of Ian Sutherland's epidemiological speculations.[51] The document included a list of short answers to Stephen's questions. These explained that after the first call from MacQueen, SHHD officials took the initiative in keeping in daily contact. MacQueen never informed SHHD that the outbreak was reaching epidemic proportions: this had become clear from the press. But these comments cannot be construed as anything more than mild criticisms. As for assistance offered and provided, SHHD accepted MacQueen's view that anyone unfamiliar with his department would be more of a hindrance than a help.[52]

There is little indication that SHHD officials were interested in using their evidence as an opportunity to criticise MacQueen. Likewise, they were wary of criticising other departments. When preparing for his interview, Sutherland told the deputy CMO that he might be asked to comment on meat plant water treatment. He believed that neglect of stages of effective water treatment other than chlorination arose from the views of a veterinary officer 'who did not . . . have the support of a public health officer'. If he was asked to comment he feared that he might be driven to make 'adverse comments which . . . could

A. M. Stephen to G. Pike, 12 June 1964, NAS HH 64/378; G. O. Lace to Mr Bird, 12 June 1964, NAS HH 64/228.

[49] A. M. Stephen to R. E. C. Johnson, 24 June 1964, NAS HH 64/352.

[50] A. M. Stephen to J. Winnifrith, 25 June 1964; M. Stephen to B. Fraser, 25 June 1964, NAS HH 64/380.

[51] 'Committee of Inquiry into the Aberdeen typhoid outbreak', 1 July 1964, NAS HH 64/352.

[52] 'Replies to specific questions', 1 July 1964, NAS HH 64/352.

be interpreted as an implied or even direct criticism of professional colleagues and others in a sister department'.[53] There was no sign of interest in pursuing a professional or departmental agenda. Stephen's attitude seems to have been similar. He told Milne that, in his day-to-day work, the connection made between corned beef and typhoid in 1963 had not come to his attention. But he merely remarked: 'This of course may be indicative only of a lack of liaison between the Ministry of Health and ourselves [SHHD].'[54] There was apparently no thought of pressing the Ministry on this point.

Once the terms of reference were settled, the ministries maintained a united front. MAFF and the Ministry of Health exchanged and discussed draft documents and sent drafts to the SHHD.[55] Their final versions of the action taken in 1963, after Grace's report about Establishment 1A, and in connection with Establishment 1819, were consistent with one another and with the narrative prepared in June, discussed in Chapter 5.[56] Potentially problematic areas were presented in a matter-of-fact manner. The Ministry of Health simply stated that in March Dr Ross believed there were no grounds for withdrawing Establishment 1A produce in circulation, giving no details of his reasoning.[57] This was explored, however, in oral witness sessions, and the draft report included some criticisms of the Ministry's reasoning. However, after a meeting between officials, Milne and other members of the committee in early November, these criticisms were softened by drawing out additional points. The Ministry had no legal powers to withdraw the suspect corned beef in circulation. Withdrawal could only be affected by persuasion of the trader, but until 20 April International Packers' directors in London denied that Establishment 1A had been using untreated water. A further recommendation was added, proposing that powers be provided for the compulsory withdrawal of suspect food in the hands of traders.[58] The published report stated that the decision that the 'already distributed produce of Establishment Argentina 1A did not constitute such a health hazard that they should be withdrawn' could be 'justified in the light of the information available . . . at the time'. However, the committee had formed the view that typhoid was endemic in Argentina and therefore there was 'no doubt that this decision has proved in retrospect to be a mistaken one'. However, the committee softened even this mild rebuke by adding that they would have reached the same decision as the Ministry under the circumstances of the time.[59]

MAFF policy was to be as helpful as possible and not to object that,

<hr>

53 I. N. Sutherland to J. Smith, 2 July 1964, NAS HH 58/352.
54 A. M. Stephen to D. Milne, 5 August 1964, NAS HH 64/378.
55 G. O. Lace to M. Macdonald, 9 July 1964, NAS HH 64/352.
56 'Memorandum by the Ministry of Agriculture, Fisheries and Food', NAS HH 64/352.
57 'Memorandum by the Ministry of Health answers to questions 1–3', PRO MH 148/354.
58 K. A. Bird to Mr Lace, 17 November 1964, PRO MAF 282/96.
59 Milne, p. 44.

for example, Establishment 1819 had nothing to do with Aberdeen,[60] but questions concerning the stockpile caused some anxieties. Humphreys-Davies thought that they needed to be 'careful to avoid giving information which could be useful to an enemy'. It was now common knowledge that a stockpile existed, but Humphreys-Davies thought that they need go no further than they might in answering parliamentary questions. But the 'insider' status of Milne and Stephen would help. Milne would readily appreciate the issues at stake, and a private word with Stephen would be in order.[61] The question on the proportion of stockpile corned beef manufactured using chlorinated water was particularly problematic. N. J. P. Hutchison, of Meat and Livestock division, was not only concerned with the security issue. He was also worried by the implication that:

> there is a simple division between chlorinated and unchlorinated. I am inclined to suppress the 'true' answer – which is, I think, about one half in water not claimed to be either of potable quality or chlorinated, or in water otherwise dubious – and say merely that we have very substantial quantities from establishments as in the question, but that at some of these potable water was used. To add proportionate figures . . . would disclose classified defence information.[62]

In their evidence, MAFF admitted that if the question was taken literally, 'most' of the stockpile corned beef would fall into the 'unchlorinated' category.[63] (By this time Hutchison had concluded that the actual proportion was about 75 per cent.[64]) If, on the other hand, the potability of the water was the criterion of acceptability, then no more than one-third of the stockpile corned beef would be unsatisfactory. The stock produced using unchlorinated water included pre-1955 and some recent South American produce, and a substantial quantity of Commonwealth stock. Exact proportions by origin were not given because such details 'if linked with information commercially available' would 'disclose the total size of the stockpile, a fact which is kept secret in the interest of national security'.[65] In connection with the question about the criteria used in monitoring the stockpile, MAFF prepared a response jointly with the surveyors, Perfect, Lambert & Co, whose questions covered the same ground. The seven-page document consisted of a frank account of the methods of monitoring the stockpile and the results obtained,[66] but no details appeared in the Milne report.

---

[60] P. Humphreys-Davies to Mr Hensley, 1 July 1964, PRO MAF 246/242.
[61] Ibid.
[62] N. J. P. Hutchison to Secretary, 10 July 1964, PRO MAF 246/242.
[63] 'Memorandum by the Ministry of Agriculture, Fisheries and Food', NAS HH 64/352.
[64] N. J. P. Hutchison to Mr Cann, 15 July 1964, PRO MAF 246/242.
[65] 'Memorandum by the Ministry of Agriculture, Fisheries and Food', NAS HH 64/352.
[66] 'Memorandum by the Ministry of Agriculture, Fisheries and Food and Messrs. Perfect, Lambert & Co.', NAS HH 64/352.

In early November, Hutchison checked the draft report, which stated that a 'not inconsiderable proportion' of the stockpile consisted of meat canned before the general introduction of chlorinated cooling water. In fact, there was 2800 tons of pre-1955 stock but 5630 produced recently at Argentine Establishments 1A and 25 and Uruguay 5. Hutchison wondered whether the existing wording would reinforce the mistaken idea that 'age is somehow linked with danger'. On the other hand, he did not want to invite attention 'to the kind of establishment we have more recently been patronising'.[67] At a meeting between Winnifrith and Milne Committee members, it was agreed to accept some amendments suggested by Hutchison. The final version stated vaguely that 'part of the Government stockpile of corned beef consists of meat about which, because of the time and place of canning, a doubt exists or will be created by our findings'.[68]

The evidence presented by the ministries made no attempt to suggest recommendations, which seem to have come largely from the committee, several reflecting the interests of Howie. One concerned the public health laboratories in Scotland. Before the end of June, Howie obtained from Stephen a copy of the 1957 report of the Scottish Health Services Council Laboratory Services Committee on the organisation of the Scottish laboratory services.[69] This supported the provision of laboratories by Regional Hospital Boards, the system established when the National Health Service was founded.[70] A briefing paper by SHHD officials commented that Howie thought that the report 'reached the wrong conclusion', and warned Brotherston that he would try and persuade him that the laboratories should be reorganised along English lines.[71] The final report compared the Scottish system unfavourably with the PHLS, noting that in England, bacteriologists were more commonly involved in fieldwork, and advising on tracing infections, taking samples, cleaning and disinfection.[72] Among the recommendations was a proposal for a reexamination of the organisation of the Scottish laboratory services. This was underway by the time of publication of the report, and led to the establishment of the Communicable Disease (Scotland) Unit in 1969.[73]

Questions about whether the SHHD might behave more like the Ministry of Health may also have arisen from Howie's concerns. On 23 June, he asked Brodie whether he would prefer the system in England, in which the Ministry

---

⁶⁷ N. J. P. Hutchison to Miss Herbert, 3 November 1964, PRO MAF 282/96.

⁶⁸ Annotated copy of draft report (doc 1A), PRO MAF 282/96; Milne, p. 39.

⁶⁹ A. M. Stephen to J. W. Howie, 30 June 1964, NAS HH 64/378.

⁷⁰ For files on the Scottish Health Services Council Laboratory Services Committee on desirability of separate laboratory service organisation in Scotland, see NAS HH 102/910 and HH 102/993.

⁷¹ J. Hogarth to CMO, 4 September 1964, NAS HH 64/352.

⁷² Milne, p. 66.

⁷³ See pp. 197–8.

of Health provided assistance at the beginning of any outbreak.[74] This theme was continued on 9 September, when the committee explored with Brotherston the relationship between SHHD and MOsH, and the differences between Scottish and English practices.[75] Scottish Office Under-secretary James Hogarth advised Brotherston that while the principles were similar, in England the Ministry of Health were 'more forceful or persuasive' in offering assistance, and that their medical staff quickly visited the scene of local outbreaks.[76] The published report commended the Ministry of Health's practice, and implied that a SHHD medical officer should have been sent to Aberdeen sooner.[77] But the committee also accepted MacQueen's criticism that the visits to Aberdeen by different SHHD officers had wasted time because of the need to brief each of them separately.[78]

Another matter probably raised by Howie was the subject of a memorandum by Mrs Hauff, after she and her Ministry of Health colleagues gave evidence on 23 July. The committee floated the idea of a 'committee of experts to advise . . . on future occasions of unprecedented bacteriological risks from a particular kind of food'. She thought one problem would be that such a committee might 'scarcely ever have any work to do', and that, when needed, there would be insufficient time to summon it. But she also pointed out strategic advantages. The government would be able to 'demonstrate that they had independent advice both in advance of an emergency and in an awkward situation'.[79] The idea was explored further with Godber and Brotherston, and a recommendation to form such a committee appeared in the final report, leading to the establishment of a bacteriological panel of the Committee on Medical Aspects of Food Policy.[80] However, the implementation of this recommendation, like several others, was tokenistic. The panel soon fell inactive, and was mentioned only once in Godber's annual reports.[81]

The investigation in Aberdeen

Difficulties arose when Aberdeen's Town Clerk enquired about the powers under which the committee operated, when Stephen telephoned on 18 June

[74] 'Dr J. Brodie re-draft of evidence', 22 August 1964, NAS HH 64/228.

[75] A. M. Stephen to J. H. F. Brotherston, 1 September 1964, NAS HH 64/380.

[76] J. Hogarth to CMO, 4 September 1964, NAS HH 64/352.

[77] Milne, p. 63.

[78] Ibid., p. 65.

[79] J. A. Hauff to Mrs Pearson, 30 July 1964, NAS HH 64/352.

[80] Committee on Medical Aspects of Food Policy, standing panel on hazards from microbiological contamination of food, minutes of first meeting, 28 September 1965, PRO MH 148/355.

[81] *RCMO 1966*, p. 142.

to arrange the preliminary visit to the city. Before authorising officials' participation, the Corporation wanted to be satisfied that they were under obligation to do so. They had gathered that 'the M.O.H. . . . might feel difficulty about disclosing medical records unless the Committee were in effect requiring him to do so under statutory powers'.[82] This may not be a sign of unwillingness by MacQueen to co-operate at this stage because he had already sent his 'Rough notes' to Stephen,[83] although later he did appear reluctant to produce further papers.

Earlier, the Scottish Office had been anxious to ensure that the committee's authority to pursue enquiries in England was clear. Rather than the committee being appointed solely by Noble, they sought to identify the powers of the three ministries to be cited in the warrant of appointment. MAFF, however, doubted whether their minister possessed relevant powers.[84] It was therefore agreed to dispense with a preamble citing powers, and the warrant was signed by the three ministers on 12 June.[85] The query of Aberdeen Corporation reopened the question of what powers of MAFF might be cited.[86] SHHD thought that for reasons of 'policy and presentation' it was important for MAFF not to withdraw. They suggested citing powers under the Food and Drugs Act, even if they were not relevant, but MAFF's legal adviser could not be moved.[87] Noble and the Minister of Health therefore signed a new warrant alone on 29 June, which mentioned the Public Health (Scotland) Act, 1897 and the Public Health Act, 1936.[88] The following day, Stephen wrote to the Town Clerk, requesting the preparation of evidence and to interview witnesses in Aberdeen on 29 July.[89]

The problem raised by the Town Clerk was not immediately important, because there was no intention to take formal evidence from Corporation employees on 23 June, and MacQueen was, in any case, on holiday. But the committee did take evidence from Dr Beddard of the North-Eastern Regional Hospital Board and Dr Brodie, the regional bacteriologist, and obtained strong impressions of how the outbreak had been handled, long before interviewing and receiving evidence from MacQueen and his colleagues. According to Beddard, as the number of cases rose, he felt it essential to 'have a forecast of the likelihood of further cases so that a close watch could be kept on the

<hr>

[82] J. Hogarth to Secretary, 19 June 1964, NAS HH 64/352.

[83] I. N. S. to Deputy C. M. O., 19 June 1964, NAS HH 61/1073.

[84] A. M. Stephen to J. A. Hauff, 4 June 1964, NAS HH 64/379; J. Hogarth to Secretary, 10 June 1964, NAS HH 64/352.

[85] Mr McCabe to Mr Baird, 10 June 1964, NAS HH 64/379; Minute of appointment, 12 June 1964, NAS HH 64/352.

[86] R. E. C. Johnson to A. J. D. Winnifrith, 19 June 1964, NAS HH 64/352.

[87] J. Hogarth to Secretary, 24 June 1964, NAS HH 64/352.

[88] Milne, p. 5.

[89] A. M. Stephen to Town Clerk, 30 June 1964, NAS HH 64/380.

availability of beds'. He made four telephone calls to the health and welfare department and visited MacQueen twice, but implied that MacQueen should have been proactive in supplying information. In the morning of 30 May, Beddard suggested that the three branches of the health service should meet to discuss and co-ordinate action and that bacteriological advice should be available. The first meeting, that afternoon, was attended by Dr Birnie of the local medical committee, and Sandy MacDonald, professor of bacteriology. Brodie attended the next meeting at Beddard's suggestion.[90] According to Brodie he had no direct contact with MacQueen until 31 May when he advised closing the shop, but no action was taken. He was not invited to visit the shop, or to advise on disinfecting, sampling or contact testing.[91] Stephen summarised the evidence of Beddard and Brodie and sent it to them for checking. In some paragraphs submitted as joint evidence, they stated that before the end of May there had been insufficient contact between MacQueen and the other branches of the health service.[92]

Stephen requested from the Town Clerk a document addressing nine questions. These covered the history of the outbreak and actions taken to determine the source of infection. Details were also required of the examinations carried out on stock, staff and possible sources of infection, and the method by which corned beef was established as the likely source, including a summary of the original case histories. Further questions covered action taken to prevent the spread of infection.[93] The Corporation's health and welfare committee set a deadline of 17 July for MacQueen to prepare the documents,[94] but MacQueen rejected this timetable. There was much outstanding collation of information, and he could not guarantee to produce the document in time for the committee's visit.[95] Stephen was irritated. The Town Clerk had told Stephen that MacQueen would need about four weeks to prepare his information. Stephen pointed out that by 29 July he would have had six weeks (from the date of Stephen's first telephone call).[96]

Despite his protestations, MacQueen signed the first instalment of his evidence on 24 July, but he did not send it to Stephen until 10 August, explaining that he had waited until the document was approved by the health and welfare committee. Attached were an appendix prepared by the superin-

---

[90] 'Oral evidence taken on 23 June 1964. Dr F. D. Beddard', NAS HH 64/228.

[91] 'Dr J. Brodie re-draft of evidence', 22 August 1964, NAS HH 64/228.

[92] 'Redraft of final three paragraphs of draft evidence taken in Aberdeen on 23rd June, 1964 from Dr James Brodie and Dr F. D. Beddard', NAS HH 64/228.

[93] A. M. Stephen to Town Clerk, 30 June 1964, NAS HH 64/380.

[94] Minute of meeting of the Health and Welfare (General Purposes) Sub-committee, 8 July 1964, ACA TH 7/6/7.

[95] I. A. G. MacQueen to J. Hunter, 14 July 1964; J. F. C. Hunter to A. M. Stephen, 17 July 1964, ACA TH 7/6/7.

[96] A. M. Stephen to D. Milne, 27 July 1964, NAS HH 64/378.

tendent health visitor, and two appendices by the chief sanitary inspector. A further appendix, by MacQueen, dated 4 August, gave his responses to thirty-one additional questions handed to him on 29 July.[97]

During the morning of 29 July, the committee were exposed to further adverse views about MacQueen's performance when they interviewed representatives of the meat products company, Robert Lawson and Sons (Dyce) Ltd, who had volunteered evidence.[98] Lawson's expanded upon the themes introduced by Beddard and Brodie – problems of communication between MacQueen and others – and criticised his media strategy. Lawson's claimed that they had great difficulty obtaining advice from the public health authorities and explained the circumstances of a closure of their factory. After a worker was admitted to hospital following a positive blood test, the management prepared a carefully worded statement announcing a precautionary closure. But when journalists collected the statement, they were already aware of the issue, from MacQueen's press conference. Subsequently, reports appeared that the employee was 'a confirmed typhoid case' although the high level of antibodies in his blood was probably due to a TAB vaccination. The man was not even a contact: he had simply been tested when accompanying his wife to a clinic, after she was advised to have a test because she was a GP's cleaner. Lawson's claimed that the case illustrated the 'haphazard, not to say casual, system of investigation of contacts'. The memorandum also noted that MacQueen's press conferences presented 'innumerable opportunities for misunderstandings, unguarded utterances and, indeed contradictions and inconsistencies', and suggested that press handouts would avoid such pitfalls.[99]

Records of the afternoon sessions have not been located. As for MacQueen's written evidence, it was clearly defensive on certain sensitive points. Regarding the action taken at Low's, he claimed that he merely accepted the recommendation of the senior assistant medical officer, Dr Brunton, after the initial investigations. According to MacQueen, Brunton felt that since the infected meat had been consumed days earlier, there was no need to close the shop. The only action necessary was to stop cold meat sales, test the employees and disinfect the premises. MacQueen also claimed that Sutherland of SHHD agreed with this decision.[100] This strategy was not lost on Brunton. In an oral history interview, he painted a picture of his former chief as someone inclined

<hr>

[97] I. A. G. MacQueen to A. M. Stephen, 10 August 1964, NAS HH 64/380. Later, additional material was forwarded to the enquiry. 'Further appendix to evidence of medical officer of health statement by Dr A. Wilson McIntosh'; H. B. Parry to I. A. G. MacQueen, 28 August 1964; W. Jackson 'Typhoid Outbreak,' 24 July 1964, NAS HH 64/228.

[98] Brander & Cruikshank (solicitors) to A. M. Stephen, NAS HH 64/380.

[99] 'Memorandum on behalf of Robert Lawson & Sons (Dyce) Ltd in regard to Aberdeen typhoid epidemic May/June 1964', NAS HH 64/228.

[100] MacQueen, 'Evidence', p. 10.

to eschew responsibility for unfavourable turns of events. Pointedly, he recalled that when he took samples to the regional laboratory, Brodie remarked that MacQueen should close the shop.[101]

Some of the questions handed to MacQueen sought further information on these issues. MacQueen was asked whether he had considered closing Low's, to which he replied that he did not believe that he possessed relevant powers. He reiterated his original explanation and argued that if he had closed Low's, he would have had to close all food premises in which typhoid victims worked, causing panic. Different businesses, he claimed, were dealt with differently according to the degree of risk.[102] However, MacQueen's after-the-event rationalisation probably exaggerates the extent to which his dealings with the food trade amounted to a thought-out policy.

A few days after the 29 July interviews, a letter from Stephen to Semple indicates the scepticism with which some of MacQueen's evidence was viewed. They regarded MacQueen's idea of 40,000 people at risk as an 'over simplification and, perhaps, an exaggeration'. The letter also discussed the question of powers to close the shop. Stephen thought the power to close premises, 'if in fact it exists', derived from the Public Health (Scotland) Act, 1897 which allowed temporary closures for disinfection by order of a magistrate.[103] The general powers of MOsH for dealing with outbreaks were taken up when the committee met Ministry of Health officials and Brotherston on 9 September. An SHHD briefing document discussed a range of powers in Scotland and England. Besides the closure of premises, the Scottish provision for securing the examination of suspected carriers was more complicated than in England, and in Scotland there were no powers for excluding children from places of entertainment. MacQueen, however, had suggested that having formal powers in the latter respect may have been 'an embarrassment rather than a help'. If he had relied upon compulsion, the Corporation might have become liable for large compensation claims. But he felt that clearer powers would be helpful in connection with the closure of premises and the submission of specimens from patients discharged from hospital,[104] and the final report took up both points.[105]

In his original evidence, MacQueen referred to the 'long standing tradition of good co-operation' with hospital and university staff and GPs as one of the advantages enjoyed by his department.[106] This optimistic view did not satisfy the committee, and several supplementary questions addressed these matters.

[101] D. P. Brunton , interview, 27 October 1999, Aberdeen, ATO/32.

[102] I. A. G. MacQueen, 'Evidence submitted to Committee of Enquiry', July 1964 (main evidence) and August 1964 (further questions), EMR, pp. 59–60.

[103] A. M. Stephen to A. B. Semple, 5 August 1964, NAS HH 64/378.

[104] J. Hogarth to CMO, 4 September 1964, NAS HH 64/352.

[105] Milne, p. 8.

[106] MacQueen, 'Evidence', p. 8.

In response to a question about how liaison between the health services was achieved, MacQueen wrote that it was initially:

> by telephone and personal meetings, e.g. I can recall a long telephonic conversation with Dr. Birnie . . . on, I think, Sunday, 24th, and two meetings with Dr. Beddard . . . about the same time, one in either his office or mine and the other in my house.[107]

No notes on these conversations were taken, 'since officers of the various services already knew each other well and worked in harmony'.[108] According to MacQueen, the formation of the special liaison committee was a consequence of the realisation of the large size of the outbreak.[109] He gave no indication of discontent about communication and co-ordination, and to the question, 'What liaison existed between your Department and the Regional Board Laboratory?', responded: 'Relationships were excellent from the beginning. My first telephone call to Dr Brodie was on 20th May.'[110]

As for the control measures and use of the press, MacQueen made some mention of these in his 'Rough notes' as well as his main evidence. In the 'Rough notes' he referred to 'Advice about Travel' as a 'controversial point'. He explained that besides stressing 'complete personal hygiene', he advised the public not to travel needlessly, and not to go on holiday to 'centres of population', and continued:

> Some have maintained that this advice . . . was not stringent enough; others have claimed that it helped to create outside Aberdeen the idea of an isolated leper-colony. In actual fact the advice was a sustained attempt to walk a tight-rope – on the one hand to minimise risk of spread of infection . . . and on the other hand to allow life . . . to proceed as normally as possible.[111]

In his main evidence, MacQueen explained that the health education campaign and travel advice were implemented because there was no easy way of identifying the quarter to one-third of Aberdeen's citizens at risk. He was helped by existing relationships between his health education section and the press, and was advised by the section that 'the most successful short-term results would be achieved by the continual appearance of a single person' in the media. It was recognised, however, that ensuring the full co-operation of the media:

---

[107] MacQueen, 'Evidence', p. 62.
[108] Ibid.
[109] Ibid., pp. 12–13.
[110] Ibid., p. 61.
[111] I. A. G. MacQueen, 'Rough notes on typhoid outbreak', 16 June 1964, ACA TH 7/6/6.

involved (both as a *quid pro quo* to reporters etc., concerned primarily with items of news value and as a means of keeping the outbreak prominently before the citizens) also giving reporters and television interviewers in large measure the information they wanted.[112]

MacQueen claimed that the campaign had achieved its aims but admitted that 'some newspapers far from Aberdeen . . . selected only the more flamboyant and eye-catching sentences and sometimes distorted even these'.[113]

MacQueen was asked whether the media had hindered his work, and if he could suggest how problems could be overcome. He admitted that initially the press was 'a bit of a nuisance' but stated that thereafter they were 'extremely helpful'. His advice to any MOH facing an outbreak was to adopt his policy of twice-daily press conferences and no interviews at other times.[114]

The epidemiological investigation fell largely to Semple, who gathered information during his extra trips to Aberdeen with Stephen. On one visit they had lunch at MacQueen's home[115] and there are some signs that, as a fellow MOH, Semple was relatively sympathetic towards MacQueen. In interview, Semple said that he was impressed by MacQueen's handling of the outbreak, and he had little sympathy with Brodie's criticisms. He recalled that he found Brodie 'a little bit gloomy' and, in his view, suffering from 'bridesmaid's syndrome'. Semple told Brodie that the epidemiology was MacQueen's affair and that he was sure MacQueen would have sought his advice if he had needed it.[116] As a result of Semple's investigations, by early September he had produced for the committee a note on the epidemiology of the outbreak.[117]

The final full meetings in Aberdeen, on 14/15 September, included interviews with a wider range of staff of the Corporation,[118] local businessman R. A. Williamson, and a GP. Williamson had been involved in producing the *How to Stamp Out Typhoid* brochure.[119] Following his interview, he summarised his evidence, and his perceptions of the committee's reactions. He claimed there had been a 'crying need' for the brochure, and that it 'saved a tremendous amount of time on the part of Doctors and the medical authorities in answering

---

[112] MacQueen, 'Evidence', p. 36.

[113] Ibid.

[114] Ibid., p. 63.

[115] Town Clerk Depute to I. A. G. MacQueen, 6 August 1964, ACA TH 7/6/7; A. M. Stephen to A. B. Semple, 5, 7 and 12 August 1964, NAS HH 64/378; Semple, interview.

[116] Semple, interview.

[117] A. M. Stephen to D. Milne, 1 September 1964, NAS HH 64/378.

[118] A. M. Stephen to J. F. Watt, 2 September 1964, NAS HH 64/380. The final list of the Corporation's witnesses comprised four medical officers, two sanitary inspectors and two health visitors, and four members of the water and drainage departments, and two deputy town clerks. Milne, p. 72.

[119] A. M. Stephen to R. A. Williamson, 24 August 1964, NAS HH 64/380.

routine questions'. It also 'relieved public anxiety' and 'raised morale'. Williamson mixed sympathy towards MacQueen with criticisms. He thought MacQueen had had an 'unnecessarily complicated task' in being responsible for fighting the outbreak and acting as press relations officer, at the same time as educating the public and the trade in preventive measures. He suggested that a small committee representing the food trade could assist in the management of outbreaks, and envisaged it meeting with the MOH and a medically qualified press relations officer. Such committees could determine '*accurately* [emphasis in original] the number of people at risk' which was 'grossly exaggerated' in Aberdeen. He gathered that the Milne Committee appreciated these points and agreed that it was important 'not to create undue alarm, whilst at the same time there was a great need to frighten people locally, if necessary, into adopting the highest possible standard of hygiene'.[120]

The GP Dr K. L. Lipp was one of the first to realise that there was typhoid in the city. He only gave oral evidence, of which no record has been recovered, but in view of the remarks in the report about MacQueen's lack of communication with GPs, his views were probably in line with some that reached SHHD informally. Hogarth reported that he met the clerk of the Aberdeen Executive Council (responsible for administering the GP service) at a conference, according to whom Aberdeen's GPs were 'highly incensed by the way in which Dr MacQueen had failed to keep them informed'.[121]

Unlike the ministries, MacQueen received no opportunity to check the draft report, but some changes were made because the government's publishers thought they might be liable for a claim for damages for defamation. The Scottish Office's solicitor advised that since the report did not criticise anyone else by name, MacQueen might feel obliged to take action to protect his reputation. The most dangerous passage referred to MacQueen's alleged lack of up-to-date knowledge of typhoid, which could be construed as an attack on his competence.[122] In view of these anxieties the reference to lack of 'up-to-date knowledge' was removed.

A letter sent by Howie to SHHD, after MacQueen claimed on television that the committee's criticisms of his publicity campaign were outside their terms of reference, suggests that he was responsible for the judgement about MacQueen's lack of 'up-to-date' knowledge. In Howie's view, the part of the remit concerning the dissemination of typhoid covered the publicity, since MacQueen held that the campaign had limited the spread of the disease. Howie felt that the last-minute deletions made it less clear that the committee was against MacQueen's publicity because he was not well informed about typhoid, remarking, 'If he had known more or taken more advice he would

---

[120] 'Summary of evidence given by Mr R. A. Williamson to the committee of inquiry into the Aberdeen typhoid outbreak 15 September 1964', NAS HH 64/228.

[121] J. Hogarth to Miss Macdonald, 25 September 1964, NAS HH 61/1074.

[122] M. K. Macdonald to Mr Hogarth, 1 December 1964, PRO MH 148/357.

have talked less that was nonsensical; and probably he would have talked less'.[123] In a further letter he regretted that the report might be misinterpreted as 'MOsH should not talk very much to the Press' rather than 'MOsH should know the ins and outs of what they are talking about before they say very much to the Press'. He thought it essential to oppose MacQueen's view that the outbreak had been cut short by the publicity, to prevent a 'false view of typhoid and its degree of communicability' from being propagated.[124]

The firms: the retailer and the manufacturers

On 24 June, Stephen invited William Low and Co to send representatives to appear before the committee, and included questions as a guide for the preparation of evidence.[125] However, since none of Low's evidence has been located we must rely upon the report for details of what the committee found out about the supermarket. A chapter in the section on the dissemination of the infection gave an account of how canned meat was stored, handled and sold, and the committee's conclusions about how so many people became infected. It was explained that at the shop, the cold meat counter was beside a large window. After cans of corned beef were opened, the contents were cut in half. Half was placed in the window, and half on a shelf behind the counter, from where it was lifted down for slicing. Cold meats left at the end of each day were stored together on a tray in a refrigerator.

It was concluded that the corned beef contaminated with typhoid germs had been stored in conditions favourable to rapid growth, especially in view of the warm weather. Furthermore, the infection spread to other meats via the shop assistants' hands, the slicing machine and work surfaces. Following these conclusions, a chapter on food hygiene regulations was the basis of several recommendations. Admitting the circumstances leading to the outbreak could have occurred anywhere, the report recommended new codes of practice or regulations covering the hygienic handling of cold cooked meats, and the maximum temperature at which cooked meats could be displayed.[126]

On 24 June Stephen wrote to Armour and Co Ltd (International Packers (London) Ltd), whose corned beef was believed to be responsible for the Aberdeen outbreak, and Liebig's Extract of Meat Co Ltd, whose ex-stockpile produce had been placed under suspicion by MacQueen. He invited them to prepare evidence and send witnesses.[127] Both firms were asked to comment

[123] J. W. Howie to R. E. C. Johnson, 18 December 1964, NAS HH 64/351.
[124] J. W. Howie to R. E. C. Johnson, 1 January 1965, NAS HH 64/399.
[125] A. M. Stephen to Messrs. William Low & Company, 24 June 1964, NAS HH 64/380.
[126] Milne, pp. 52–3.
[127] A. M. Stephen to Messrs Liebig's Extract of Meat Co Ltd, International Packers (London) Ltd, 24 June 1964, NAS HH 64/380.

upon their meat inspection, slaughter, processing and packaging arrangements, the treatment and sampling of cooling water, and the location of their packing stations in relation to sewer outfalls to rivers. Some weeks later, Stephen approached the Argentine Meat Producers (CAP), whose corned beef had been associated with the 1963 outbreaks, holding a preliminary meeting with them, before sending a list of questions. They were asked whether, in the light of Aberdeen, they still rejected the link between CAP corned beef and the 1963 outbreaks.[128]

None of the Armour and Co evidence survives in the National Archive of Scotland, but in preparing their evidence the company submitted a series of questions to the Aberdeen city and county corporations, and the PHLS. From these we may infer the kinds of arguments that the company attempted to construct. As for Liebig's, there is a unique verbatim record of their encounter with the committee, and CAP's written evidence also survives.

The manufacturers' witnesses all appeared before the committee in September, by which time the committee had formed the view that it was possible for typhoid germs to enter cans from cooling water, and to survive undetected. Among the key witnesses in this connection was the Metal Box Company expert T. E. Bashford, who advised that bacteria which were generally thought of as gas producers could behave differently within cans.[129] Such cans could thereby pass through quality control undetected. Another witness, Dr A. J. H. Tomlinson of the PHLS laboratory at County Hall, London, advised on the results of experiments which demonstrated that *Salmonella typhi* could grow in corned beef while the meat remained normal in appearance.[130]

The chain of reasoning justifying the view that typhoid organisms could survive in cans involved many steps, one of them concerning the question of whether or not the residual heat within the can would kill any typhoid organisms that entered. On this matter, Messrs James Barnes, Pty Ltd, an Australian company, volunteered evidence via their Glasgow agent. Initially, they suggested that the residual heat would kill the organisms, but later arranged experiments which demonstrated that a suggestion made by Howie was correct: the bottom corners of the can remained sufficiently cool for typhoid bacilli to survive.[131]

An important witness in reinforcing the contamination-during-manufacture theory was Howie's colleague, E. S. Anderson, director of the PHLS's Enteric

---

[128] A. Stephen to Argentine meat producers, 6 August 1964 and 26 August 1964, NAS HH 64/380.

[129] T. E. Bashford to J. W. Howie, 23 June 1964, NAS HH 64/228.

[130] A. J. H. Tomlinson, Evidence, HH 64/228.

[131] A. M. Stephen to S. Kerr, 6 August 1964, NAS 64/380; P. Barnes to Secretary of the Committee of Enquiry, 20 August 1964, NAS HH 64/228; A. M. Stephen to D. Milne, 1 September 1964, NAS HH 64/378.

Reference Laboratory.[132] He had carried out the phage typing in connection with the outbreak and discussed the implications of the finding that phage type 34 was involved. His evidence also included a reinvestigation of the 1948 outbreak at Oswestry, in which he had recently shown that phage type 34 had been responsible.[133] Anderson also prepared papers on the incidence of typhoid in Argentina, arguing that the WHO data were inaccurate. On the basis of the mortality figures he estimated that the true incidence was 500 per million of the population per year, leading to about 300 new carriers per year. He discussed the South America river system and argued, from the speed of the current of the river Paraná, and the location of Establishment 1A downstream from Rosario (population 600,000), that when Establishment 1A was using untreated river water it was certainly polluted with *Salmonella typhi*. He also submitted a letter which testified that at the time of the Pickering outbreak, which was also associated with Establishment 1A produce, the typhoid bacillus had been present in the river water used for cooling.[134]

After seeking permission from the committee, Armour and Co submitted a series of questions to MacQueen and the PHLS.[135] MacQueen received twenty-three questions,[136] but objected to some that required 'opinionative answers' on matters on which he was unwilling to commit himself.[137] The only questions which introduced an 'unusual note' were three which suggested that 'some form of floodwater penetrated Low's basement early in May', and which appear to have originated with Armour's own investigations at the shop. MacQueen could recall nothing of the matter, but it emerged that the city engineer's staff had visiting Low's on 8 June to investigate 'seepage of water causing dampness on parts of the wall and floor'. Samples were taken which showed no traces of faecal bacteria, and tests showed no seepage from drains.[138] Armour and Co's line of questioning suggests that they were interested in finding grounds for proposing sources of infection in the shop other than their corned beef. The committee examined this matter further when they took evidence in Aberdeen in September, by which time further reports were available, which concluded that the problem was caused by inadequate

[132] E. S. Anderson to A. M. Stephen, 23 June 1964, NAS HH 64/380.
[133] A. M. Stephen to D. Milne, 17 July and 1 September 1964, NAS HH 64/378; Milne, pp. 26–7.
[134] E. S. Anderson to A. M. Stephen, 27 August 1964; 'Additional observations for the Committee of Inquiry', NAS HH 64/228.
[135] Slaughter & May to A. M. Stephen, 15 July 1964; A. M. Stephen to Slaughter & May, 22 July 1964, NAS HH 64/380.
[136] Town Clerk Depute to I. A. G. MacQueen, 6 August 1964, ACA TH 7/6/7.
[137] A. M. Stephen to D. Milne, 17 August 1964, NAS HH 64/378.
[138] 'Replies to questionnaire enclosed with letter dated 24th July 1964 from Messrs. Slaughter & May, Solicitors, London to Dr. I. A. G. MacQueen', 21 August 1964, ACA TH 7/6/7.

drainage of rain-water.[139] Armour and Co also asked detailed questions about typhoid cases among Low's staff, overseas travel, the food history of patients, cases at Lawson's factory, and links between Lawson's and the supermarket, all, no doubt, in the hope of being able to develop alternative hypotheses accounting for the outbreak.[140] They asked Anderson at the PHLS for details about the prevalence of *Salmonella typhi* phage type 34 cases and carriers in Britain. Anderson listed dates of isolation of the phage type and the numbers of cases involved, but knew of no carriers.[141]

There is no indication in the report that Armour's enquiries generated any significant and lasting doubts about the source of the outbreak. The report did leave a degree of uncertainty, however, by stating that the can of corned beef which was the 'most probable cause' of the outbreak was 'most probably manufactured' at Argentine Establishment 1A, but other possible sources were discussed and rejected in turn. The report expressed surprise that the management of Establishment 1A had proceeded with canning after their chlorination plant broke down because it had been installed in 1955, ahead of other South American canners and as a direct result of the Pickering outbreak, which was suspected to have been caused by Establishment 1A canned tongue. However, the report then softened the criticism:

> Presumably they were not fully convinced of the need for chlorination as a safeguard for human health. The three episodes . . . in 1963 were not publicised and we must admit that those who believed in a causal relationship between undrinkable river water, cans of corned beef, and human typhoid did not find that there was unquestioning acceptance of their evidence or arguments. Moreover we think that canners relied on their belief that any contamination would be revealed if their methods of incubation and inspection were followed.[142]

It was only with the Aberdeen outbreak that 'responsible medical and scientific opinion' became 'fully aware of the nature of the issues involved' and, although the Establishment 1A management made a wrong decision, it was only after the Aberdeen outbreak that the use of unchlorinated river water could be judged as 'negligent' rather than 'merely unwise'.

---

[139] Statements by Andrew Gray Laing, senior drainage engineer, Charles Tennant, senior plumbing and drainage inspector, Dennis Fergus Anderson, distribution engineer, Harold Taylor, sewerage inspector, and John William Cruikshank, senior water inspector, 11 September 1964, ACA TH 7/6/7.
[140] 'Replies to questionnaire enclosed with letter dated 24th July 1964 from Messrs. Slaughter & May, Solicitors, London to Dr. I. A. G. MacQueen', 21 August 1964, ACA TH 7/6/7; Slaughter & May to Town Clerk, 27 August 1964, NAS HH 64/228.
[141] 'Answers to Questionnaire from Messrs. Slaughter & May'; E. S. Anderson to A. M. Stephen, 15 August 1964, NAS HH 64/228.
[142] Milne, p. 28.

As for the evidence of the other manufacturers, CAP's evidence was based on the argument that corned beef could not become contaminated during cooling 'without subsequently showing signs of spoilage', and they retained this view even following the Aberdeen outbreak. They had carried out research which convinced them that typhoid bacilli entering a tin would always be accompanied by other organisms that would decompose the contents and distort the tin. In view of this, they believed that in Aberdeen the corned beef must have been contaminated after the can was opened.[143] Their document gave full details of the company's quality control systems. Cans contaminated by gas-forming bacteria via pin-holes which resealed on cooling were easily identified as 'blown'. Those contaminated by non-gas-forming bacteria, or which remained unsealed, were identified by percussion. The research involved experimental autoclaves that used water with different concentrations of contaminating flora, including typhoid bacilli. Before autoclaving, pin-holes were introduced by drilling, and were either sealed or left open before incubating. In was shown that typhoid bacilli could survive within cans but contamination was invariably detectable by cans blowing, by percussion, or from the obviously putrefied nature of the contents.[144] A week prior to their appearance before the Milne Committee, the CAP representatives met Ministry of Health and MAFF officials for a discussion of their projected responses to the committee. The minutes show that CAP's expert clung resolutely to the position that entry of a pure culture of typhoid during corned beef manufacture was impossible.[145]

The transcript of the session of the committee with Liebig's witnesses shows that their lawyer attempted to argue a similar line as CAP but from microbiological and canning principles rather than experimental results. As part of his opening remarks he claimed that the possibility of canned meat becoming contaminated by typhoid bacilli but not spoilage organisms was so remote that it could be excluded 'as a matter of practical reality'. Once the company's experts were introduced, however, and Howie took over the questioning, there was considerable backtracking. Howie asked the experts to concede that contamination of cans with typhoid bacilli accompanied by coliform bacteria was likely to be less rare than contamination with typhoid alone, but that coliforms were not necessarily gas producers within cans. The works bacteriologist was prepared to accept this point, but stated initially that he would expect to see some liquefaction of the gelatine within the can. Howie, however, asserted that the consumer would not necessarily throw out such a can, and that coliforms were not particularly good at liquefying gelatine. At this point Borthwick interjected, and after obtaining an estimate of 100 million for the number of cans of corned beef imported to the UK

[143] 'August 24th, 1964' (CAP written evidence), NAS HH 64/228.
[144] 'Technical report', 22 September 1964, NAS HH 64/228.
[145] 'Notes of a meeting held on 21st September, 1964', PRO MH 148/200.

annually, drew attention to the possibility of even a very rare event actually occurring. This part of the transcript reads as if the Milne committee, having already made up their minds, were attempting to persuade the witnesses of the viability of their own views, rather than taking evidence.

A large proportion of the meeting was devoted to discussion of the telephone calls between Liebig's and the health and welfare department in Aberdeen, which led to MacQueen's announcement that the corned beef associated with the outbreak might have passed through the stockpile. A series of confusions and miscommunications were discussed, but Semple expressed sympathy for the difficulties that MacQueen faced. Liebig's witnesses were very much against MacQueen, not only because he had mentioned their product, but because he had dogmatically stated that the outbreak was caused by corned beef.[146]

The witnesses spent some time detailing the damage that had been done to the corned beef trade. Sales were running at about 10 per cent of those of the previous year. Liebig's had been forced to tell their factories in Africa that they could accept no more product than had already been manufactured and, as a result, the 'whole of the cattle economy in Kenya' was 'falling to pieces'. Liebig's witnesses hoped that the publication of the Milne committee's report would form the basis for the revival of the corned beef trade, and it may be that their representations prompted some remarks in the final chapter of the report, which sought to re-establish confidence in corned beef. The chapter drew attention to the dramatic fall in corned beef consumption on account of the publicity given to the Aberdeen outbreak. The financial losses of canneries, and of meat producers in countries unconnected with the outbreak, were noted. Finally, after declaring that when produced under satisfactory conditions, canned meat is among the safest foods available and a source of inexpensive first-class protein, the report concluded that if, in future, 'only water of a suitable bacteriological standard' were used in canning, it would be almost impossible for any further cans to become contaminated.[147]

Publication and reaction

The report was signed and delivered to the Secretary of State for Scotland and the Minister of Health on 19 November. Printing was expected to take three to four weeks and officials suggested a publication date during the Christmas parliamentary recess. At MAFF, however, under-secretary Hensley advised that propriety favoured publication before the recess, with a statement that the government accepted and had or would take action over the findings.[148]

---

[146] A. M. Stephen to Alsop, Steven Beck & Co, 3 July 1964, NAS HH 64/228.
[147] Milne, pp. 70–1.
[148] J. Hensley to Mr Humphreys-Davies, 19 November 1964, PRO MAF 282/96.

Deputy secretary Humphreys-Davies disagreed. Since there was little criticism of the ministries he thought that they could not 'be accused of trying to hush the thing up'. On the other hand, he observed:

> there is some severe criticism of the ridiculous antics of Dr MacQueen, springing partly from professional ignorance and partly (though it does not say so in so many words) a desire for personal aggrandisement. And some pretty strong words are said about the serious social, economic and financial consequences at home and abroad which flowed from his inept handling of the epidemic and its attendant publicity.[149]

He thought that if the report appeared just before or after Christmas, the recess would exert a 'deflationary effect', and when Parliament reconvened the Secretary of State could issue a statement.

The Scottish Office thought it unlikely that the report would attract 'lively comment', since its 'main thesis', that corned beef caused the outbreak, had been 'widely canvassed'. They agreed that the criticisms of government were weak, doubted whether the report would revive the compensation issue, and thought that the main interest would centre on MacQueen's 'handling of the publicity and his imperfect liaison with the Hospital Board and general practitioners'.[150] Opinion at the Ministry of Health, in contrast, was that if there was a news shortage the report might receive significant attention, since the outbreak had attracted interest and 'people are interested in food'. They favoured publication during the recess as 'a time when most people have other things to think about'.[151]

Winnifrith, MAFF's Permanent Secretary, informed his minister, Fred Peart (the former Labour Party spokesman on agriculture – the Labour Party having won the general election in October), that the report would appear during the recess. He advised that Peart could be 'reasonably complacent' about the minor criticisms, 'since the faults occurred at the time of the previous administration'.[152] Peart, however, minuted on 25 November that he would like to see 'positive action'.[153]

On the same day as Peart's minute, a junior Scottish Office minister stated, in response to a parliamentary question, that the report would be published before the end of the year, but possibly not before Christmas, due to printing difficulties.[154] However, on 3 December, Lady Tweedsmuir, Conservative MP for South Aberdeen, asked Willie Ross, the Secretary of State in the new

---

[149] P. Humphreys-Davies to Secretary, 20 November 1964, PRO MAF 282/96.

[150] To Secretary of State, 'Report of the Departmental Committee of Inquiry into the Outbreak of Typhoid Fever in Aberdeen' (Draft); M. K. Macdonald to Mr Lace, 16 November 1964, PRO MAF 282/96.

[151] J. A. Hauff to M. K. Macdonald, 17 November 1964, PRO MAF 282/96.

[152] A. J. D. Winnifrith to Minister, 23 November 1964, PRO MAF 282/96.

[153] E. J. G. Smith to Mr Hensley, 25 November 1964, PRO MAF 282/96.

[154] *PD(C)*, vol. 702, col. *1276* (25 November 1964).

government, for a statement, because some details of the report had appeared in the press. Ross was satisfied that the leak was not from an official source, and declined Tweedsmuir's request.[155] The news item, in the *Glasgow Herald*, claimed that the report exonerated corned beef as the source of the Aberdeen outbreak.[156] Tweedsmuir and other MPs for North-East Scotland began to lobby the government for the early release of the report, arguing that if imported corned beef was exonerated, foods produced in the area were placed under suspicion.[157] Because of the 'leak', and a ruling by the Prime Minister's office that the week between Christmas and New Year was not suitable for the release of the report, the civil servants had to set aside their preferences and rapidly prepared the necessary briefing documents for a publication date of 17 December.[158]

Ross' statement on the day of publication consisted of a written answer to a question from Hughes. He began by recording that 'in general' the government accepted the findings. He summarised the main findings and remarked that he was glad to note that when produced under proper conditions corned beef is safe and nutritious. He observed that some recommendations had been acted upon and explained that the others would be discussed with the parties concerned.[159] The press coverage was, as predicted, only transitory, even in the local press, but the newspapers highlighted the criticisms of the ministries, and defended MacQueen, to a greater extent than the officials might have imagined.

Aberdeen's *EE* greeted the report with the headline 'It's bouquets and brickbats for Dr MacQueen/He should have shut shop quickly', with MacQueen's response reported under the heading '"It is most pleasing," says city MOH'. MacQueen welcomed the conclusion that typhoid had been imported in corned beef, which 'completely exonerated' the city, but he complained that the media were outside the committee's remit, and that they had taken no evidence from 'TV, radio or pressmen' or his health education staff. He explained that for years his department's policy had been to 'take the public into our confidence and to co-operate with the media', and claimed that the publicity had contributed to the 'remarkable achievement whereby the all-clear could be given after only 28 days'.[160]

The following morning the local *P&J* led with the headline 'MacQueen hits back/"Too much publicity? – I should do same again"'. Rather than the publicity having 'unfortunate results' nationally, MacQueen claimed the results

---

[155] Ibid., vol. 703, col. *73–4* (2 December 1964).

[156] 'Corned beef not source of outbreak', *Glasgow Herald*, 26 November 1964, p. 9c.

[157] Baird to McCabe, 7 December 1964, NAS HH 64/399.

[158] T. L. Spiers to Miss Macdonald, 1 December 1964; M. A. J. Pearson, 'Revised notice of meeting', NAS HH 64/399.

[159] *PD(C)*, vol. 704, cols *131–2*.

[160] 'It's bouquets and brickbats for Dr MacQueen', '"It is most pleasing," says city MOH', *EE*, 17 December 1964, pp. 1a, 1c.

had been 'very fortunate'. Attention had been drawn to corned beef as a possible source of typhoid, which had been 'hushed up' in earlier outbreaks. In addition, he declared that the use of the media in raising food hygiene to 'something approaching perfection' was 'the big new weapon forged by the Aberdeen outbreak' which had drastically cut the period of infection compared to the other outbreaks.[161] But the newspaper also referred to other opinions. The city's director of publicity, Harry Webber, agreed with the Milne report and claimed that it was only because of his own efforts that Aberdeen had had what was, in the end, one of the best holiday seasons ever. He felt that 'a public relations expert could comfortably have avoided the world-wide publicity, without detracting from the seriousness of the situation'.[162]

The responses of Michael Noble, the former secretary of state for Scotland, were also given. Noble wished that he had overridden MacQueen's objections and sent an officer to Aberdeen at the start of the outbreak. In order to safeguard Aberdeen, he felt that MacQueen had thrown Scotland 'to the winds', and presented a picture of 'greater alarm and despondency than was justified'. But Hughes objected, arguing that if MacQueen had treated the outbreak lightly, typhoid might have spread throughout Britain.[163] A *P&J* editorial agreed that MacQueen should have closed the supermarket immediately, but thought that the criticisms regarding the publicity were 'grossly unfair'. The results should be the 'only arbiter' in assessing MacQueen's methods. *P&J* made no apology for their own role and concluded that it was 'less than generous to carp at what was, after all, merely an aptitude for the telling phrase'.[164] *EE* also defended MacQueen, declaring that they could not see how he could have handled the outbreak any more effectively.[165]

Most newspapers rejected the criticisms of MacQueen. The *Daily Mirror* described MacQueen's treatment as a 'raw deal' and the criticism of his press strategy as 'nonsense'. It was 'far more sensible than the bad old medical principle that the less you tell the patient, the better it will be'.[166] The *Sun* commented similarly that the advice to MOsH to limit themselves to press statements would reinforce the attitude that the less the public know the better. It was 'unfair and silly' that the heaviest criticisms fell upon MacQueen, because the 'real error of judgement was the failure of the Ministry of Health

---

[161] 'MacQueen hits back', *P&J*, 18 December 1964, p. 1a. MacQueen had already rehearsed these arguments in his department's *Health and Welfare* bulletin, which was also the basis for an item in the *Municipal Journal*. I. A. G. MacQueen, 'Random reflections on the outbreak', *Health and Welfare*, 1964, No. 23, pp. 1–6 (NHSA); 'Good communications helped beat typhoid', *Municipal Journal*, 1965, vol. 72, p. 2798.
[162] 'Praise from Lord Provost: criticism from Noble', *P&J*, 18 December 1964, p. 1a.
[163] Ibid.
[164] 'It's unfair to Doctor MacQueen', *P&J*, 18 December 1964, p. 6a.
[165] 'Lessons to be learned', *EE*, 18 December 1964, p. 6a.
[166] 'Doctor's dilemma', *Daily Mirror*, 18 December 1964, p. 2e.

to recall the suspect tins of corned beef'.[167] The *Daily Record* commented similarly that controversy about MacQueen's publicity should not obscure the 'main finding' that 'the failure by two ministries to have suspect stocks withdrawn was the basic reason for the outbreak'.[168] Only Glasgow's *Evening Times* supported the view that the publicity had had 'needless consequences for Aberdeen and all Scotland', although they accepted that MacQueen had 'erred on the right side in seeking publicity'.[169] Most newspapers had inside-page stories which developed criticisms of the ministries. For example, the *Daily Express*, *Glasgow Herald* and *Daily Telegraph* included articles headed 'Blunder on typhoid/Ministry error caused Aberdeen outbreak',[170] 'Ministry error in typhoid outbreak/Suspect corned beef should have been withdrawn'[171] and 'Ministry corned beef decision "mistaken"'.[172] But from 19 December onward there was little further coverage.

While the Milne report soon fell from the public eye, it was discussed in professional meetings over the next few weeks, and in the professional press. *Municipal Engineering*, a journal read largely by sanitary and public health inspectors, observed that the work of the sanitary inspectors during the Aberdeen outbreak had gone largely unnoticed by the Milne Committee. As for the publicity generated by MacQueen, the journal thought that MacQueen 'probably erred on the right side'.[173] In a later issue of the journal, H. L. Hughes, chief public health inspector for Harlow, expressed surprise that in view of the publicity given to the Harlow outbreak in 1963, doctors and the public were apparently unaware of the link that had been made between corned beef and typhoid until the publication of an article in the *BMJ* in June 1964. This implied, he thought, that 'both the public and public health department personnel either are singularly lacking in interest in current affairs or have very short memories indeed'.[174] He also observed that nothing was said in the report about the responsibility of the Ministry of Health to keep public health personnel abreast of food hygiene problems.

Aberdeen's GPs' Medical Committee resolved on 6 January 1965 that, in general, it agreed with the report. It disputed, however, the account of the initial communications between MacQueen and the GPs. According to the report, after abandoning his draft letter to GPs when the outbreak appeared in the press, MacQueen wrote to them on 24 May. The Committee pointed out, however, that 'no such letter was in fact received'. They also found that

---

[167] 'Carry on doctor!', *Sun*, 18 December 1964, p. 2g.

[168] 'The record says the experts must decide', *Daily Record*, 18 December 1964, p. 2e.

[169] 'Clean bill of health', *Evening Times*, 18 December 1964, p. 4a.

[170] 'Blunder on typhoid', *Daily Express*, 18 December 1964, p. 15a.

[171] 'Ministry error in typhoid outbreak', *Glasgow Herald*, 18 December 1964, p. 7a.

[172] 'Ministry corned beef decision "mistaken"', *Daily Telegraph*, 18 December 1964, p. 17c.

[173] 'Typhoid report', *Municipal Engineering*, 1964, vol. 141, p. 2554.

[174] H. L. Hughes, 'Typhoid outbreak showed importance of liaison', *Municipal Engineering*, 1965, vol. 141, p. 59.

'the comments made in the report on the question of publicity are not over-stated'.[175] However, Dr Beddard of the North-Eastern Regional Hospital Board found the criticisms based on his evidence too strong. He commented that the notion that it had been impossible for him to discuss the outbreak with MacQueen in the early stages was nonsense, and that he merely thought the liaison meetings should have started earlier.[176]

MacQueen used the January 1965 number of the *Medical Officer* to mount a counter-attack against the report. He contrasted the Croydon and Aberdeen enquiry findings and repeated the points about the remit of, and witnesses to, the committee. He also asserted that a committee consisting of:

a retired Civil Servant, a representative of the meat trade, an administrative bacteriologist, a housewife and an MOH of a city with notoriously poor health statistics – was obviously incompetent to consider health education and publicity.[177]

MacQueen was supported by the Scottish branch of the Society for the Medical Officers of Health. They set up a subcommittee which concluded that the report had treated MacQueen unfairly and that 'the Medical Officer of Health did his work well. It should be noted that there were very few secondary cases. Publicity played a part in this and helped to have the cases detected earlier.'[178] MacQueen continued this argument later in 1965, in his annual report for 1964,[179] and twenty years after the outbreak was still arguing that his strategy had allayed rather than created public alarm.[180]

Some support for MacQueen was expressed at a conference of the Royal Society of Health on the safety of canned food held in January 1965. The MOH of Pickering at the time of the 1955 to 1956 outbreak commented that 'if he [the MOH] had been as successful as Dr MacQueen in obtaining publicity, this Conference would have been held in 1956 instead of 1965'. He also remarked that due to the lack of publicity, the achievement of himself and his collaborators in tracing the infection to contaminated cooling water at an Argentine canning factory had met with 'official indifference'.[181]

---

[175] J. A. Birnie, 'Typhoid outbreak – the Milne report. Report by the Local Medical Committee', 6 January 1965, NHSA GRHB D6\1\17.

[176] A. M. Stephen to Milne Committee members, 3 December 1964, NAS HH 64/399.

[177] I. A. G. MacQueen, 'Reflections on the typhoid report,' *Medical Officer*, 1965, vol. 113, pp. 31–3.

[178] Society of Medical Officers of Health (Scottish Branch), Minutes of Meeting of Special Sub-committee to study report on Aberdeen typhoid outbreak, 7 January 1965, GUABRC.

[179] I. A. G. MacQueen, *Report of the Medical Officer of Health for Aberdeen for 1964*, 1965, p. 18.

[180] AULSCA, MS 3628 interview with Ian MacQueen in *A City under Siege*, a BBC radio programme broadcast on 13 April 1984.

[181] Royal Society of Health, *The safety of canned foods. Report of the Royal Society of Health Conference on the safety of canned foods*, London, 1966, pp. 144–5.

The shaping of the Milne report

In this chapter we have seen that while the Milne Committee was initially established with one main objective in mind, namely to exonerate former stockpile corned beef of blame for the outbreak, it interpreted its remit broadly and covered a wide range of issues. As more and more details of the story came to light during the days after the announcement of the committee, and as concerns were voiced about many aspects of the way that the outbreak was being handled, these all became matters for the committee to investigate. Political and public opinion demanded nothing less, and the debate about restricting the remit of the committee became irrelevant.

The 'insider' status of the secretary and chairman provided some scope for officials to privately steer the committee away from sensitive issues, such as the origins and amount of corned beef in the stockpile. Here MAFF could rely upon the well-understood and shared culture of official secrets in the interests of state security. Stephen, in particular, had a broad role in setting the agenda and steering the committee, since he made the original suggestions as to who would be called as witnesses, prepared lists of questions and summaries of evidence, and drafted the report. Of the other members of the committee, the two experts Howie and Semple played the most active and important roles.

Howie's professional interests may have prompted the inclusion of a recommendation on the establishment of a standing expert committee on the bacteriological aspects of food safety. Likewise, the recommendation about the review of the laboratory service in Scotland may have been, from Howie's point of view, a potential opportunity to extend the remit of the PHLS into Scotland. Crucially, it was probably Howie's judgement as to MacQueen's knowledge and understanding of the problems posed by a typhoid outbreak which underpinned the committee's rationale for condemning much of MacQueen's strategy, and particularly his use of the media. MacQueen's media performance was criticised by a variety of witnesses, while the testimony of local witnesses led to criticisms of his dealings with the laboratory, the Health Board and the GPs.

The ministries' carefully constructed evidence suggests that they played little part in proposing recommendations to the committee. The archival material available suggests that ideas for recommendations came from the committee members and witnesses other than the ministries, but they were tried out on later witnesses, including the ministries' representatives. The ministries appear to have played little part in developing the critique of MacQueen's performance. But there also seems to have been no effort on the part of the ministries to defend MacQueen even though, as we saw in Chapters 4 and 5, at the time of the outbreak, key personnel at the SHHD were, like MacQueen, worried about the danger of successive 'waves' of infection, and blamed the media excesses on the media rather than MacQueen.[182]

---

[182] See pp. 124–6, 128–32.

Among the officials there was at least a sense of satisfaction that while the criticisms of MacQueen were strong and evident, the criticisms of the ministries where weak and hidden. The ministries had a number of advantages. Their officials had the time and staff to prepare their evidence carefully, and, unlike MacQueen, they were also given an opportunity to comment on the draft report – comments which had the effect of softening some of the passages critical of themselves. MacQueen and his staff, in contrast, were still recovering from the outbreak and were busy with its aftermath when preparing their evidence, and were reluctant to work to the committee's timetable. There is a defensive tone to parts of MacQueen's evidence. There were some attempts by MacQueen to head off criticism in some areas by frankness about the problems he faced: but regarding relationships and communication with the laboratory and the hospital board, for example, he simply pretended that there were no problems.

The different ministries made sure that their evidence was consistent, and, after the debate about the terms of reference, appear to have maintained a united front: there was no sign of competition for departmental advantage. There seems to have been some initial tension over the membership, the concern being to safeguard the Scottish interests. But the members appointed seemed to have been quite prepared to point to English examples of good practice as possible models for Scotland. One such issue concerned the organisation of the laboratory services, as already mentioned. Another was the question of procedures adopted by the health departments when local outbreaks of infectious diseases occurred.

Howie's authority as director of the PHLS to speak on matters bacteriological appears to have been important in the committee's handling of their sessions with the manufacturers. These sessions seem to have been construed by the committee as opportunities to persuade the manufacturers of the validity of the findings they had already arrived at, based upon the testimony of expert witnesses. The industry was reluctant to be convinced that it was possible for corned beef, contaminated during cooling, to be a source of typhoid. However, as with the ministries, the report dealt very gently with the firms, including the retailer, and took on board their concerns about the economic damage caused by the publicity given to corned beef as a source of typhoid.

The passages dealing with the culpability or otherwise of the manufacturer of the corned beef associated with the Aberdeen typhoid outbreak noted, by way of mitigation, that the possible link between typhoid and corned beef manufactured using non-chlorinated water revealed by earlier outbreaks had not been well publicised. No attempt, however, was made to explore and explain why greater publicity had not occurred. Such questions, which would require consideration of matters of international politics and economics, and civil service culture and procedure, which were discussed in Chapter 2, probably would not have occurred to Stephen and his colleagues as suitable topics for the committee, even with its expanded remit. There are also other matters considered by the Milne committee, such as the inspection and improvement of the conditions in overseas meat plants and the disposal of the withdrawn suspect corned beef that we have not dealt with in this chapter, since they will be discussed in the chapters that follow.

The implementation of the Milne Committee's recommendations

The Ministry of Health took the lead in considering the response to the Milne report. From January 1965, the views of trade, local government, professional organisations and government bodies were canvassed, and the tabulated responses were discussed interdepartmentally.[183] The Ministry of Health officials then generated a briefing document for ministers, and drafted a statement for one of them to deliver in Parliament. By the autumn there had been only a few questions on various recommendations, but in view of the intense interest in the disposal of suspect stock at that time, more were expected. Officials therefore favoured placing a progress report in the parliamentary record as a point of reference for later responses. They agreed that the report would be best presented by Ross, since he had made the original statement on the Milne report, and that a written statement in response to a parliamentary question immediately prior to Christmas 1965 would minimise publicity.[184] Ross' statement was given on 22 December.[185]

Ross reported that in connection with the recommendations concerning shop hygiene, interested parties considered they could best be tackled by means of non-statutory codes of practice.[186] According to the table of responses to the consultation exercise, all organisations consulted were amenable to the idea of a new general code on handling cold cooked meats, and many expressed a willingness to help prepare one, or a wish to be consulted.[187] An early draft of the briefing document, however, suggested that a new code was probably not necessary. A code on hygiene in the retail meat trade already existed and had been published in 1959. If the guidance relating to cleanliness of surfaces and equipment, and keeping meat products at less than 50°F and away from direct sunlight, had been applied in Aberdeen, such a major outbreak would probably not have occurred.[188] However, the final draft was more favourable

---

[183] The Ministry set up a series of files on the various recommendations but most appear to have been lost or destroyed, the 'co-ordinating' file (PRO MH 148/355) being the main one surviving.

[184] *PD(C)*, vol. 705, cols *170–1* (26 January 1965), 889–90 (2 February 1965), vol. 718, col. *1002* (3 February 1965); 'Submission to ministers', to Mr Dodds, 29 October 1965; Secretary to Minister, 16 November 1965; A. F. Reid to T. E. Nodder, 1 December 1965; M. J. O. Francis, 'Action on Milne statement', 6 December 1965, PRO MH 148/355.

[185] *PD(C)*, vol. 722, cols *439–41* (22 December 1965).

[186] Ibid.

[187] 'Comments on recommendation (vi)', PRO MAF 282/87.

[188] 'Joint submission to ministers' (early draft), PRO MH 148/355.

and explained to ministers the process of consultation with interested parties and the Food Hygiene Advisory Council that would be involved in the preparation of a new code.[189]

The Milne Committee's recommendation specifically on detergents and sterilisers was that these cleaning agents should be subject to approval by the central health authorities. According to the briefing document, although the trade was amenable to this idea in principle, the proposal would be impractical, since detailed instructions on methods of use for different purposes would also have to be included.[190] The tabulated responses show that some professional organisations such as the BMA supported the recommendation, but the Association of Public Health Inspectors pointed out the need for additional guidance. The British National Committee on Surface Active Agents also highlighted the complexity of cleaning and sterilising operations, and argued that an approved list of detergents was impractical. Several organisations representing food manufacturing were content for an approved list of cleaning agents to be applied to retailers but felt that manufacturers should be free to develop their own methods. The National Association of Multiple Grocers thought that the cleaning agents already on MAFF's approved list for the dairy industry should be used as the basis of a list for other food businesses, and the PHLS made a similar point. If a new list was constructed, the 'necessary bacteriological testing' would be a 'formidable undertaking' and 'obtaining agreement on testing methods would be difficult and time-consuming'.[191] However, the Aberdeen typhoid outbreak and the Milne report did stimulate some research at the PHLS on methods of cleaning slicing machines, carving knives and surfaces, which was published from 1968 to 1970.[192]

The Milne Committee also proposed that a maximum temperature of 40°F for the display of cold cooked meat should be embodied in statutory regulations, but acknowledged that this would present practical difficulties. According to the briefing document, there was opposition to the recommendation from the trade because of the difficulties that would be created for small shops, especially those in rural districts. The officials therefore suggested that, as a first step, 50°F should be laid down in a code of practice. They described this temperature as 'acceptable for the protection of public health in the present circumstances'. It was a temperature that could be maintained without

---

189 'Joint submission to ministers', PRO MH 148/355.

190 Ibid.

191 'Comments on recommendation (x)', PRO MAF 282/87.

192 R. J. Gilbert and I. M. Maurer, 'The hygiene of slicing machines, carving knives and can-openers', *Journal of Hygiene*, 1968, vol. 66, pp. 439–50; R. J. Gilbert, 'Cross contamination by cooked-meat slicing machines and cleaning cloths', *Journal of Hygiene*, 1969, vol. 67, pp. 449–53; R. J. Gilbert, 'Comparison of materials used for cleaning equipment in retail food premises, and of two methods for the enumeration of bacteria on cleaned equipment and work surfaces', *Journal of Hygiene*, 1970, vol. 68, pp. 221–32.

refrigeration.[193] However, the tabulated responses to the consultation exercise show that the PHLS and all the professional associations supported the 40°F recommendation. The Association of Public Health Inspectors argued that it should be extended to 'other vital states of storage and distribution' and introduced without delay. But strong opposition came from the Parliamentary Committee of the Co-operative Union, which pointed out that the 40°F standard would mean that cold meat would have to be displayed in a refrigerated cabinet, and this would 'lead to an appreciable reduction in the number of sales outlets'. As far as the committee was aware, 50°F was a satisfactory standard. The food manufacturers' organisations raised similar objections and the National Association of Multiple Grocers found the recommendation too 'sweeping'.[194]

The problems surrounding the cleaning of slicing machines and use of cleaning agents were discussed in the CMO's reports for 1965 and 1967,[195] and guidance on the handling of cold meats was eventually published in a new voluntary code of practice, *Hygiene in the Meat Trades*, in 1969. This code covered two areas, the first being the retail trade, including cold cooked meat and meat delicatessen, the second being the transport of meat and meat products. Guidelines were included on the cleaning of surfaces, equipment and machinery, and how to avoid cross-contamination. In particular, the code called for 'wider recognition of the fact that cold cooked meats, uncooked cured meats and raw meats present a hazard of contamination one to another and should therefore be handled in complete separation'.[196] The code advised that it was 'preferable to use refrigerated display cabinets' for cold cooked meats in which the temperature was maintained at 40°F or below. However, the code stated later that windows used to display cold cooked meats 'should be refrigerated so that all the products displayed are held at a temperature below 50°F', and that display cabinets 'should be capable of holding the foods at a temperature below 50°F'.[197] Revised Food Hygiene (General) Regulations, issued in 1970 after consultations with the trade, made no changes to the statutory requirements on temperature control. Foods were to be brought below 50°F upon arrival at food premises. However, this did not apply to food exposed for sale, or food kept for the replenishment of food exposed for sale.[198] This was hardly what the Milne Committee had in mind.

Ross' statement noted that the Milne Committee's recommendation that

---

[193] 'Joint submission to ministers', PRO MH 148/355.

[194] 'Comments on recommendation (x)', PRO MAF 282/87.

[195] *RCMO 1965*, pp. 130–1; *RCMO 1967*, pp. 136–8.

[196] *RCMO 1969*, p. 126.

[197] Department of Health and Social Security, Ministry of Agriculture, Fisheries and Food, Welsh Office, *Hygiene in the Meat Trades*, London, 1969, pp. 15, 25.

[198] Food Hygiene (General Regulations) 1970, *Statutory Instruments 1970*, part II, section 2, London, 1970, pp. 3940–55, at pp. 3949–50.

training for food operatives in food hygiene should be examined with a view to improvement had been referred to the Food Hygiene Advisory Councils.[199] But numbers attending courses in food hygiene for the Royal Society of Health examinations at twenty-one colleges in England and Wales were already buoyant during 1964 and 1965, perhaps in view of the climate of opinion generated by the typhoid outbreaks.[200] The report of the council for England and Wales, which was published in February 1966, pointed out that family and sporadic outbreaks had shown a less marked decline than general food poisoning incidents and placed greatest emphasis on public apathy as the main cause of poor food hygiene. Four of the recommendations simply covered the intensification of existing food hygiene education. The others favoured the organisation of a meeting with trade organisations to discuss the enhancement of food hygiene education and publicity, and the preparation of short codes of practice, one for the trade and one for the public.[201] Meetings were subsequently held in October 1966 with representatives of national trade and women's organisations to discuss 'ways of stimulating and maintaining public interest in food hygiene'.[202] In 1967 two ten-point codes were approved by the Council, one for workers and one for housewives, and published by the Central Council for Health Education. The codes covered such points as hand-washing before and not smoking while handling food, the need to reheat leftovers thoroughly, and to keep the lid on the dustbin.[203]

In Scotland, the enhancement of food hygiene education appears to have been tackled, for a time, with considerable enthusiasm. The SHHD report for 1966 explicitly linked new initiatives to raise awareness of food hygiene with the Aberdeen typhoid outbreak:

> Every effort has been made to maintain the concern for the improvement in food hygiene which received such a powerful stimulus at the time of the Aberdeen outbreak. There is evidence that this interest has been maintained.[204]

A similar comment was included in the report for 1967.[205] The Scottish Food Hygiene Advisory Council suggested that in view of the shortage of sanitary inspectors, domestic scientists might be recruited to help educate food trade

---

[199] *PD(C)*, vol. 722, cols 439–41 (22 December 1965)

[200] 'RSH food hygiene courses are playing a vital role', *Municipal Engineering*, 1965, vol. 142, p. 1385.

[201] Food Hygiene Advisory Council, 'Food Hygiene Education and Publicity Report to the Minister of Health', *Monthly Bulletin of the Ministry of Health and Public Health Laboratory Service*, 1966, vol. 25, pp. 31–3; B. D. Allen, 'Ideas and action are needed to get this message across', *Municipal Engineering*, 1966, vol. 143, p. 773.

[202] *RMH 1966*, p. 66.

[203] *RMH 1967*, p. 67; 'Codes of housewives and food-handlers', *Municipal Engineering*, 1967, vol. 144, p. 409.

[204] *RSHHD 1966*, p. 9.

[205] *RSHHD 1967*, p. 11.

staff in food hygiene, and some local authorities made such appointments. Conferences for domestic science teachers interested in intensifying food hygiene education in schools were held in Scotland's major cities.[206] Courses were also held for sanitary inspectors, and caterers, including hospital caterers, involving the Royal Sanitary Association for Scotland, and the Royal Institute of Public Health and Hygiene, higher education institutions and local authorities.[207] However, even in Scotland the efforts to improve the training of food workers in food hygiene appear transitory. The SHHD report for 1970 only mentioned a course for sanitary inspectors,[208] and the Food Hygiene (General) Regulations 1970 (which applied to England and Wales) included no provisions relating to training.[209]

As for the recommendations that MOsH should be given powers to examine persons who might reasonably be suspected of carrying infectious diseases, Ross reported that legislation would be introduced.[210] The briefing document explained to ministers the existing gap in the law, and referred to forthcoming legislation in which an appropriate clause might be included.[211] The tabulated comments show that all those consulted favoured the proposal, but some made additional suggestions, for example, that exclusion of suspected carriers from the workplace and compensation for such persons should be included. Ross' promise for a change in the law was fulfilled in England and Wales by the Public Health (Infectious Diseases) Regulations 1968.[212] As regards the recommended enhancement of the powers of MOsH to close premises, the briefing document explained that while trade bodies, local authorities and professional associations favoured the proposal, there was little evidence of MOsH finding their powers inadequate. Existing powers to deal with suspect food and to order the closure of premises for disinfection were considered sufficient.[213] But the main reason why officials opposed statutory powers was to avoid the question of compensation, which was raised by the trade organisations during the consultation exercise. The Association of Public Health Inspectors again argued for additional action beyond the Milne committee's recommendation. They wanted the power to disqualify proprietors from operating food premises to also be available.[214]

---

[206] *RSHHD 1965*, p. 92; *RSHHD 1966*, p. 100; *RSHHD 1967*, p. 111.

[207] *RSHHD 1966*, p. 100; *RSHHD 1967*, pp. 110–11; *RSHHD 1968*, p. 11; *RSHHD 1969*, p. 19.

[208] *RSHHD 1970*, p. 21.

[209] Food Hygiene (General Regulations) 1970, *Statutory Instruments 1970*, part II, section, 2, London, 1970, pp. 3940–55.

[210] *PD(C)*, vol. 722, cols 439–41 (22 December 1965).

[211] 'Joint submission to ministers', PRO MH 148/355.

[212] Public Health (Infectious Diseases) Regulations, 1968, *Statutory Instruments 1968*, part II, section 2, pp. 3800–11, at pp. 3808–9.

[213] 'Joint submission to ministers', PRO MH 148/355.

[214] R. Hillenbrand to Mrs Pearson, 17 March 1965, PRO MH 148/355; 'Comments on recommendation (x)', PRO MAF 282/87.

On the recommendation that persons engaged in food handling should be obliged to declare whether they had suffered from a gastro-intestinal infection, Ross intimated that this was not considered practical.[215] The briefing document explained that the phrase 'gastro-intestinal infection' was vague and, in any case, under existing regulations employees were already obliged to inform their employer if they were suffering from or carrying a *Salmonella* or staphylococcal infection.[216] However, Ross endorsed the intention of the recommendation, and approved of voluntary screening as already practised by some larger employers. Ross also stated that the recommendation that powers should be introduced allowing for the compulsory withdrawal of suspect food already distributed had been considered, but it had been decided to continue to rely upon voluntary methods.[217] According to the briefing document the trade had not been consulted on this because they could be expected to support the recommendation if compensation was payable, but otherwise to oppose it. Officials expected the trade to continue to accept their responsibilities as in the past, but in the event of their refusing to respond to a request to withdraw stock, 'Departments could almost certainly achieve the desired effect by publicly advising medical officers of health of details of the stock which it was advised should be withdrawn, or by alerting the public to a hazard from the particular food'.[218]

Finally, on the recommendation on the possible reorganisation of the Scottish laboratory services, Ross stated that he had reached the view that the present organisation was most suitable. However, in order to ensure that the service was seen to be available to all users, a subcommittee of the Standing Advisory Committee on Laboratory Services had been established.[219] The briefing document explained that the subcommittee would encourage interaction between the laboratories, invite MOsH to participate in periodical meetings, and report on the preparation of collected periodic epidemiological reports.[220] This led to the publication of *Communicable Diseases Weekly Report* from 1967 and the establishment of the Communicable Disease (Scotland) Unit (CDSU) at Ruchill Infectious Diseases Hospital, Glasgow, in 1969. Initially administered by the Western Regional Hospital Board, the unit was transferred to the Common Services Agency with the NHS reorganisation in 1974. The staff originally consisted of one consultant and two administrative staff, but during the 1980s an interdisciplinary team began to be established. By 1994, when the CDSU merged with the Environmental Health (Scotland) Unit to form the Scottish Centre for Infection and Environmental Health,

[215] *PD(C)*, vol. 722, cols 439–41 (22 December 1965).
[216] 'Joint submission to ministers', PRO MH 148/355.
[217] *PD(C)*, vol. 722, cols 439–41 (22 December 1965).
[218] 'Joint submission to ministers', PRO MH 148/355.
[219] *PD(C)*, vol. 722, cols 439–41 (22 December 1965).
[220] 'Joint submission to ministers', PRO MH 148/355.

the professional staff included nine doctors, two environmental health officers and a veterinarian.[221]

On the evidence presented thus far, the typhoid outbreaks of 1963 to 1964 clearly had some impact upon food safety policy making, but there is no evidence of any wholesale changes in approach. In particular, it seems that officials were very willing to take account of the views of industry bodies and to disregard the views of professional bodies such as the Association of Public Health Inspectors, which reduced the impact of the Milne Committee's proposals. The strategy of Ross delivering the progress report on the Milne recommendations immediately prior to Christmas 1965 proved effective. Apart from questions concerning the disposal of suspect stock, MPs and the press took little further interest in the detail of the implementation of the recommendations. During January 1966 there was only one parliamentary question on hygiene education.[222] The Ministry of Health press office returned the notes that had been prepared for them, reporting that they had not been needed.[223]

[221] D. Reid, 'The Scottish Centre for Infection and Environmental Health', in *RSSH 1994*, pp. 74–9.
[222] *PD(C)*, vol. 723, cols 42–3 (25 January 1966).
[223] Mr Harding to Mrs Pearson, 12 January 1966, PRO MH 148/355.

7

The recommendation on the inspection of overseas meat plants

The roles of existing policy agendas, and interdepartmental and inter-professional tensions

Introduction

Three recommendations in the Milne report concerned the system whereby Britain protected itself against the importation of human disease in meat and meat products. One suggested the development of an international inspectorate, and Willie Ross, Secretary of State for Scotland, reported in December 1965 that further consideration of this would await a report on meat and meat products by the WHO/FAO Codex Alimentarius Commission.[1] The briefing document that the officials prepared for ministers showed that while they were happy for the commission to develop international standards, they were sceptical about, and uninterested in, the possibility of its replacing national inspectorates.[2] Subsequently, overseas meat inspection did not evolve in the direction envisaged by the Milne Committee. Instead, the inspection of meat plants exporting to Britain, and other members of the European Community, has been transferred to the European Commission Food and Veterinary Office.[3]

The second recommendation concerned the point at which responsibility for the safety of foreign meat and meat products passed from MAFF to the Ministry of Health. While legally MAFF and the Ministry of Health were jointly responsible, in practice MAFF inspected foreign meat plants and granted 'official certificates', and handed responsibility to the Ministry of Health only after the process of importation, including the inspection of consignments by port health authorities, was complete. The Milne Committee,

---

[1] *PD(C)*, vol. 722, cols 339–441 (22 December 1965).

[2] 'Joint Submission to Ministers Recommendations of the committee with notes of action taken or proposed', PRO HH 148/355.

[3] FAO Information Division, 'Understanding The Codex Alimentarius', internet http://www.fao.org/docrep/w9114e/W9114e00.htm, accessed 31 March 2004; European Commission, Food and Veterinary Office, internet http://europa.eu.int/comm/food/fs/inspections/index_en.html, accessed 31 March 2004.

however, suggested that the Ministry of Health should be responsible from the point of unloading. Making this adjustment proved relatively unproblematic. By the time of Ross' December 1965 statement, it had been agreed that at the point of importation MAFF would only remain responsible for questions regarding the authenticity of official certificates.[4]

This chapter will concentrate, however, upon the recommendation which concerned the number and qualification of those involved in the overseas inspections, the first part of which was already implemented by the time the Milne report was published. As Ross observed in his statement on 17 December 1964, two additional veterinary officers had been assigned to the work,[5] which was formerly undertaken only by Leo Grace, the chief technical adviser on meat inspection, and Roger Blamire, his deputy. But implementation of the other part of the recommendation, namely that the inspection team should include a medical officer, especially when a country first applied for an official certificate, proved altogether more problematic.[6] An analysis of the process of implementation of this recommendation will form the main substance of this chapter. At the time of Ross' statement of December 1964, the issue was still the subject of discussion between MAFF and the Ministry of Health, and consensus had yet to emerge. It will be shown that existing professional differences and policy preferences between the departments, the resolution of which also involved the Treasury, as well as fear of adverse publicity, were important factors conditioning the decision-making process.

The origins and reception of the recommendation for medical involvement in overseas meat inspection

Following the 1963 outbreaks, MAFF began to plan an expansion of their overseas meat inspection programme and these plans were well advanced by mid-June 1964, when they were reviewed in a memorandum by Ken Bird, chief executive officer of MAFF's Food Standards, Hygiene and Slaughterhouse Policy division. According to Bird, in 1962 eighteen countries had each sent more than 1000 tons of canned meat to Britain and sixteen others sent smaller quantities, but the great majority of these countries had not been visited within the past five years. With the additional two experienced officers who had been appointed, all the slaughterhouses and canneries could be covered in two

---

[4] *PD(C)*, vol. 722, cols *439–41* (22 December 1965); 'Joint submission to ministers', PRO MH 148/355; K. A. Bird to R. Hillenbrand, 26 August 1965, PRO MAF 148/335; Scottish Home and Health Department, *The Aberdeen Typhoid Outbreak*, Edinburgh, 1964 (Milne report), p. 33.
[5] *PD(C)*, vol. 704, cols *131–2* (17 December 1964).
[6] Milne, pp. 7–8.

years.[7] A programme was drawn up and approved by the Minister by early September.[8] Soon, however, the possibility of a medical officer joining the visits would be under discussion, following the Milne Committee's recommendation.

The origins of the recommendation for medical involvement in overseas meat inspection are unclear, although, as we noted in Chapter 6, Ian Sutherland of the SHHD remarked on 8 June that the recent emphasis upon chlorination of meat plant water had arisen from the opinion of 'a veterinary officer who did not . . . have the support of a public health officer and a water engineer'.[9] Sutherland later expressed concern that if asked for an opinion by the Milne Committee, he might be driven to make comments that 'could be interpreted as an implied or even direct criticism of professional colleagues and others in a sister department'.[10] It may be that, despite his misgivings, Sutherland did air his views, and that the implication that a medical officer might be involved, in future, in the official certification procedure appealed to the committee.

There is no evidence to suggest that the Ministry of Health was enthusiastic about this idea during the preparation of the report, such as might suggest that their officials were the source of the recommendation. Some comments on a draft of the report, dictated at the beginning of November by Sir George Godber, the CMO, display ambivalence about what could be achieved by inspections of foreign canning establishments. Godber remarked that the passage of the report on this matter had been written as if such inspections were 'a real insurance against unhygienic inspection methods'. In his view, such inspections could only provide a 'commentary on the way in which the inspectors of the country of origin do their work'.[11]

Within MAFF, the Milne report's comments and recommendations on overseas inspection were under discussion by early October. Animal Health division II (until recently part of the Food Standards, Hygiene and Slaughterhouse Policy division), which was responsible for the overseas inspections, explained in a memorandum that Grace and Blamire were also concerned with home meat inspection and slaughterhouse hygiene. In recent years the latter work had taken priority, and overseas visits had been confined mainly to countries that had applied to export meat to Britain for the first time. As for the necessity or otherwise of implementing the proposal that overseas visits

[7] K. A. Bird to G. O. Lace, 'Imported Meat and Meat Products', 16 June 1964, PRO MAF 282/90.

[8] A. J. D. Winnifrith to Minister, 25 August 1964; K. A. Bird to Mr Kelsey, 1 September 1964, PRO MAF 282/89.

[9] I. N. Sutherland to Deputy CMO, 8 June 1964, NAS HH 58/160. See also p. 167.

[10] I. N. Sutherland to J. Smith, 2 July 1964, NAS HH 58/352.

[11] 'CMO's dictated comments on seeing first draft of the Milne Report, 3rd November', PRO MH 148/355.

should include a medical officer, this would depend on the Ministry of Health's attitude:

> If the Ministry of Health are in favour of implementing this recommendation, as they can be expected to be, it would be impossible to oppose it, since even the most stringent precautions cannot be entirely secure for all time and failure to take the committee's recommendation would leave the minister without defence, if despite sound precautions, a further connection between imported canned meat and disease should be established in the future.[12]

When the full draft report was made available for comment, MAFF objected to the paragraph concerning the activities of veterinary officers. The draft stated that while the primary concern of veterinary officers was to prevent the importation of animal diseases, 'an equal if not greater regard must be paid to the human health aspects'.[13] This was a reference to the role of the veterinary attaché to the British Embassy in Buenos Aires in monitoring animal health problems, especially foot-and-mouth disease. MAFF officials felt that the committee had conflated the veterinary attaché's role with the public health concerns of the veterinary meat inspectors who were sent periodically from Britain.[14] In response to MAFF's representations, a redraft of the paragraph placed greater emphasis upon the continuing importance of protection against animal diseases, before observing 'that in the light of recent experience there is now a need for intensifying measures to safeguard human health'. The original draft went on to suggest the involvement of medical officers in inspections of meat plants as follows:

> It appears to us . . . that in the field of hygiene, requiring as it does a comprehensive knowledge of bacteriology and having its basis in preventative medicine, someone with a medical training is required to oversee this part of the inspecting team's duties.[15]

The emphasis on medical and bacteriological training suggests, perhaps, that whatever the origins of the recommendation, it probably appealed to Semple and Howie. But the substitution agreed after MAFF's representations, which appeared in the final published report, conveyed an entirely different point:

[12] 'Aberdeen typhoid outbreak report of the Milne Committee', 10 October 1964, PRO MAF 282/97.

[13] Draft copy of the Milne report with alterations agreed by David Milne and members of the committee, 3 November 1964, PRO MAF 282/96.

[14] 'Milne report note of points to be taken up with Sir David Milne'; G. O. Lace to Mr Hensley, 2 November 1964, PRO MAF 282/96.

[15] Draft copy of the Milne report with alterations agreed by David Milne and members of the committee, 3 November 1964, PRO MAF 282/96.

the course for the Diploma in Veterinary State Medicine, which the Minister's Advisers hold . . . [provides] a full grounding in Bacteriology, particularly in relation to food hygiene, similar to the specialised instruction which a medical graduate undergoes if he takes the Diploma in Public Health. We think nevertheless that there might be an advantage in medical participation in the duties of the inspection team.[16]

This conceded the recommendation, but safeguarded the sensibilities of MAFF's veterinary officers.

MAFF, Ministry of Health and SHHD officials met on 24 November to discuss the report and action required in preparation for its publication. The Minutes suggest no conflict on the question of medical involvement in overseas inspections at this stage, and merely record that senior medical officer Dr John Ross undertook to obtain the CMO's view.[17] But at MAFF it soon became clear that the veterinarians, lay officials, and even the Minister were sceptical about the involvement of doctors.[18] During the final preparations for publication of the report, MAFF commented to the Ministry of Health that since the notion that 'veterinary officers were not so well trained in bacteriology as medical officers' had been eliminated, there was now no supporting argument for medical participation in inspections. MAFF would therefore have to consider the recommendation very carefully before accepting it.[19]

On 10 December, at an interdepartmental meeting that aimed to provide advice to ministers as to how to respond to the report, there was no agreement as to whether it was desirable for a medical officer to join the overseas inspections. It was decided to advise ministers to state, if questioned, merely that this recommendation was under consideration.[20] This was the line adopted in a briefing paper, agreed jointly between the departments, which also stated, along the lines of Godber's view, that the committee had failed to take on board the point that overseas inspections could not offer a complete safeguard. The document told ministers that the inspections were 'in the first instance to explain our hygienic requirements and thereafter there is a check on the standard of inspection carried out in the country of origin'.[21]

The general media showed no interest in the recommendation, while the *Lancet*, in a leading article on 2 January 1965, which pointed to the failure of past overseas inspections, made no attempt to reinforce the recommendation

---

[16] Milne, p. 40.

[17] 'Note of a meeting held on 24th November at the Ministry of Health', PRO MAF 282/97.

[18] E. J. G. Smith to Mr Hensley, 30 November 1964, PRO MAF 282/96.

[19] G. O. Lace to J. Hensley, 7 December 1964, PRO MAF 282/97.

[20] J. Hauff to G. O. Lace, 5 January 1965, PRO MAF 282/97.

[21] Joint submission to ministers, 'Recommendations of the committee with notes on the action proposed', PRO MH 148/355.

for medical involvement.[22] In contrast, there were immediate signs of resistance within the veterinary profession to the suggestion that medical personnel might encroach upon the responsibilities of its members. The President of the British Veterinary Association, D. F. Oliver, wrote to *The Times* about the matter, commenting that the Milne Committee had failed to accord sufficient credit for Grace's achievement in discovering and reporting that Argentine Establishment 1A had been using unchlorinated river water. He further argued that the number of veterinary inspectors needed to be increased, since they were 'the best qualified to safeguard our imported meat supplies . . . having the long experience and specialised knowledge'.[23] The *Veterinary Record* continued and broadened the argument, by bringing in questions about the control of home meat inspection in an editorial at the beginning of January 1965:

> What must be criticised is the system under which the inspection of meat and meat products remains – in this country almost alone in the western world – primarily a medical and not a veterinary matter. The minds of successive Governments have remained obstinately closed on the subject, and here it appears again as misconceived as ever. In making its recommendation about the inclusion of a medical officer in future overseas inspection teams the Report gives no reason; it does not suggest what part the medical officer could usefully play, nor how the Chief Adviser's survey could have been improved by medical advice.[24]

These remarks point to the professional issues at stake. Within MAFF, K. A. Bird, chief executive officer of Animal Health division II, commented to assistant secretary G. O. Lace that the *Veterinary Record* editorial seemed to 'herald a lively interest in future meat inspection arrangements on the part of the profession', while the letter in *The Times* indicated that the recommendation for medical involvement in overseas meat inspection would arouse 'keen professional opposition'.[25] Mixed up with these professional issues were questions concerning the division of responsibilities between ministries, as we will see in the following section.

Professional and departmental issues

The *Veterinary Record*'s reaction to the Milne Committee's recommendation is connected to a long-term campaign by the veterinary profession in Britain for the creation of a centralised meat inspection service under veterinary

<hr>

22 'Typhoid: neglect and action', *Lancet*, 1965, vol. 1, pp. 36–7.
23 D. F. Oliver, 'Meat inspection', *The Times*, 29 December 1964.
24 'The Aberdeen typhoid outbreak', *Veterinary Record*, 1965, vol. 77, p. 3.
25 K. A. Bird to G. O. Lace, 4 January 1965, PRO MAF 282/97.

control.[26] In Britain, in contrast to the state veterinary meat inspection services in Europe, meat inspection was the responsibility of local authority public health departments, and under the control of medical officers of health. In Scotland, where there were relatively few large slaughterhouses, meat inspection was generally supervised by veterinarians employed by public health departments. In England and Wales, in contrast, where there were many more small slaughterhouses, a similar arrangement pertained in very few areas. In most local authorities, meat inspection was supervised directly by the medical officer of health, and carried out by public health inspectors (formerly sanitary inspectors) who had taken a special qualification.

MAFF and the Ministry of Health were formally jointly responsible for the slaughterhouse hygiene and meat inspection regulations. As we have seen, home slaughterhouse hygiene and meat inspection occupied part of the time of the two technical advisers on meat inspection, but there was very little involvement of other MAFF veterinary staff. Only in the inspection of overseas meat plants exporting to Britain had British veterinarians achieved a leading position in a public health function, under the system established within the Public Health (Imported Food) Regulations, 1948, and following the report of the Interdepartmental Committee on Meat Inspection in 1951. Since the merger of the Ministry of Agriculture and Fisheries and the Ministry of Food to form MAFF in 1955, recognition of the official certificates for the import of meat and meat products had been the responsibility of MAFF veterinary officers. Grace was certainly aware of and determined to protect the small and specialised niche he occupied on behalf of the veterinary profession from alternative claims to expertise. In Chapter 2, we saw that during the preparations for his trip to South America following the 1963 typhoid outbreaks, he reacted angrily to the suggestion that he might be accompanied by a canning expert.[27]

Besides the determination of MAFF veterinarians to protect their position, the implementation of the Milne Committee's recommendation was influenced by two recent policy review exercises that dealt with aspects of meat hygiene and inspection. These raised questions of divisions of responsibility between departments, especially the Ministry of Health and MAFF. The first was the Committee of Enquiry into Fatstock and Carcase Meat Marketing and Distribution, which had been appointed in 1962, and reported in February

---

[26] P. A. Koolmees, 'The development of veterinary public health in Western Europe, 1850–1940', *Sartoniana*, 1999, vol. 12, pp. 153–79; P. A. Koolmees, J. R. Fisher and R. Perren, 'The traditional responsibility of veterinarians in meat production and meat inspection', in F. J. M. Smulders (ed.), *Veterinary Aspects of Meat Production, Processing and Inspection. An Update of Recent Developments in Europe*, Utrecht, 1999, pp. 7–31; C. W. Schwabe, *Veterinary Medicine and Human Health* (3rd edn), Baltimore, MD, 1984; J. Swabe, *Animals, Disease and Human Society: Human–Animal Relations and the Rise of Veterinary Medicine*, London, 1999.
[27] See p. 54.

1964. This committee, chaired by Sir William Verdon-Smith, consisted mainly of businessmen and academic economists, and recommended the establishment of a fatstock meat authority with a wide range of functions.[28] These functions were to include the development and operation of a central meat inspection service that would carry out ante- and post-mortem inspection throughout the country. This proposal was intended to improve standards in England and Wales in particular, where there was little ante-mortem inspection, and some meat also escaped post-mortem inspection. In October 1963, new meat inspection regulations had already been introduced in England and Wales which allowed the local authorities to charge for their services, and which were intended to secure 100 per cent post-mortem inspection within two years.[29]

The other exercise was an internal working party of civil servants, the Lees working party, chaired by Mr Stanley Lees, director of organisation and methods at the Treasury, which was formed at around the same time as the Aberdeen typhoid outbreak. It was appointed by the Treasury to investigate the division of responsibilities regarding food hygiene and related matters, as part of a review of the machinery of government that the Conservative government had instituted in 1962. Since January 1964 the Treasury had been investigating the 'Social Service Departments', which included MAFF and the Ministry of Health.[30] Its intention was to make proposals to streamline government and to make the division of responsibilities under the Imported Food Regulations, the Food and Drugs Act (1955), and other legislation, more logical and economical. The transfer of functions between departments had long been part of the process of government in Britain, especially since the Second World War. There had been 142 transfers into or out of departments between 1946 and 1963, and agriculture ranked third in the frequency of shifting responsibilities, due to its complex relation with other ministries.[31]

The Permanent Secretary of the Ministry of Health, Sir Bruce Fraser, favoured the review that Lees was charged with, submitting a memorandum to the Machinery of Government Committee which stated that the present division of responsibilities was inefficient. He claimed that there was a 'strong case for a complete review of functions on some rational basis, e.g. so as to give Health a clear responsibility for food safety and hygiene and nutrition, and Agriculture a clear responsibility for production, supply, labelling etc'.[32]

---

[28] Ministry of Agriculture, Fisheries and Food, *Fatstock and Carcase Meat Marketing*, London, 1964.

[29] The Meat Inspection Regulations, 1963, SI No. 1229.

[30] See PRO CAB 21/5081–2, Re-organisation of machinery of government, 1962–1964, and T 277/1371–4, Committee on Machinery of Government Social Service Departments, January to December 1964.

[31] R. Rose, *Ministers and Ministries A Functional Analysis*, Oxford, 1987, pp. 45–52.

[32] 'Memorandum by the Permanent Secretary, Ministry of Health', 10 April 1964, PRO MAF 260/356.

But this was not the view of many within MAFF. One MAFF official, looking ahead to the future creation of a centralised veterinarian-led meat inspection service, thought that MAFF's veterinarians would be able to take such an initiative in their stride, but claimed that if the Ministry of Health assumed the responsibility they would have to develop their own competing veterinary service.[33] In June, the Meat Hygiene and Slaughterhouse Branch of MAFF's Food Standards, Hygiene and Slaughterhouse Policy division prepared a memorandum in connection with the Lees working party, discussing their responsibilities in the field of food hygiene, including their shared responsibilities with the Ministry of Health, such as the making of meat inspection and slaughterhouse hygiene regulations. The paper favoured the preservation of the status quo, arguing that any changes would be no more logical than the current system. As for overseas meat inspection and the official certificate procedure, the document argued that there were advantages to retaining this within the same ministry as was responsible for the parallel animal health precautions.[34]

Nevertheless, the Lees working party sought to create a clear-cut division, with all hygiene and public health matters being transferred to the Ministry of Health. Some senior MAFF officials were sympathetic towards making such adjustments, including Deputy Secretary Peter Humphreys-Davies,[35] and the Permanent Secretary Sir John Winnifrith. Winnifrith remarked in July that he had no doubt that MAFF:

> should agree that responsibility for the hygiene of imported meat and meat products should go . . . to the Ministry of Health, with such veterinary assistance and advice as the Ministry of Health need being provided by our veterinary establishment.[36]

However, as regards home-killed meat, Winnifrith wanted to reserve judgement in view of the consideration that needed to be given to the Verdon-Smith recommendation for a centralised meat inspection service. While MAFF was opposed to a meat inspection service connected to a meat commission, a body which would aim to further the interests of the meat trade, Winnifrith thought that so long as there was:

> any possibility of such an organisation with a strong element of vets supervising . . . it would be madness to transfer responsibility to the Ministry of Health. The fact is that this department alone has the necessary nucleus of full-time and part-time staff up and down the country.[37]

[33] J. G. Carnochan to Mr Hensley, 23 April 1964, PRO MAF 282/95.
[34] Meat Hygiene and Slaughterhouse Policy Branch, June 1964, PRO MAF 260/356.
[35] P. Humphreys-Davies to Secretary, 17 July 1964, PRO MAF 260/356.
[36] A. J. D. Winnifrith to P. Humphreys-Davies, 21 July 1964, PRO MAF 260/356.
[37] Ibid.

The report of the Lees working party was completed in August and recommended that the certification and inspection of overseas meat plants should become the responsibility of the Ministry of Health, but should be carried out on their behalf by MAFF veterinary officers. The report went on to state, however, that the final decision should be deferred until policy for home meat inspection was settled.[38]

A meeting held at the Treasury on 15 September to discuss the report was attended by Winnifrith, Fraser, Lees, and Sir Phillip Allen, the second Secretary at the Treasury. The Minutes suggest that Winnifrith was still reserving judgement on home meat inspection but actively seeking to shed his department's overseas responsibility, while the Ministry of Health was attempting to use the latter position as a lever for acquiring both responsibilities:

> The Ministry of Health did not think that departmental responsibility for overseas meat inspection should be transferred to them ... if the responsibility for inspection at home were not transferred. The Ministry of Agriculture, on the other hand, considered the two jobs were essentially different. Overseas it was a question of supervising a factory process, and this involved medical rather than veterinary skills.[39]

This view of overseas inspection as a medical job was soon under challenge within MAFF. Under-secretary John Hensley minuted to Humphreys-Davies that it seemed to him the discussion had become muddled. No department could be responsible for overseas meat inspection as such – rather the issue was one of responsibility for the hygiene of imported meat which included checking the standard of hygiene at overseas meat plants. This was as much a veterinary as a medical task, the inspection of meat plants relying on knowledge of bacteriology common to both professions. Furthermore,

> Veterinary experience is better background to this side of the work than medical experience, and there can be little doubt that veterinarians are more acceptable to overseas countries in this work than doctors would be. Naturally, there is a strong medical interest in the work, but I do not think that we could recommend that doctors should do it. The reason why we thought that the Ministry of Health could take over the responsibility was not that we thought the work was medical but that we thought that our veterinarians could advise the Ministry of Health on it in the same way as their doctors at present advise us.[40]

---

38 Report of the Working Party on Departmental Responsibility for Food Hygiene and related matters, 25 August 1964, PRO MAF 260/356.

39 'Note of a meeting held in Sir Phillip Allen's room', 16 September 1964, PRO MAF 282/95.

40 J. Hensley to Mr Humphreys-Davies, 7 October 1964, PRO MAF 282/95.

Hensley's Minute accompanied a paper on the future of meat inspection that he had prepared for Winnifrith. This assumed that neither the Verdon-Smith proposal for a meat inspection service attached to a fatstock commission, nor centralisation under either ministry, would proceed in the near future. Hensley envisaged that the most likely next step towards 100 per cent post-mortem inspection would be granting local authorities the right to control the hours of slaughter, a power which had been under discussion in 1963, but which was not included in the 1963 regulations. But he anticipated that 100 per cent inspection would still not be achieved due to continuing staffing difficulties, and a centralised system would then be contemplated. In the meantime, transfer of responsibility for meat inspection to the Ministry of Health could not be recommended.[41]

Winnifrith responded on 13 October that he found a 'lack of realism' in Hensley's paper. He thought that it had been agreed not to oppose the Verdon-Smith recommendation for a centralised service, and his further comments reveal that if such a service could be secured, he would be prepared to concede more to the Ministry of Health than he was prepared to admit during the negotiations at the Treasury. He remarked that as 'the main problem in the end is to ensure the safety of human beings', he could not see why meat inspection should be MAFF's responsibility, since 'responsibility for the hygiene of food generally is recognised as one for the Ministry of Health'. And as for the hygiene of imported meat, Winnifrith was 'firmly of the view that there is no ground whatever for making the responsibility for the hygiene of this form of food a responsibility of our minister when the responsibility for all other forms of food rests firmly and squarely with the Ministry of Health'. Winnifrith declared that he could not understand Hensley's 'apparent back-tracking', and wanted a full discussion of the issues because soon he might have to give advice to a new minister: the election was to take place two days later.[42]

At a further meeting on 16 October between Winnifrith, Fraser and Allen at the Treasury, Fraser again attempted to link overseas work and home meat inspection. He argued that if the Ministry of Health was to take over the hygiene of imported meat, it followed 'as night followed day' that they should also be responsible for the hygiene of home-grown meat. But Winnifrith now probed for more details of the Ministry of Health plans, and recorded that Fraser was 'clearly shaken' when he was asked how he would organise control of home-grown meat hygiene. It was clear to Winnifrith that the Ministry of Health had given the matter no thought and that they and the Treasury were assuming that meat inspection would continue to be run by local authorities. Winnifrith urged them both to think in terms of a central government service, and how full ante-mortem as well as post-mortem inspection could be

<hr>

[41] J. Hensley, 'Lees working party Note for the Secretary', 7 October 1964, PRO MAF 282/97.

[42] J. Winnifrith to P. Humphreys-Davies, 13 October 1964, PRO MAF 282/95.

achieved. It was agreed to think again about a centralised service and the personnel that would be needed to run it, and Winnifrith asked Humphreys-Davies to prepare papers exploring these issues.[43]

John Reid, Director of veterinary field services, developed the argument that if a centralised veterinarian-led meat inspection service were to be established, it would be most efficient and economical for it to be attached to MAFF and to be served by the existing corps of local veterinary inspectors, and a limited number of new recruits.[44] This argument was supported by the CVO and adopted in subsequent briefing documents.[45] The new Minister of Agriculture, Fred Peart, also favoured the creation of a central meat inspection service, and shortly before Christmas, Winnifrith wrote to Sir Phillip Allen at the Treasury modifying the views he had expressed earlier. He now declared that if there was to be a centralised meat inspection service, it would be most economically provided by the MAFF, and that it would also be better for imported meat hygiene to remain with MAFF, as the department with the veterinary staff appropriate to the task.[46]

The stage was set for a period of difficult negotiations with the Ministry of Health, which, as we will see below, complicated the decision making on the Milne Committee's recommendation.

Interdepartmental negotiations

Despite their apparent earlier ambivalent attitude towards medical involvement in overseas inspections, Godber and his colleagues at the Ministry of Health soon began to see attractions in the proposal, or at least the advantages of pressing the point upon MAFF. A draft letter to MAFF even suggested that, in view of medical officers' routine duties in connection with water supplies, it was possible that 'if a medical officer had joined the inspectorate earlier, certain defects at canning establishments might automatically have come to light'. Perhaps, in this case, the four typhoid outbreaks over the previous eighteen months may have been avoided.[47] The final version, however, sent by Ministry of Health Assistant Secretary Mrs J. A. Hauff to Lace, was subtler and showed awareness of the veterinarian's sensibilities. Godber was now said to feel that the Milne Committee's recommendation was one that it would be 'wise to accept in principle', although it would not be necessary for a medical

---

43 A. J. D. Winnifrith to Mr Humphreys-Davies, 16 October 1964, PRO MAF 282/95.

44 T. Reid, 'Meat inspection', 22 October 1964, PRO MAF 282/95.

45 G. O. Lace, 9 November 1964; G. O. Lace to Mr Hensley, 10 November 1964; J. Hensley to Mr Humphreys-Davies, 27 November 1964, PRO MAF 282/95.

46 'Draft letter for the Permanent Secretary to send to Sir Phillip Allen' [note that this dates from around August 1965, but refers back to the earlier letter], PRO MAF 282/97.

47 Draft letter for G. O. Lace, PRO MH 148/355.

officer to be included in every visit. He also accepted that the medical officer would not be there to 'usurp the functions of the veterinary inspectors'. But the letter pointed out that after similar basic training in bacteriology, the work of veterinary and medical officers differed greatly: the latter being responsible for food hygiene and oversight of water supplies, which was experience of 'special value' in connection with the overseas inspections. But beyond these points, the letter emphasised the political dimension:

> Although inspection from this country can never be a safeguard in itself . . . if we had another major outbreak . . . the Government's inspection arrangements would be almost bound to come under fire (however unjustified). . . . If it then transpired that one of the recommendations of . . . [the Milne] report had been rejected, against the advice of the C. M. O., I feel sure that both your department and mine would find themselves in difficulty.[48]

MAFF was reluctant to accept either of these arguments. In considering the response to be made to the Ministry of Health, Lace commented to his colleagues that the Milne report merely stated that it would be a 'good thing' for a doctor to be involved in inspections with no supporting arguments. He thought that this could be grounds for rejecting the recommendation. In addition, while the argument that medical officers were more knowledgeable regarding water was superficially attractive, Lace thought that the principles of water hygiene in canning establishments was a specialised matter of which Ministry of Health doctors were likely to have little experience. He continued:

> A further point which ought to be made although it may strike at the pride of the medical profession is that throughout the world outside this country and a few Commonwealth territories who march in step with us, these matters are universally under the control of veterinary services and the intrusion of medical men into an already delicate field of extra-territorial enforcement of our standards would only serve to make for bad feeling and poorer efficiency.[49]

Negotiations concerning the implementation of the Lees working party and Verdon-Smith reports were underway at that time. MAFF was about to tell the Ministry of Health that it considered that, in future, meat inspection in Britain should be supervised centrally by a corps of MAFF veterinarians. It was felt that there was no need to hurry a reply to Mrs Hauff, and that conceding the Milne recommendation on overseas inspection of canneries at this point would weaken MAFF's general case on the organisation of meat inspection.[50]

[48] J. Hauff to G. O. Lace, 5 January 1965, PRO MAF 282/97.
[49] K. A. Bird to G. O. Lace, 13 January 1965, PRO MAF 282/97.
[50] Lace to Hensley, 7 January 1965, PRO MAF 282/97; 'Meat inspection Note for the Minister's meeting on 7th January 1965', PRO MAF 246/254; G. O. Lace to K. A. Bird, 14 January 1965, PRO MAF 282/97.

The Ministry of Health were against the establishment of a centralised veterinary meat inspection service, and they invoked probable staffing difficulties and the likely responses of the Treasury, as well as the opposition of the Society of Medical Officers of Health, the Association of Public Health Inspectors, the British Medical Association, and the local authorities.[51]

By mid-January 1965, Godber's position had shifted firmly in favour of medical involvement in overseas inspections. In a telephone conversation with Sir John Ritchie, the CVO, he suggested an additional advantage. The medical officer, he thought, would be able to consult with local health authorities regarding the health conditions in the area under inspection. Ritchie told his colleagues he was convinced that this was 'nothing but setting up a front'. Nevertheless, he could see 'considerable difficulties' with the Ministry of Health if implementation of the recommendation was opposed by MAFF.[52] Later in the month, after a further conversation between Godber and Ritchie, Hauff asked for a meeting with MAFF representatives to discuss the practicalities.[53]

Within MAFF, Lace now told Hensley, his immediate superior, that he thought they would now have to respond to Mrs Hauff's request because although they did not think the recommendation was 'useful or of practical importance' they could not delay dealing with it 'without holding up the Milne and Lees considerations which link up with Verdon-Smith'. But he now raised the question of costs, the greater administrative difficulties in arranging joint visits, and the objections of the veterinary officers. Concerning the notion that the medical officer might usefully check on local health conditions, he thought that this could introduce a whole new set of criteria for assessing the fitness of imported foods. The whole purpose of the recent efforts regarding the quality of cooling water had been to ensure that food was safe even when imported from countries like Argentina, where diseases such as typhoid were endemic. He also remarked that it would be illogical for the medical officer to visit on the first occasion only, since health conditions could change. Finally, he intimated that his feeling was that Ministry of Health officials were 'embarrassed by the recommendation, but are playing safe in supporting it'.[54]

Lace thought that the argument with the Ministry of Health should not be allowed to drag on, but it did. About a month later a meeting between the two ministries took place at Under-secretary level, Hensley representing MAFF. However, rather than considering the practicalities of joint overseas inspections, the meeting was concerned with matters of principle and the whole field of meat inspection. Minutes prepared at MAFF after the meeting suggested that the Ministry of Health were now unlikely to object to MAFF rather than

[51] J. P. Dodds to J. Hensley, 20 January 1963, PRO MAF 246/254.
[52] J. N. Ritchie to J. Hensley, 18 January 1965, PRO MAF 282/97.
[53] J. Hauff to G. O. Lace, 26 January 1965, PRO MAF 282/97.
[54] G. O. Lace to J. Hensley, 3 February 1965, PRO MAF 282/97.

themselves taking full control of meat hygiene, although they were 'sceptical about the value of it'. After further exploration of possible staffing problems, a joint submission to the Treasury was anticipated. As for overseas inspections, the Ministry of Health did not contend that medical participation in overseas inspections had any great merit, but felt it was difficult to reject 'for fear of criticism later if anything went wrong'.[55] It was agreed that MAFF would suggest a form of words which, while not accepting the recommendation, would say that:

> medical participation would be considered in individual cases where it appeared that there were medical problems which might call for it. In this way we should maintain the principle that veterinarians were in charge of the job and were qualified to do it, and avoid any unjustified contention that they could not do it without medical advisers breathing down their necks.[56]

Hensley asked Lace to consider a suitable formula,[57] and a few days later Lace sent a paragraph to colleagues for their comments. Lace proposed that the agreement would state that the 'existing close collaboration' between MAFF's veterinary inspectors and the Ministry of Health's medical staff would continue, but 'if special circumstances were thought to warrant it the need for medical participation in overseas visits would be considered'. Lace remarked that 'In trying to satisfy all, I expect to please none',[58] but a few days later recorded that Blamire was happy with the proposal, and Bird suggested only a minor amendment. Lace put the formula to Hensley, commenting that he hoped it would satisfy the Ministry of Health without 'weakening the position' of MAFF's veterinary staff,[59] and it was then communicated to Mrs Hauff.[60] She responded in mid-April with an alternative, more positive wording for the final phrase of the sentence, which she wanted to read: ' . . . where special circumstances are thought to warrant it medical participation in overseas visits will be arranged.' She also thought that an agreement along these lines 'should be supported by an actual joint visit in the near future' and asked Lace to consider an opportunity for such a visit.[61] Lace advised Hensley that this placed the onus on MAFF to suggest when a joint visit would be appropriate, and that 'this will make it easier for us to operate the procedure and to avoid our officers being saddled with medical companions in circumstances of particular

---

[55] 'Departmental responsibility for meat hygiene', 10 March 1965, PRO MAF 282/95.

[56] 'Extract from Mr Hensley's Minute to Mr Humphreys-Davies of the discussions with the Ministry of Health on 4 March 1965 about meat inspection', PRO MAF 282/97.

[57] J. Hensley to G. O. Lace, 5 March 1965, PRO MAF 282/97.

[58] G. O. Lace to K. A. Bird and R. Blamire, 10 March 1965, PRO MAF 282/97.

[59] G. O. Lace to J. Hensley, 23 March 1965, PRO MAF 282/97.

[60] G. O. Lace to J. Hensley, 23 March 1965; J. Hensley to G. O. Lace, 24 March 1964; G. O. Lace to J. Hauff, 25 March 1964, PRO MAF 282/97.

[61] J. Hauff to G. O. Lace, 14 April 1964, PRO MAF 282/97.

embarrassment to them'.[62] Hensley asked Lace to consider some special item in the forthcoming programme, which could be made as a joint visit 'without undue embarrassment'.[63]

In mid-April, negotiations over home meat inspection progressed to a meeting between the two ministers and their chief officials. The MAFF side argued that Britain's meat inspection arrangements lagged far behind other countries and could only be improved by instituting a centralised system under veterinary control, but the Ministry of Health favoured only minor changes to the present local authority system. The Ministry of Health was willing to concede a greater extent of veterinary supervision, but argued that if local authorities were given the power to regulate the hours of operation of slaughterhouses, 100 per cent post-mortem inspection could be achieved. They also pointed out that there were plenty of examples of unsatisfactory meat being imported into Britain from countries with centralised veterinary meat inspection services.[64] The Treasury were then consulted, but were not convinced that centralisation would make for a more efficient service and expressed concerns about the probable shortage of veterinary officers to run a centralised scheme. They favoured improving the current scheme by means of increased charges on the meat trade.[65]

The final agreement on overseas inspections was not struck until the two permanent secretaries met in July and negotiated, in the light of the Treasury's opinion, an agreement on hygiene and meat inspection in home slaughterhouses, which was subsequently endorsed by the two ministers. They agreed that these matters would remain the joint responsibility of the two ministers, and that inspection would continue to be carried out by the local authorities. The local authority would be given powers to regulate the hours of slaughter and MAFF's veterinarians would become more involved in providing advice on meat inspection. This was not to say that MAFF had given up the idea of a centralised service altogether: they would revive the issue if the local authority service failed to improve.[66] MAFF's response to the Verdon-Smith report, a white paper proposing the creation of the Meat and Livestock Commission published in August, simply stated that while the new body would advise on slaughterhouse licences, the government's view was that slaughterhouse hygiene and meat inspection should remain under government control.[67] The meat inspection regulations of 1963 were extended for a further

[62] G. O. Lace to J. Hensley, 23 April 1965, PRO MAF 282/97.

[63] J. Hensley to G. O. Lace, 26 April 1965, PRO MAF 282/97.

[64] 'Note of a meeting between the Minister of Agriculture, Fisheries and Food and the Minister of Health on Wednesday, 14th April, 1965', PRO MAF 246/54.

[65] R. F. Briterstone to J. Hensley, 12 July 1965, PRO MAF 246/54.

[66] A. J. D. Winnifrith to Minister, 19 July 1964, PRO MAF 246/54.

[67] Ministry of Agriculture, Fisheries and Food, *Marketing of Meat and Livestock*, London, 1965, p. 6.

year from October 1965, and a year later the control of hours of slaughtering and a greater degree of veterinary supervision were introduced.[68] As for overseas inspections in connection with the official certificate procedures, the permanent secretaries agreed that medical participation would be accepted on 'any suitable occasions', but it was to be 'quite clear' that the MAFF veterinary officers 'would continue to be in charge'.[69]

Other tensions between the two ministries over the division of responsibilities as envisaged by the Lees report came to a climax at about the same time as the permanent secretaries' agreement. By the autumn of 1964, MAFF officials had realised that there were innumerable problems in trying to achieve the kind of strict division of responsibilities that the Lees working party had imagined: for example, the difficulties in drawing distinctions between food additives (which were supposed to become the responsibility of the Ministry of Health) and ingredients (which were supposed to be the responsibility of MAFF).[70] MAFF officials began to favour retaining the double signature of regulations, with informal agreements that each ministry would take the lead in particular areas.[71] By April 1965, they were trying to persuade their Ministry of Health counterparts that the best course of action was to reject the Lees working party findings and to preserve the status quo.

Humphreys-Davies observed that during the previous year within parts of MAFF there had been 'a strong feeling . . . that any question of food hygiene which might give rise to public controversy or other difficulties should be got rid of wherever possible', but that this view had now faded. It is likely that the earlier sentiment to which Humphreys-Davies referred, and which we saw expressed in the views of Winnifrith in particular, was encouraged by the experiences of the Ministry in connection with the Aberdeen and earlier typhoid outbreaks. Humphreys-Davies also claimed that the Lees review had originated as an attempt by the Ministry of Health to expand their responsibilities after losing many functions over the years to other ministries such as to the Ministry of Housing and Local Government.[72] But Winnifrith did not accept the latter notion, commenting that the review had arisen from a conversation between himself and the Permanent Secretary of the Ministry of Health, during which Winnifrith had agreed that they ought to prevent the confusion caused by two ministers having joint responsibility for regulations. Nevertheless, Winnifrith now agreed that the Lees proposals should be dropped.[73] The Ministry of Health initially resisted this suggestion,[74] but soon

[68] G. O. Lace to Mr Hensley, 25 October 1965, PRO MAF 282/93.
[69] A. J. D. Winnifrith to Minister, 19 July 1964, PRO MAF 246/54.
[70] J. H. V. Davies to J. Hensley, 16 October 1964; H. R. Barnell to Mr Hensley, 27 November 1964, PRO MAF 260/357.
[71] J. Hensley to Mr Wadham-Smith, 29 January 1965, PRO MAF 260/357.
[72] P. Humphreys-Davies to Secretary, 7 April 1964, PRO MAF 260/357.
[73] A. J. D. Winnifrith to Mr Humphreys-Davies, 13 April 1965, PRO MAF 260/357.
[74] Celia Herbert to Mr Hensley, 6 July 1965, PRO MAF 260/357.

agreed that, as MAFF wished, any adjustment of responsibility could be arranged informally rather than as a formal transfer of function orders.[75] The only significant adjustment of responsibilities which eventually followed from the Lees review was the transfer of the pharmacology subcommittee of MAFF's Food Additives and Contaminants Committee to the Ministry of Health's Committee on Medical Aspects of Food Policy.[76]

After the permanent secretaries' deal was finally approved, no immediate progress could be made in arranging a joint overseas inspection, since Grace was in the USA.[77] In August, however, after Grace had returned, Lace pressed him to suggest a suitable visit. He told Grace that 'the hard fact is that ministers are being advised to announce some measure of acceptance of this bit of Milne, and that it will have to be seen to have been accepted by a joint visit or visits having been made'.[78] Grace reported that all his colleagues 'dislike the idea intensely' of being accompanied by a medical officer whom they would regard as an 'encumbrance' who would 'merely embarrass the veterinary officer when dealing with other veterinarians'. He stated that, looking back over the years, he could identify no situation in which the involvement of a medical officer would have been useful. He further commented that the Milne Committee produced 'no evidence that I or my colleagues have failed in any aspect of our investigations in the past'. Nevertheless, he realised that the decision had been taken to 'pay token respect to Milne recommendation (ii)' and suggested that a medical officer might be invited to a forthcoming visit to Yugoslavia, as information about deficiencies of Yugoslavian pasteurised canned meat had been received by the Ministry of Health from local health authorities and forwarded to MAFF.[79]

Hensley advised Humphreys-Davies, Deputy Secretary at MAFF, that while no one thought much of the idea of medical participation in overseas visits, it was a necessary part of the 'package deal' agreed with the Ministry of Health.[80] Humphreys-Davies subsequently told Winnifrith that it was proposed to offer the Yugoslavia visit 'by way of a gesture, and to anticipate more embarrassing demands'.[81] Winnifrith agreed that the 'gesture' of a joint visit to Yugoslavia would 'do no harm'. A medical officer could accompany Blamire, Grace's deputy, to Yugoslavia, but Blamire would be in charge of the expedition.[82] On 25 August, Sir Arnold France, who had now replaced Fraser as Permanent Secretary of the Ministry of Health, pressed MAFF to push ahead with organising a joint inspection. He told Winnifrith that 'the participation

[75] J. Hensley to Mr Humphreys-Davies, 13 July 1965, MAF 260/357.
[76] A. J. D. Winnifrith to P. Allen, 7 January 1966, PRO MAF 282/95.
[77] G. O. Lace to L. Grace, 25 June 1965, PRO MAF 282/97.
[78] G. O. Lace to L. Grace, 12 August 1965, PRO MAF 282/97.
[79] L. Grace to J. Hensley, 20 August 1965, PRO MAF 282/97.
[80] J. Hensley to P. Humphreys-Davies, 20 August 1965, PRO MAF 282/97.
[81] P. Humphreys-Davies to Secretary, 23 August 1965, PRO MAF 282/97.
[82] To P. Humphreys-Davies, 25 August 1965, PRO MAF 282/97.

of our medical staff in the overseas work should be put into actual effect on at least one occasion soon, and should not be left simply as an agreement on paper. Otherwise I fear we may incur criticism.'[83]

MAFF sent an official invitation to the Ministry of Health for a medical officer to join the visit to Yugoslavia on 6 September 1965,[84] but negotiations about the timing of the trip were already underway. Dr John M. Ross, the senior medical officer who would be involved, was unhappy about the proposal. He felt that it was not the sort of visit that had been envisaged as a joint venture, but realised that the Ministry of Health would have to be represented. Otherwise MAFF might claim 'that we rejected their first request for a medical officer to join their veterinary inspector'.[85] He complained to Godber about the short notice of the invitation and told Godber that there would be a clash with an important meeting. This was the first meeting of a committee established to implement another of the Milne Committee's recommendations, namely the panel on the Microbial Hazards in Food of the Committee on Medical Aspects of Food Policy. Ross suggested that it would be undiplomatic to send someone to Yugoslavia until the panel had had an opportunity to give their advice on the inadequacies of Yugoslavian canned meat. With these considerations in mind, the departure date was delayed from late September until 11 October 1965.[86] The lay policy makers of the Ministry of Health who had been involved in the negotiations saw the trip more positively. One expressed satisfaction that 'We have at last succeeded in persuading MAFF . . . that a medical officer should accompany veterinary staff in the inspection of overseas meat establishments'.[87]

During the two-week visit of Ross and Blamire to Yugoslavia, they inspected twenty establishments, the central control laboratory, and held discussions with the Yugoslav authorities. The collaboration between the two during the trip appears to have been unproblematic, but tensions between MAFF and the Ministry of Health resurfaced during the production of a report. While Ross was able to comment on a draft,[88] Blamire alone signed the report. Ross commented to a colleague that 'since "we" is used throughout the report "we" should have signed it'.[89] However, Ross sympathised with MAFF's 'desire to maintain procedures'[90] and felt that now that the 'ice has been broken' similar proposals in the future should not cause any 'heart-burning'.[91] Some time after

[83] A. France to A. J. D. Winnifrith, 25 August 1965, PRO MH 148/272.

[84] A. J. D. Winnifrith to A. France, 6 September 1965, PRO MH 148/272.

[85] J. Ross to G. Godber, 2 September 1965, PRO MH 148/272.

[86] Foreign Office to Belgrade, 2 September 1965, PRO MH 148/272.

[87] R. Hillenbrand to Pearson, 24 September 1965, PRO MH 148/272.

[88] R.V. Blamire to J. Ross, 10 February 1966, PRO MH 148/272.

[89] Addendum, 11 March 1966, Ross to Hauff, 7 March 1966, PRO MH 148/272.

[90] J. Ross to J. Hauff, 7 March 1966, PRO MH 148/272.

[91] Ibid.

the trip, when Grace asked Blamire for his opinion of the value of joint visits, Blamire replied:

> All I can say is that during our trip there was no friction whatsoever between us and I am quite sure that Dr Ross now has a fuller appreciation of the work involved in these overseas visits of inspection. I still hold the view, which I held before the visit and I know you share, that we are quite capable of doing these jobs on our own.[92]

A few weeks later, Bird recorded that while Grace thought medical involvement in overseas meat inspection a waste of time, and that this was supported by Blamire's experience in Yugoslavia, Grace agreed that the exercise would have to be repeated during 1966.[93] Ross and Blamire collaborated on a number of inspections over the next few years, visiting Ethiopia and Eritrea. MAFF contrived to avoid Ministry of Health involvement in the next visit to South America in 1967, but Ross was later involved in a trip to Argentina and Uruguay.[94] The reports of these trips show little evidence of specific contributions from the medical officer.[95] On average there would be ten to fifteen overseas trips per year by a member of the veterinary staff but they would be accompanied by a medical officer on only one.[96]

Conclusions

The account given of the discussion and action on one recommendation of the Milne report highlights a number of factors which may condition food safety decision making. The issue, in this case, was essentially that of how the best scientific advice could be obtained, and the process of implementation of the recommendation was significantly influenced by long-term professional interests and interdepartmental tensions, associated with separate but ongoing and related policy-making processes. These other factors delayed the implementation of the recommendation and encouraged a half-hearted approach: but ultimately the main stimulus to the eventual implementation was fear, mainly among senior civil servants, of possible adverse publicity. Even 'token' implementation of the recommendation would allow the government's claim to be taking the Milne report seriously.

[92] R. V. Blamire to Mr Grace, 23 March 1966, PRO MASF 282/9.
[93] G. O. Lace to Mr Hensley, 5 April 1966, PRO MAF 282/9.
[94] See pp. 281–4.
[95] Copy of files of R.V. Blamire on overseas visits, deposited with the Aberdeen Typhoid Project.
[96] Ministry of Agriculture, Fisheries and Food, *Annual Report of the Chief Veterinary Officer*, London, 1964–85.

Throughout the decision-making process described in this chapter ministers were directly involved only occasionally, although their wishes were more frequently invoked by senior officials. This was not so in the example we will be considering in Chapter 8, namely decision making on the Milne Committee's recommendation on the fate of the withdrawn suspect canned meat, which involved intervention from the highest level of politics.

8

The disposal of suspect canned meat

The priority of politics over technical advice

Introduction

In September 1964, at their session with Liebig's representatives, the Milne Committee expressed the hope that reprocessing suspect stock, and the reassurance that new stock was produced safely, would rehabilitate corned beef.[1] The committee subsequently recommended that withdrawn produce could be 'released for sale in the normal way' after 'an acceptable method of reprocessing'.[2] At that time, research on reprocessing was nearing completion, and in his statement the Secretary of State for Scotland said that consultations with the trade about reprocessing were underway.[3]

There were about 8000 tons of suspect stockpile material, but the pressing problem was disposing of commercial withdrawn stocks. These included about 500 tons from Argentine 1A, owned by the American company Armour (International Packers) Ltd, and 160 tons from Uruguay Establishment 5, owned by Weddel & Co Ltd, part of the British Vestey Group. These were withdrawn in June 1964.[4] There were also 120 tons of Establishment 25 produce, withdrawn by the Argentine company CAP in 1963, which remained in Britain when Milne reported.[5]

As detailed in Chapter 5, Argentine Establishment 1819 stock was withdrawn following the 'Wapping Dock incident', the discovery of *Salmonella typhimurium* in a can, and an adverse report by the veterinary attaché.[6] The rotting 1819 material at Wapping, imported by Canbury Ltd, was apparently

---

[1] See p. 184.

[2] Scottish Home and Health Department, *The Aberdeen Typhoid Outbreak*, Edinburgh, 1964 (Milne report), p. 39.

[3] *PD(C)*, vol. 704, cols *131–2* (17 December 1964).

[4] 'Reprocessed canned corned meat memorandum for submission to Treasury', September 1965, PRO MAF 282/113; J. A. Hauff to Mr Dodds, 29 June 1965, PRO MH 148/206.

[5] J. A. Hauff to Mr Dodds, 29 June 1965, PRO MH 148/206; 'Appendix 2 Report of the Committee of Inquiry into the outbreak of typhoid in Aberdeen Joint Submission to Ministers Action to be taken about the withdrawn and other stocks of canned meat affected by finding (XIV)', PRO MAF 282/97.

[6] Withheld canned meat from Argentine Establishment 1819, Brief for the Minister of Health, 3 January 1966, PRO MH 148/99. See also p. 154.

220

part of a consignment of American army surplus supplies. However, Foley Brothers Ltd and four other importers had imported considerable quantities of 1819 stock directly from Argentina. Foley Brothers held 117 of the 422 tons believed to be in Britain, the rest being in the hands of the other importers, distributors, retailers and various institutions.[7] Of the commercial stock, it became clear that the disposal of the 1819 material would prove most problematic. This was because the importers and distributors had no relationship with the South American suppliers, unlike those holding stock from Argentine establishments 1A and 25, and Uruguay 5.

In this chapter we will follow the story of the eventual disposal of the suspect stock. As a result of interventions by sections of the food trade, the reaction of the press and public, and fear of adverse publicity and political repercussions, the implementation of the Milne Committee's recommendation on reprocessing as originally envisaged proved impossible. The major manufacturers re-exported their suspect stock back to South America. The 1819 material, however, was eventually exported elsewhere for human consumption, mostly in its original form. As for the government-owned suspect stock, economic considerations eventually overcame the risks of reneging on commitments not to release it. By the early 1970s, the bulk of the stockpile suspect stock had been exported for reprocessing and consumption abroad. In concluding this chapter, we will reflect on the features of food safety policy making in the 1960s that are illustrated by this episode.

Suspect stockpile stock 1963 to 1964

Among the issues discussed by MAFF officials following the first 1963 outbreaks were the implications for stockpile policy of the link between Establishment 25 and typhoid. Initially, they thought that changes were unnecessary but later suspended releases of Establishment 25 stock, while new shipments continued to be accepted.[8] In November 1963, when the Ministry of Health advised the withdrawal of Establishment 25 stock produced after 30 May 1962, the stop on stockpile releases was made indefinite and further shipments rejected. The stoppage applied to all Establishment 25 stock, since the plant had always used untreated cooling water.[9]

In February 1964, it was decided that the 1953/54 Establishment 25 stock could be released, while CAP would be asked to replace the 1100 tons produced after 30 May 1962 with sound stock. Over 5000 tons produced between

---

7 R. Hillenbrand to Mrs Pearson, 2 February 1965; R. Hillenbrand, 3 February 1965, PRO MH 148/202.
8 See p. 50.
9 R. E. J. Goodman to Dr Barnell, 18 November 1963, PRO MAF 282/75.

1959 and 1962 would be held, pending investigations (there were no purchases from any source between 1955 and 1958). In April, it was decided to keep it until it was unfit, and for use only in a nuclear war, when any risk would be 'infinitesimal compared with all other risks to the survivors'.[10]

Following the publicity given to the stockpile in early June, the Minister of Agriculture, Christopher Soames, sought details from his officials about the rationale for stockpiling corned beef. He was informed that it gave 'a better balance of ready-to-eat food as against what otherwise would be a disproportion of starch', and was assured that the turnover policy was more economical than 'storage until destruction'.[11] In early June, due to the Aberdeen outbreak, MAFF suspended all sales of South American stock, but continued selling pre-1955 Australian and New Zealand produce.[12] MAFF's agent for the sale of stockpile corned beef gave their customers the opportunity of cancelling orders,[13] but most honoured their contracts. By mid-June, 800 tons of non-South American canned meat had been released.[14]

In mid-June, the Ministry of Health realised that, besides the 1963 typhoid outbreaks, some earlier outbreaks had been associated with corned beef (such as those at Oswestry and Crowthorne[15]). Sir George Godber, the CMO, now advised that only meat manufactured at establishments using clean cooling water should be released. Without information about the water employed at factories in Australia and New Zealand,[16] Soames decided to suspend releases of Australian and New Zealand stock. Urgent telegrams were sent to the High Commissioners asking them to investigate.[17]

If the pre-1955 Australian and New Zealand stock was suspect, this would have major implications: sales of £5.5 million over the next two years were forecast, and the proceeds were earmarked for new purchases.[18] Prolonged suspension of disposals was undesirable. It might suggest that MAFF did not believe their own claim that Aberdeen was not linked with ex-stockpile meat. There were commitments to regular customers, and the probability that deferment would result in more stock deteriorating to the point at which it

[10] 'Notes of a meeting held in Mr. Taylor's room at 3 p.m. on Thursday 2nd April 1964', MAF 246/44; A. J. D. Winnifrith to Mr Hensley, 3 June 1964, PRO MAF 246/39.

[11] W. C. T., 'Canned meat stockpile', 5 June 1964; Emergency Services division, 'Canned corned meat stockpile Note for the Minister', 15 June 1964, PRO MAF 246/178.

[12] A. R. Parselle to W. C. Tame, 4 June 1964, PRO MAF 246/39.

[13] W. S. Wallin to A. R. Parselle, 10 June 1964, PRO MAF 246/39.

[14] W. C. Tame to Mr Hutchison 17 June 1964, PRO MAF 246/178.

[15] See pp. 20–1.

[16] A. J. D. Winnifrith to Minister, 16 June 1964; W. C. Tame to Mr Hutchison, 17 June 1964, PRO MAF 246/178.

[17] A. J. D. Winnifrith to Mr Hensley, 17 June 1964, PRO MAF 246/178; 'Text of cable to H. M. High Commissioner Canberra H. M. High Commissioner Wellington', PRO MAF 282/88.

[18] 'Canned meat stockpile: disposal policy', 19 June 1964, PRO MAF 246/178.

was unsaleable. But the information from Australia was not reassuring. Two plants, accounting for 6000 6lb-cans in the stockpile, had used untreated river water. MAFF, however, argued that since thousands of tons had been consumed without apparent ill-effect, it could be regarded as safe.[19]

Officials were anxious to offer corned beef for sale at the beginning of July according to usual practice, but Godber again advised releasing no stock before the Milne Committee reported. However, he set out an 'order of safety':

(1) meat of cans of any size cooled with water of potable quality – age and size no object. (2) Meat cooled with water from a source not likely to be specifically polluted. (3) The residue of large batches of which much has been consumed without harm, 12oz tins being probably safer than 6lb. (4) Meat produced more recently from plants using heavily polluted water – 12oz tins safer than 6lb.[20]

The greater safety of small cans was 'partly theoretical', and it was thought unlikely that small cans could cause an 'Aberdeen incident'. In general, Godber thought the risks 'not great' and 'political' rather than 'medical', because if 'an outbreak from Ministry stocks took place before the Milne committee had reported it would be very difficult to expound . . . our reasons for having released from the stockpile'.[21]

A MAFF memorandum prepared for a ministers' meeting on 10 July developed arguments for resuming disposals. The trade had not been informed of the suspension of releases, so there was a chance to avoid putting 'Commonwealth corned beef under a cloud'. Furthermore, suspending sales might increase the price of fresh meat. MAFF therefore favoured releasing New Zealand and Australian stock other than that from Australian Establishments 4 and 7 in July, in the hope that the latter stock could also be released later.[22] The ministers approved.[23] Subsequent consultations with Godber provided the basis for the release of Establishments 4 and 7 stock from August. Godber now advised:

Even with dirty river water the chance of an Aberdeen type can is very small; at plants 4 and 7 it is much smaller than this . . . I think the risk is one Ministers could accept insofar as I can appraise it, but, if challenged, they could not say that the water was from a pure and wholesome public supply or chlorinated. I am quite ready

[19] 'Canned meat stockpile: disposal policy', 25 June 1964, PRO MAF 246/178.
[20] J. Hauff to N. J. P. Hutchison, 6 July 1964, PRO MAF 246/178.
[21] Ibid.
[22] 'Canned meat stockpile: disposal policy Note by the Minister of Agriculture, Fisheries and Food, 6 July 1964'. The final version of the memorandum was C. Soames to Lord Privy Seal, 9 July 1964, PRO MAF 249/178.
[23] 'Note of a meeting held at the Privy Seal's Room', 10 July 1964, PRO T 227/1656.

to be quoted as advising that the risk is so small as to be negligible, but it seemed to me that Ministers would wish to decide whether this was sufficient defence if they are challenged on the basis that they have released some meat which falls below the safety standards they intend to set.[24]

Stockpile disposals were depressed after the Aberdeen outbreak. It had been expected to realise £1 million during the six months from July, but only £400,000 was achieved.[25] Some 2100 tons of stock was sold by November, by which time demand was increasing.[26] Stockpile policy formed part of the discussion on the Milne report between the ministries, but MAFF also consulted the Ministry of Health separately about whether disposals could continue on the basis of Godber's advice. The Ministry of Health assented, but the pre-1955 and suspect post-1958 South American stock would remain withheld, pending investigations of reprocessing. Officials advised ministers that all that needed be said publicly was that no unsafe stockpile meat would be released without reprocessing.[27]

The problem of Argentine Establishment 1819

W. S. Foley, Managing Director of Foley Brothers, became well known to officials. On 23 June he took the news that MOsH had been asked to advise that 1819 corned beef should be withdrawn, 'more in sorrow than in anger',[28] but he later challenged the Ministry of Health's advice. On 17 August he revealed that bacteriological tests of his stock had all been negative, that the Argentine authorities claimed the official certificate was sound, and that according to Establishment 1819, their cooling water had been chlorinated. He concluded: 'Whatever justification may . . . have been thought to have existed for imposing this Ban, we think it is now clear that it was based upon incorrect information.'[29] Later, he commissioned a chemist to visit Establishment 1819, who found the plant hygienic. The chemist also challenged the *Salmonella typhimurium* finding, explaining:

the sampling of an apparently sound can of corned beef . . . is . . . a very difficult operation, and during the opening of the can it is almost impossible not to contaminate the meat with material lying on the outside . . . where there have been

---

[24] A. Barber to C. Soames, July 1964, PRO MAF 246/178.

[25] A. R. Parselle to Mr Hutchison, 18 February 1965, PRO MAF 246/178.

[26] C. Soames to Lord Privy Seal, 9 July 1964, PRO MAF 249/178; A. R. Parselle to N. J. P. Hutchison, 4 December 1964, PRO MAF 246/178.

[27] 'Joint submission to Minister, Appendix 2', PRO MAF 282/97.

[28] J. Hauff to Mr Pater, 24 June 1964, PRO MH 148/98.

[29] W. S. Foley to Ministry of Health, 17 August 1964, PRO MH 148/202.

blown cans in a consignment, contents may be dispersed all over the outside of the sound cans.[30]

He was not prepared to accept the finding without confirmation by a second laboratory.

Prior to writing to MOsH about Argentine 1A and Uruguay 5, the Ministry secured the co-operation of the importers, but this had not been possible in the case of Establishment 1819. Only one importer agreed to take back stock from their customers while most, including Foley Brothers, refused.[31] Officials were anxious to avoid becoming involved in disputes between retailers, distributors and importers. All they could tell 1819 stockholders was that it had yet to be decided whether the withdrawal would be permanent. Further decisions would have to await the Milne Committee's findings.[32]

By August, some officials were uncomfortable with placing so much emphasis on the Milne Committee. Dr Ross told his colleagues: 'In my view the Department is tending to lean too much on the Milne Committee to get out of an awkward situation.'[33] He did not expect that the committee's report would have any bearing on the decisions to be taken on the Establishment 1819 stock. He hoped, however, that the importer of stock via the USA could be 'taught a sharp lesson' for handling produce in such poor condition.[34] On the other hand, those importing from Argentina were 'acting in good faith'. He suggested that the firms be advised that their stock be returned to Argentina, and that the ministries should support them in any argument. Other officials agreed that the present position was unsatisfactory. Faced with questions about the authority under which the 1819 corned beef was withheld, they wanted to say more than reiterating previous advice.[35] However, Ross also thought that no reputable company would release suspect stock against the advice of the Ministry, because they would risk substantial claims for damages and loss of reputation if 'anything untoward should result'.[36]

Mrs M. A. J. Pearson, Principal Secretary at the Ministry of Health, thought the Argentine government would decline to pay for the withdrawn Establishment 1819 produce. In this eventuality it might prove impossible to persuade the 1819 stockholders to continue to withhold their stock. She therefore asked the Ministry's legal adviser to explore the possibility of preventing the marketing of 1819 stock by regulation.[37] It emerged that the regulations

---

[30] R. F. Milton to Parker, Garret & Co, 5 October 1964, PRO MH 148/98.

[31] 'Schedule A', PRO MH 148/98.

[32] M. A. J. Pearson to W. W. Howitt, 1 July 1964, PRO MH 148/98.

[33] J. M. Ross to Mr Davidson, 12 August 1964, PRO MH 148/98.

[34] Ibid.

[35] J. B. Davidson to Mr Watson, 13 August 1964; E. H. Watson to Mr Davidson, 14 August 1964, PRO MH 148/98.

[36] M. A. J. Pearson to Mr Davidson, 19 August 1964, PRO MH 148/98.

[37] Ibid.

under the Food and Drugs Act, 1955 could only be prospective, but there was a possibility of using the Consumer Protection Act, 1961 operated by the Home Office.[38]

Assistance to stockholders in claiming compensation from Argentina was the subject of discussion between the ministries on 1 October. The Ministry of Health suggested that MAFF could threaten the withdrawal of the official certificate if the Argentine government failed to respond, but MAFF thought this would be improper. The meeting agreed that the Foreign Office should be consulted about an official approach after the Milne Committee had reported. Ministers would at least be able to assure traders that 'all possible steps had been taken on their behalf'.[39] Nothing of immediate significance for the 1819 stockholders emerged from all these deliberations, and all officials could do was to send more elaborate letters explaining the reasons for the advice to withdraw the stock.[40] This information was reiterated at a meeting between MAFF and Ministry of Health officials, with Foley's solicitor and analyst.[41]

Consideration of using the Consumer Protection Act continued, but shortly before the publication of the Milne report, ministers were advised that it would be unnecessary to consider such a step. The officials thought that the 'practical possibility' of the firms disregarding the government's advice would be 'remote after the publicity now likely to be attendant on the views of the Milne Committee'. The firms would not risk marketing a food that the Milne Committee deemed to carry a degree of risk.[42] Officials now placed more emphasis on reprocessing,[43] and argued that the Establishment 1819 stockholders should be given the same chance to reprocess their stock as the others.[44] A further submission on public compensation noted that there were no relevant precedents. On publication of the report, a letter was sent to all known stockholders, making it clear that the government's view was that the suspect stock should remain withheld. The firms were also asked what proposals they had for reprocessing, return of stock to South America, or disposal by other means.

---

[38] Mr Davidson to M. A. J. Pearson 20 August 1964; J. C. Hales to Mrs Hauff, 3 September 1964, PRO MH 148/98.

[39] 'Meeting held on 1st October to discuss the future of canned meat from Establishment 1819', PRO MH 148/200; K. A. Bird to Mr Lace, 5 October 1964, PRO MAF 148/98.

[40] R. Hillenbrand to W. S. Foley, 18 September 1964, PRO MH 148/202; R. Hillenbrand to Produce Distributors Ltd, 26 October 1964, PRO MH 148/200; R. Hillenbrand to Dear Sir, October 1964, PRO MH 148/201.

[41] 'Note of a meeting held on 2nd November 1964', PRO MH 148/202.

[42] 'Submission to Ministers Report of the departmental committee of inquiry into the Aberdeen typhoid outbreak', 15 December 1964, PRO MAF 282/97.

[43] 'Note of a meeting held on Wednesday 25th November to discuss the future of stocks from Argentina Establishment 1819', PRO MH 148/98.

[44] 'Withdrawn commercial stocks of canned meats from Argentina Establishment 1819 of which production was faulty in certain other respects', PRO MAF 282/97.

Recommendations of a working party on reprocessing would be available shortly.[45]

The impact of the Milne report upon the definition of suspect stocks

A meeting of officials on 24 November raised the question of whether the Milne report implied any broadening of the definition of suspect stock.[46] The report stated that 'meat canned by a process in which water not of a potable nature was used in the cooling process presents an unacceptable risk'.[47] It would have to be considered whether this applied to sizes other than 6lb cans.[48] MAFF subsequently commented that any proposal to withdraw all canned meat 'not cooled in satisfactory water' would meet two difficulties. First, they could not establish for every establishment whether and for what period unsatisfactory water had been used. Second, it would be impossible to identify the date of manufacture of some small cans.[49]

Ministers were informed of this conclusion. Besides precluding any attempt to identify further suspect stock, it meant that remaining earlier production, and non-6lb cans, from Argentine establishments 1A and 25, and Uruguay 5, would be left on the market. This was justified on the grounds that much had been consumed without ill-effect, and little such stock remained. The risk was 'small and a further withdrawal would cause public alarm out of all proportion to the risk'. As for Australian Establishments 4 and 7, officials thought that it would be 'an excessively meticulous interpretation' of the Milne report to ask MOsH and the trade:

> to search for and withdraw stocks which were tacitly (or in the case of the Government stockpile, explicitly) allowed to be marketed over the last 6 months. There would be particular confusion and alarm . . . if, at this date, corned beef of Commonwealth origin was declared to be suspect.[50]

However, Milne confirmed the 'suspect' status of one category of stock, namely pre-1955 South American produce, because they implied that

---

[45] 'Joint submission to Minister, Appendix 3; Submission to Ministers Report of the departmental committee of inquiry into the Aberdeen typhoid outbreak', 15 December 1964, PRO MAF 282/97.

[46] 'Note of a meeting held on 24th November at the Ministry of Health', PRO MAF 282/97.

[47] Milne, p. 39.

[48] 'Note of a meeting held on 24th November at the Ministry of Health', PRO MAF 282/97.

[49] G. O. Lace to J. Hensley, 7 December 1964, PRO MAF 282/97.

[50] 'Joint submission to Minister, Appendix 2', PRO MAF 282/97.

chlorination had not been commonly practised in South America until 1955.[51] As noted above, sales of this corned beef from the stockpile had been suspended in June 1964. but there were about 100 tons or £25,000-worth of this material in private hands (CAP and International Packers held £20,000-worth), sold prior to June. MAFF officials sought authority to repurchase it.[52]

The stock had been sold on the basis that MAFF believed each parcel suitable for consumption, but with no warranty. However, in view of the government's acceptance of the Milne report, MAFF's legal department thought that they must accept liability. MAFF told the Treasury that if this stock was returned to their stores there would be less risk of it entering consumption, and argued that:

> the longer any stuff which we could get back is at risk of being put into the distributive channels the greater the possible danger to health through typhoid and the claims resulting therefrom. This is a real risk on the financial front; the risks on the political front are even more serious.[53]

The Treasury were not convinced. Since no warranty had been given, they suggested that 'the responsibility not to allow the meat to go for consumption' fell upon the firms, and that MAFF held no responsibility, 'moral, or otherwise'.[54] MAFF claimed that Sale of Goods legislation made the validity of the disclaimer doubtful. The Parliamentary Secretary to the Ministry of Health had already said in Parliament that holders of condemned goods should look to the supplier for compensation, and in this case the supplier was the government.[55] If MAFF refused to take back suspect stock they would be in a defenceless position, because they would have failed to do what commercial suppliers had done voluntarily at the behest of the Ministry of Health.[56] Finally, the Treasury gave in.[57] MAFF invited traders to deliver the stocks to a MAFF store, whereupon a refund would be paid.[58] By January 1966, 97 tons had been repurchased.[59] Small parcels were still turning up, which officials attempted to deal with 'as quickly and simply as possible to avert confusion resulting in either the consumption of suspect stock or another

---

[51] Milne, p. 28.

[52] A. R. Parselle to W. F. C. Clark, 31 December 1964, PRO MAF 246/50.

[53] W. F. C. Clark to S. Barraclough, 3 February 1965, PRO MAF 246/50.

[54] S. Barraclough to W. F. C. Clark, 17 March 1965, PRO MAF 246/50.

[55] W. F. C. Clark to S. Barraclough, 24 March 1965, PRO MAF 246/50. The Parliamentary Secretary made his remarks during an adjournment debate. *PD(C)*, vol. 708, cols *1433–43* (17 March 1965). See also p. 230.

[56] K. A. Bird to Mr Lace, 23 March 1965, PRO MAF 246/50.

[57] S. Barraclough to W. F. C Clark, 9, 14 April 1965, PRO MAF 246/50.

[58] A. R. Parselle to Arley Foods and eight other traders, 14 April 1965, PRO MAF 246/50.

[59] W. F. C. Clark to A. R. Parselle, 13 January 1966, PRO MAF 246/50.

round of public anxiety about corned beef generally'.[60] The repurchased stock accounted for a very small proportion of the suspect stockpile material, the eventual fate of which will be discussed below.

Reprocessing proposals

The working party on reprocessing, set up in July 1964, consisted of representatives from MAFF, six governmental and industry bodies,[61] and the Metal Box Company. They arranged laboratory trials of a method of pasteurisation, based upon the advice of the former director of the PHLS. The Central Public Health Laboratory conducted tests using cans inoculated with *Salmonella typhi*, *Escherichia coli* and *Streptococcus faecalis*,[62] and Metal Box Company translated the method into cannery practice.[63] Ambassador Foods, near Liverpool, conducted trials using non-suspect 6lb cans from the stockpile, the results proving acceptable in terms of taste and other qualities of the meat.[64]

The working party completed their report shortly after the publication of the Milne report, and recommended a method which would ensure that the centres of cans were maintained at over 80°C for thirty minutes. On 12 January 1965, the Ministry of Health sent the basic specifications to the stockholders and other interested parties,[65] and among the responses were the first indications that sections of the trade would oppose reprocessing. The National Association of Multiple Grocers thought that reprocessed stock would be 'valueless', 'whether or not reprocessing was effective'. They strongly recommended that 'express notice should be given to prospective purchasers that such goods have been re-processed'.[66]

On 12 January, Foley Brothers and officials discussed methods of marking reprocessed cans to prevent confusion with unreprocessed stock. Foleys were in negotiation with Samor Pure Foods of Didcot, who could treat their stock over three months.[67] Two days later, Foleys informed the Ministry of Health that they had arranged a trial, but were asked not to proceed until a code of practice had been agreed by MAFF.[68] At this time, Foleys anticipated that reprocessing would solve all their problems, and informed their customers that

---

[60] M. A. J. Pearson to A. R. Parselle, 27 January 1966, PRO MAF 246/50.

[61] These were the Agriculture Research Council, British Food Manufacturing Industries Research Association, Central Public Health Laboratory, Ministry of Health, Perfect Lambert Ltd and the United Kingdom Atomic Energy Authority.

[62] B. Hobbs to Mr Hearne, 23 October 1964, PRO MH 148/206.

[63] 'Report of working party on the reprocessing of canned corned beef', MH 148/206.

[64] RH to Mrs Pearson, 18 December 1964, PRO MH 148/206.

[65] M. A. J. Pearson to Dear Sir, 12 January 1965, PRO MH 148/202.

[66] J. C. Inglis Gillett to M. A. J. Pearson, 1 February 1965, PRO MH 148/206.

[67] 'Note of a meeting held on 12th January 1965', PRO MH 148/202.

[68] W. S. Foley to Ministry of Health, 14 and 27 January 1965, PRO MH 148/202.

they would soon accept stock back if they were able to reprocess and dispose of it.[69]

Stories in the press added to the pressure to settle the fate of the withdrawn corned beef. According to one, a wholesale firm released 151 cases of suspect corned beef between September and December, the first being noticed in Hartlepool on 18 December. By 11 January, the firm had retrieved only eighty cases, and the MOH for Newcastle therefore wrote to GPs, neighbouring MOsH and hospitals.[70] When the codes were inspected carefully, however, it emerged that only a few of the cans had been manufactured using untreated water.[71] On 22 January, the Ministry of Health wrote to all stockholders and reminded them of the necessity for strict stock control. They were also asked not to proceed with reprocessing until the MAFF code of practice was issued.[72] But at least the fate of the Establishment 1A stock was soon settled. During February it was shipped back to Argentina for reprocessing and consumption locally, which took place with little publicity or opposition.[73]

The Newcastle scare formed the basis for a House of Commons adjournment debate,[74] in which the local MP confronted the Parliamentary Secretary of the Ministry of Health. He asked for warehouse security to be tightened and suggested that powers to destroy foodstuffs be extended. He proposed compensation for the trade and emphasised the need for public reassurance about canned meat. The Parliamentary Secretary hoped the debate would not revive fears about corned beef safety. He estimated that since 1955 there had been about 550 non-fatal cases of typhoid from eating corned beef, or one per 6,500,000 6oz portions, while, during the same period, 65,000 people had been killed and 3,400,000 injured in traffic accidents. He added that the final decision on the fate of the suspect stocks was a matter for the firms, and that compensation did not arise. This was also when he remarked that traders should look to their suppliers for recompense.[75]

MAFF's code of practice was ready by March, but before printing it they decided to wait until after a reprocessing trial involving 1819 stock owned by Henry Lane & Co, one of the smaller importers, at Ambassador Foods at

---

[69] C. F. Williamson to M. A. J. Pearson, 25 January 1965, PRO MH 148/202.

[70] J. A. Hauff to Mr Pater, 15 January 1965, PRO MAF 282/97.

[71] 'Accidental releases of corned beef from a Newcastle warehouse'; Mrs Pearson to Mrs Hauff, January 1965, PRO MAF 282/97.

[72] M. A. J. Pearson to Dear Sir, 22 January 1965, PRO MH 148/205.

[73] 'Corned beef to be re-exported', *Daily Telegraph*, 9 February 1965, cutting in PRO MH 148/207; A. B. Semple to J. Ross, 19 February 1965; A. B. Semple to G. Godber, 19 February 1965; R. M. Harris to Secretary, 19 March 1965, J. M. Ross to A. B. Semple, 30 March 1965, PRO MH 148/207.

[74] Topics for adjournment debates, which are limited in duration to half an hour, are chosen by ballot, and provide opportunities for MPs to raise matters which otherwise might not be debated, and to receive a response from a minister.

[75] *PD(C)*, vol. 709, cols *1433–43* (17 March 1965).

Kirby.[76] The results, discussed on 12 May, were disappointing. The code included rules about the inspection of cans prior to and following reprocessing. Any showing physical damage were to be rejected, as was any case containing a burst or leaking can. In Lane's batch, 65 per cent of the cans were unsuitable. MAFF commented that part of the explanation was that the reprocessing method had been devised for soldered stockpile cans rather than unsoldered commercial cans. Lane's managers pleaded for the code to be amended but the officials offered little hope of this. Pearson also noted that bodies 'representative of public opinion' had stated that even reprocessed stock should not be allowed on the market.[77] This reflects the view taken by the Food Hygiene Advisory Council, the statutory body representing trade and public interests set up under the Food and Drugs Act.[78] On 30 April, they asked their chairman to inform the ministers that they were opposed to withdrawn stocks being released for human consumption, even after reprocessing.[79]

A further trial was carried out under ministry supervision by Foley Bothers at Samor Foods, beginning on 1 May.[80] MAFF inspectors reported that the rejection rate of the cans prior to processing was again high: 28.6 per cent of 500 cases of 6 × 6lb rectangular cans, and 42.5 per cent of the same number of cylindrical cans.[81] A second batch was treated under the supervision of the local MOH. Of the cans reprocessed, although most left the retorts in a reasonable condition, when inspected at a depot at Palmers Wharf, Deptford, 198 out of 330 selected for incubation showed some degree of damage.[82]

Foley was undeterred and on 21 May wrote to the Ministry stating that, in his opinion, the cans stood up to reprocessing well.[83] Of the cans incubated, only twenty-four were finally rejected,[84] but Foley accepted the 'necessity for greater care in handling'.[85] He considered the reprocessed cans to be 'perfectly sound and in a satisfactory condition for normal trade distribution', and proposed to resume reprocessing.[86] With the Ministry's consent reprocessing recommenced, and, in all, Foleys reprocessed 16.5 tons of corned beef.[87] On 1 June, they began to press for distribution to be allowed,[88] but were in for a

[76] A. R. Parselle to M. A. J. Pearson, 17 March 1965, PRO MH 148/206.

[77] 'Meeting held on 12th May 1965', PRO MH 148/202.

[78] See p. 31.

[79] Lord Strang to Minister of Health, 29 May 1965, PRO MAF 282/97.

[80] 'Proposals for reprocessing', PRO MH 148/206; H. W. Edis to Dr Robinson, 22 April 1965, PRO MH 148/202.

[81] J. F. Hearne and R. E. G. Thomas, 'Reprocessing canned corned beef at Samor Pure Foods Ltd', 6 May 1965, PRO MH 148/202.

[82] A. Robinson to Dr Ross, 11 June 1965, PRO MH 148/202.

[83] W. S. Foley to M. A. J. Pearson, 21 May 1965, PRO MH 148/202.

[84] A. Robinson to Dr Ross, 11 June 1965, PRO MH 148/202.

[85] W. S. Foley to M. A. J. Pearson, 1 June 1965, PRO MH 148/202.

[86] W. S. Foley to M. A. J. Pearson, 21 May 1965, PRO MH 148/202.

[87] 'Corned beef – Establishment 1819', PRO MAF 282/114.

[88] W. S. Foley to M. A. J. Pearson, 1 June 1965, PRO MH 148/202.

frustrating wait. At the end of July, Foley expressed disappointment that he had still not received the go-ahead.[89]

In June, despite the gathering opposition to reprocessing, the Ministry of Health prepared to release the code of practice. However, on the advice of MAFF, they decided to canvass the views of the food trade associations before seeking the approval of the Minister of Health, Kenneth Robinson.[90] The Ministry therefore wrote to nine trade associations, explaining that they were ready to advise the return to the market of the withdrawn corned beef after reprocessing. While the reprocessed corned beef would not be labelled as such, a mark would be added so that MOsH could recognise it. A copy of the letter to be sent to stockholders was enclosed, and the organisations were asked whether, 'having considered the implications, they had any points that they wished to bring to the minister's attention.[91]

Several organisations expressed reservations, and so the Ministry held a meeting on 16 August, attended by thirteen representatives of six trade associations, and representatives of CAP, International Packers (Armour), Weddell & Co, and Foley Brothers. The stockholders viewed reprocessing as worthwhile. Some were reluctant to mark reprocessed cans, but others thought this desirable, to avoid suspicions of accidental omission of reprocessing. Importers and distributors other than the owners of withheld stock, and the British Food Manufacturers Federation, were of a different opinion. They thought that any publicity given to the release of the withheld stock, even after reprocessing, would seriously damage the corned beef market. The officials pointed out that it was unrealistic to suppose that reprocessing could be carried out in secret, and that publicity stemming from 'apparent concealment' would do more harm than a statement that the Milne Committee recommendation was being implemented. The retail organisations were completely against putting the withdrawn canned meat back on the market. Most of their members would not handle the reprocessed product, and wanted it to be clearly marked.[92]

After the consultation exercise, Robinson agreed that, subject to the consent of MAFF and the Scottish Office, the withheld stock could be placed on the market after supervised reprocessing.[93]

---

[89] W. S. Foley to Ministry of Health, 28 July 1965, PRO MH 148/202.

[90] N. J. P. Hutchison to J. A. Hauff, 25 June 1965; N. J. P. Hutchison to J. H. V. Davies, 25 June 1965; 'Corned beef – Establishment 1819', PRO MAF 282/114; 'Withheld canned meat from Argentine Establishment 1819 brief for the Minister of Health 3rd January, 1966', PRO MH 148/199; N. J. P Hutchison to Mrs Hauff, 25 June 1965, PRO MH 148/206.

[91] M. A. J. Pearson to associations of importers and distributors of canned meat, 20 July 1965, PRO MAF 282/113.

[92] 'Note of a meeting held on 16th August, 1965 at the Ministry of Health'; 'Reprocessed canned meat Memorandum for submission to Treasury', PRO MAF 282/113.

[93] Ibid.

Reprocessing, the press and the Prime Minister

Before the final interdepartmental discussion, the press took up the re-processing story, after someone from the trade leaked details of the consultation process.[94] On 23 August, a *Times* headline declared 'Suspect tinned beef may be reissued'.[95] This caught the attention of the Prime Minister (Harold Wilson), whose 'first reaction' was that this was 'a matter to be handled with great caution'. Wilson's office informed MAFF that he wanted to be consulted before any decision was taken.[96] The ministries also came under pressure from the Australian government trade commissioner, who expressed concerns about implications for Australian canned meat sales. It had taken a long time 'to restore public confidence in canned meat' and he could not understand why action would be contemplated which 'could re-awaken the public memory to the whole unfortunate incident'. MAFF's Consumer Council also commented that reprocessed corned beef sold to the public should be openly labelled as such.[97]

As trade rather than health issues were at stake, it fell to MAFF to sort out the situation. MAFF told Wilson's office that they could be assured that their Minister, Fred Peart, realised the sensitivity of the matter.[98] He was about to visit Australia and New Zealand, but wrote to Robinson before leaving. Peart accepted that reprocessed meat was safe, but wanted to take account of:

> the likely public reaction on any decision we might take – even though that reaction is based on emotional and psychological factors. The outcry there has been since the Press got to hear of the proposed treatment of the meat – even from such informed bodies as the Australian Government, the C. W. S., [Co-operative Wholesale Society] and our own Consumer Council – to my mind shows very clearly what the reaction will be.[99]

Peart argued that they should bring all possible pressure to bear to keep the stock off the market.

MAFF officials proposed a deal whereby, if the trade arranged for their suspect stock to be permanently withheld from human consumption in Britain, the suspect stockpile stock would also be withheld. In seeking the Treasury's approval, they argued that while the effect of selling reprocessed corned beef might be considered a matter for the trade, if the outcome proved adverse, then the government would be blamed and 'the prospects of co-operation

---

94 Ibid.

95 'Suspect tinned beef may be reissued', *The Times*, 23 August 1965, p. 5c.

96 P. Le Cheminant to E. J. G. Smith, 23 August 1965, PRO PREM 13/891.

97 High Commissioner for Australia to Mr France, 24 August 1964; 'Reprocessed canned meat Memorandum for submission to Treasury', PRO MAF 282/113.

98 E. J. G. Smith to P. Le Cheminant, 25 August 1965, PRO PREM 13/891.

99 F. Peart to K. Robinson and W. Ross, 1 September 1965, PRO MAF 282/113.

... in similar future situations may be prejudiced'. The estimated cost of withholding the suspect material until it was inedible was £1.4 million. If a deal could not be secured it might be necessary to consider a compensation scheme, or buying the commercial suspect stock at an estimated cost of £250,000.[100] The Treasury agreed to the deal being proposed, but vetoed any question of compensation or purchase.[101] The deal was explained to the Prime Minister's office and a comment from Wilson showed he expected a hard line to be taken: 'The "if" sounds weak. Presumably we say this stuff must be got rid of.'[102]

A note discussing strategy at the next meeting with the trade suggests that MAFF had high hopes for their 'trump card'. It was expected to influence the big importers, because they had long been against the stockpile turnover policy.[103] However, the Ministry's offer did not elicit a decisive response. Most representatives felt that the release of reprocessed stock would damage the market, but Sir Derek Vestey argued that stockholders should be allowed to reprocess and sell the product wherever they could. The representatives of the distributive trade did not consider it practical for all sections of the trade to contribute to the cost of permanently withholding the suspect stock. It was agreed that the South American Freight Committee (which represented the large producers) would organise a meeting within the next few days and report back. A press statement was agreed, which stated that discussions were continuing and that, meantime, there would be no change in the status of the withdrawn stock.[104]

On 22 September, MAFF heard that the producers had rejected the suggestion that they might help the Establishment 1819 stockholders, but agreed that their own stock would not be placed on the market. The decision reached the press, and the *Daily Mail* commented that MAFF and the remaining stockholders were expected to follow suit. Under-secretary John Hensley thought that in view of this publicity there was little risk that the 1819 stockholders would consider reprocessing and marketing. There was no need to consider compensation or purchasing, and the proper course was to tell the trade that the remaining stock was their responsibility.[105] But Ministry of

---

[100] 'Reprocessed canned meat Memorandum for submission to Treasury', R. J. E. Taylor to Mr Jotcham, 10 September 1965, PRO MAF 282/113.

[101] R. J. E. Taylor to Mr Jotcham, 10 September 1965, PRO MAF 282/113.

[102] J. A. Anderson to D. J. Mitchell, 10 September 1965; D. J. Mitchell to J. A. Anderson, 13 September 1965, PRO PREM 13/891.

[103] N. J. P. Hutchison, 'Notes for meeting with Trade on 14th September about suspect canned meat', 13 September 1965, PRO MAF 282/113.

[104] 'Note of meeting at MAFF on 14th September 1965', PRO MAF 282/113; 'Corned beef press notice', PRO PREM 13/891.

[105] R. Hillenbrand to Dr Ross, 17 September 1965, PRO MH 148/99; J. Hensley to Mr Humphreys-Davies, 27 September 1965; 'Draft submission corned beef', PRO MAF 282/113.

Health Assistant Secretary Mrs Hauff commented that if the trade decided to pursue reprocessing they would have to co-operate, since there were no health implications. She was sceptical about Hensley's plan and predicted that it would 'entail wide publicity and subject the Government to a repetition of all the adverse publicity recently encountered'.[106]

On 6 October, Permanent Secretary Winnifrith advised Peart upon his return from abroad that the object was now to 'put the maximum pressure on that small section of the Trade which is still unwilling to get rid of these stocks'.[107] If stockholders decided to reprocess and sell their stock, it would have to bear a special mark, and it would be made 'perfectly clear' that 'no effort whatever would be made on the part of Government or the local authorities to conceal the origin of the reprocessed meat, or its channels of distribution – indeed rather the reverse'.[108]

On 14 October a further meeting took place, attended only by representatives of organisations known to have members holding suspect stocks. Since the large producers had agreed not to release their stocks, Hensley said that the government would like to announce that the Establishment 1819 stockholders would do likewise, or at least that this was the recommendation of their organisations. But no such undertaking was forthcoming, the organisations being unwilling to take a position without consulting their members. Several representatives raised questions of compensation but were advised that there was no prospect of this. The Freight Committee representatives then stated that unless all stockholders withheld their stock they would withdraw their commitment. It proved impossible to agree on a press statement.[109] Winnifrith commented that the meeting had been 'very disappointing with the position getting worse, not better'.[110]

A meeting of 1819 stockholders organised by the London Chamber of Commerce resolved to withhold their stocks only if compensation was granted. However, at a further meeting at MAFF on 25 October, Hensley repeated that there was no question of this. Fortunately, the major stockholders did not make good their threat to withdraw their undertaking. There was discussion of government help with an approach to Argentina regarding compensation for the 1819 stockholders, but little hope that this would be successful.[111] A press statement was issued, stating that the government did not intend to release its withdrawn stock and that the major importers had agreed to 'not dispose of their stocks on the home market for human consumption', while 'other

[106] J. Hauff to J. Hensley, 29 September 1965, PRO MAF 282/113.

[107] A. J. D. Winnifrith to Minister, 6 October 1965, PRO MAF 282/113.

[108] P. Humphreys-Davies, 'Third revised draft submission to Minister Corned Beef', 4 October 1965, PRO MAF 282/113.

[109] 'Note of a meeting held on 14th October, 1965', PRO MAF 282/113.

[110] A. J. D. Winnifrith to Minister, 18 October 1965, PRO MAF 282/113.

[111] 'Note of a meeting on 25th October 1965', PRO MAF 282/113.

private stockholders' were 'considering their position'.[112] MAFF told the Prime Minister's office that this outcome was better than expected. Since the press had taken the statement to mean that the smaller stockholders would follow the lead of the larger ones, it looked as if 'the worst of the episode is now over'.[113]

Unilateral action and intimidatory publicity

During the summer and autumn, the Ministry of Health considered various ways of disposing of the 1819 stock. They followed up the possibility of making a claim against the Argentine government, and sounded out the Foreign Office. But the Foreign Office thought that the 'primary manner for securing redress' was for the importers to take action against the Argentine exporter. That Establishment 1819 was believed to be in liquidation was not a reason for blaming the Argentine government. In any case, there was the 'question of goodwill'. The Foreign Office noted that Britain had been:

> pressing the Argentines to maintain a certain level of beef exports to this country which they have been trying to do in spite of more attractive prices which they have been receiving . . . on the Continent. If we are to obtain a satisfactory share of Argentine beef exports it is essential that we should not jeopardise the goodwill which we enjoy by putting forward a claim for compensation which rests on rather shaky grounds.[114]

All options were problematic, and no effective assistance from government departments for 1819 stockholders seemed to be forthcoming. Foley Brothers therefore prepared to take unilateral action. On 4 November, the Ministry of Health heard about moves by the firm to take some of their reprocessed stock to Gloucestershire, and it emerged that they had swapped reprocessed for unreprocessed stock held by a customer.[115] A further parcel was taken to another company's store in Poplar.[116] Officials feared that Foleys were about to market the reprocessed corned beef and, when challenged, Foley told them that he did not regard himself as bound by 'any alleged agreement'. At the 25 October meeting, following the refusal of compensation, he declared that he 'would not be agreeable to any further restraint', and would do his best to clear his company's liability. His earlier 'constructively helpful' suggestions

---

[112] Ministry of Agriculture, Fisheries and Food, 'Press notice corned beef', PRO MH 148/98.

[113] J. A. Anderson to P. Le Cheminant, 25 and 27 October 1965, PRO PREM 13/891.

[114] C. R. Wrigley to J. A. Hauff, 22 September 1965, PRO MAF 282/113.

[115] A. Robinson to Dr Ross, 4 November 1965, PRO MH 148/203; N. J. P. Hutchison to Mr Payne, 8 November 1965, PRO MAF 282/113; W. C. Turner to A. Robinson, 6 December 1965, PRO MH 148/207.

[116] A. Robinson to Dr Ross, 5 November 1965, PRO MH 148/203.

had been met by threats of 'intimidatory publicity'.[117] During a telephone conversation with Mrs Hauff, he agreed not to market the goods until after a meeting convened by the London Chamber of Commerce on 9 November. Mrs Hauff told him that if the cans were sold without an approved mark they would again be withheld, 'with all the publicity likely to ensue'. Foley asked for the mark to be agreed urgently.[118]

Foley was also considering other possibilities. He claimed to have interested overseas buyers and asked what the Ministry of Health would say to foreign health authorities if he was to export suspect stock. Hauff said they would write a 'simple, informal letter', explaining that the stock had been voluntarily withheld following the Aberdeen outbreak, refer to the Milne report, and give information about reprocessing if appropriate.[119] However, when supplied with details of the certificate to be attached to any consignment, Foley objected to the mention of *Salmonella typhimurium*, which would prevent him from proceeding with the order.[120]

The London Chamber of Commerce meeting only agreed to request the Board of Trade and the Argentine Embassy to accept deputations.[121] Winnifrith of MAFF briefed the Board of Trade, concluding that he hoped that whoever received the deputation would 'play for time in the hope . . . that the recalcitrants will think better of their intentions'.[122] But no such meeting was arranged.[123] The deputation to the embassy took place on 20 December. The Chamber explained that the 1819 stock could not be disposed of in Britain because reprocessing was uneconomic, and one stockholder could not complete a contract with an overseas buyer because of the Ministry of Health's insistence on mentioning *Salmonella typhimurium*. In view of such factors the stockholders requested facilities to reprocess their stock in Argentina.[124]

Meantime, it was decided that '99' should be added to the ends of reprocessed cans.[125] Pearson explained the decision to Foley Brothers, pointing out that MOsH would have to be informed of the arrangement. The Ministry also requested details of the location and movement of Foleys' stock.[126] Foley reacted sharply. He asked what legal powers the Ministry was acting under,

---

[117] W. S. Foley to J. A. Hauff, 8 November 1965, PRO MH 148/203.

[118] W. S. Foley to J. A. Hauff, 8 November 1965, J. Hauff to Mr Dodds, 8 November 1965, PRO MH 148/203.

[119] Ibid.

[120] W. S. Foley to J. A. Hauff, 29 November 1965, PRO MAF 282/114.

[121] Meat division, 'Note for the Minister', 12 November 1965, PRO MAF 282/113.

[122] R. Powell to A. J. D. Winnifrith, 25 November 1965; A. J. D. Winnifrith to R. Powell, 7 December 1965, PRO MAF 282/113.

[123] J. A. Anderson to Mr Hensley, 4 January 1966, MAF 282/114.

[124] J. G. Allanby to Economic Counsellor, 21 December 1965, PRO MAF 282/114.

[125] N. J. P. Hutchison to Mr Small, 10 November 1965; Meat division, 'Note for the Minister', 12 November 1965, PRO MAF 282/113.

[126] M. A. J. Pearson to E. W. Clack, 19 November 1965, PRO MAF 282/113.

and declined to supply the information requested. In conclusion, he told Mrs Pearson:

> you must be aware that the long drag of this sorry story must be terminated. The individual and vested interests may have to fight issues but the goods have to be disposed of into sensible channels of distribution or The Government concerned and other Parties must arrange adequate Compensation of the Stockholder.[127]

Foley was losing patience. He told a customer that he was pressing the Ministry of Health to give up their 'Extra Legal' stand, explaining that 'Together with everybody else concerned we have been "strung along" to await new events . . . which have influenced us . . . not to try and force the issue'. But Foley now had 'arrangements in hand to put our stocks back into distribution'. In addition, if possibilities of disposal to other markets proved feasible, he undertook to help his customer.[128]

Foley continued to resist providing details of distribution of reprocessed stock, on 15 December telling Pearson that he could not understand why this was necessary. But he confirmed that his company would co-operate with MOsH in applying stamps to reprocessed cans.[129] In view of the apparent impending release of reprocessed stock, on 21 December Godber wrote to MOsH to inform them about the mark,[130] and the Ministry reported to the Prime Minister's private secretary that Foleys were putting their reprocessed stock on the market.[131] The private secretary had not entirely understood the situation, since he informed Wilson that one of the importers 'of the Argentine corned beef *which was associated with the Aberdeen typhoid outbreak* [emphasis added] has told the Ministry of Health that he has processed his stock and now proposes to sell it for human consumption'.[132] Wilson's reaction was to 'insist strongly that whatever steps necessary to ensure that this beef did not enter trade for human consumption should be taken'.[133] MAFF officials sought to explain the difficulties involved, and agreed that Peart would let Wilson have a submission. They aimed to prepare, by 4 January, a document that would review MAFF's efforts, and explain why no powers could be invoked to enforce a ban, because no health hazard was involved.[134] These plans were, however, overtaken by events. The circular to MOsH set off renewed press reports,

[127] W. S. Foley to M. A. J. Pearson, 24 November 1965, PRO MAF 282/113.

[128] W. S. Foley to Messrs Wright & Green & Robinson Ltd, 24 November 1964, PRO MAF 282/114.

[129] W. S. Foley to M. A. J. Pearson, 15 December 1965, PRO MH 148/202.

[130] G. E. Godber, 21 December 1965, PRO MH 148/99.

[131] T. E. Nodder to M. H. M. Reid, 21 December 1965, PRO PREM 13/891.

[132] M. H. M. Reid to Prime Minister, 21 December 1965, PRO PREM 13/891.

[133] P. Le Cheminant to J. A. Anderson, 22 December 1965, PRO PREM 13/891.

[134] E. J. G. Smith to Mr Hensley, 23 December 1965, PRO MAF 282/114.

activated the trade organisations, drew Members of Parliament into the issue, and stimulated the intervention of the Prime Minister.

A new round of publicity

The National Association of Multiple Grocers complained to MAFF that they first heard about the special marks through the press, and that the advice of the distributive trade had been ignored,[135] while the National Grocers' Federation appealed to Mr K. Lomas, MP for Huddersfield West. Lomas sent telegrams to government departments asking them to prevent the sale of reprocessed corned beef. The Federation's secretary also telegrammed Wilson, stating that his organisation thought the reprocessed stock should be destroyed. They were 'appalled' that the government was permitting its sale.[136]

In view of the publicity and lobbying, a meeting between Peart and Foley was arranged for the late afternoon of 30 December, and Foley was persuaded to suspend sales of the reprocessed meat while he considered his position. A press notice was rapidly issued and the matter was reported on the 6 p.m. television news.[137] It was by no means clear what Foley would do. The *Glasgow Herald* reported him as saying that he had to 'go away and think further', but that 'These goods are ethically and legally fit for sale'.[138]

The press, on the whole, appear to have appreciated that commercial rather than health issues were at stake, *The Times* commenting that the row:

> does not hinge on a question of public health but on the psychology of bully-beef eaters. The bulk of the trade, probably correctly, holds that no expert guarantee of purity is enough to reconcile people to meat which seems to them to have so unappetizing a history.[139]

The Times thought the matter one of commercial tactics that should be left to the trade, a view forcibly expressed by the Conservative MP Enoch Powell. On Foley being called to an interview by Peart, Powell declared that this public summons of a private individual at the request of the Prime Minister was a 'particularly atrocious example of lawless action by this Government'.[140]

Prior to the meeting between Peart and Foley, Hensley phoned the Ministry of Health to discuss the problem. If it proved necessary to take powers to compel the withdrawal of the 1819 stock, they would have to be on either

---

135 J. C. Butler to N. J. P. Hutchison, 29 December 1965, PRO MAF 282/114.

136 'Corned beef release shocks trade', *Grocer*, 1 January 1966, p. 28; 'Corned beef "not of typhoid batch"', *Daily Telegraph*, 30 December 1965, cutting in PRO MAF 282/114.

137 J. P. Dodds to Mr Nodder, 30 December 1965, PRO MH 148/99.

138 'Reprocessed corned beef sales suspended', *Glasgow Herald*, 31 December 1965, p. 1e.

139 'A question of trade', *The Times*, 31 December 1965, p. 11c.

140 'Protest at action on corned beef', *The Times*, 3 January 1966, p. 6b.

health or trade grounds, but Hensley saw great difficulties in either course. Hauff thought the 'health grounds' option a non-starter. If provisions for the seizure of unfit food were amended so as to include suspect corned beef, the definition of 'unfit' would have to be so wide as to include, for example, 'food grown with the help of pesticides' and 'food to which "additives" have been added'.[141]

By 3 January, Hensley had drafted a submission on possible courses of action. One was fresh legislation preventing the sale of 1819 corned beef, but this would make demands for compensation difficult to resist. In addition, the option of purchasing risked setting an undesirable precedent. A labelling regulation, with publicity to explain what the label meant, was regarded as 'the least objectionable alternative'.[142] Regulations were therefore drafted to require reprocessed 1819 corned beef to be labelled with the words 'Reprocessed corned beef – Establishment 1819' in block letters half an inch in height.[143]

On 5 January, Peart met Wilson and told him that the labelling regulations threat would probably induce Foley to co-operate. Wilson thought Foley should be urged to dispose of his stock as exports or pet food, and suggested that the stock might be swapped with sound stock from the stockpile. Peart, however, explained that it was difficult to provide compensation for Foley while this had been refused to others. He also thought that public feeling about feeding suspect food to animals was likely to be as strong as about selling it for human consumption.[144]

Later on 5 January, before a further meeting with Foley, Peart and his officials agreed that the best option would be to re-export the 1819 corned beef.[145] The record of the meeting with Foley suggests that Peart did not need to threaten the labelling regulation. Foley clearly felt badly treated, and even betrayed. But when asked by Winnifrith about the lack of communication between the stockholders and ministers since October, Foley blamed this on lack of response from the Board of Trade. He had hoped that the proposed meeting would clear up questions concerning the authenticity of documents in connection with the re-export of 1819 stock (alluding to the Argentine official certificate). Winnifrith then told Foley that the stockholders should not think that they had exhausted all possibilities of assistance from MAFF. Persuaded that help with facilitating re-export would now be forthcoming, Foley agreed to maintain a standstill on his reprocessed stocks and to meet other stockholders with a view to securing their co-operation.[146]

---

141 J. Hauff to Mr Dodds, 30 December 1965, PRO MH 148/99.

142 J. Hensley, 'Reprocessed corned beef', 3 January 1966, PRO MH 148/99.

143 'Corned beef proposed draft statement', 5 January 1965, PRO PREM 13/891.

144 'Record of a meeting between the Minister of Agriculture, Fisheries and Food, and the Prime Minister, January 5, 1966', PRO PREM 13/891.

145 J. A. Anderson to Mr Hensley, 6 January 1966, PRO MAF 282/114.

146 J. A. Anderson to Mr Hensley, 5 January 1966, PRO MAF 282/114.

On 7 January, Peart and his officials met Foley and two other stockholders. Foley began by reading a statement agreed at a meeting of stockholders. They would abide by government policy, but this would involve them in considerable loss unless they received 'full support' in facilitating the return of the goods to Argentina or export to other markets. If such a solution could be achieved, Foley told the Minister that he 'could be assured of virtually a hundred per cent co-operation from the trade'. Peart undertook to 'take what action he could to assist the return of the corned beef to the Argentine'. As for exporting to other markets, after Foley explained that the main problem was the proposed 'clausing' of the export documents by the Ministry of Health, Peart undertook to discuss the matter with Robinson, if necessary.[147] Wilson was pleased, commenting to Peart that he was 'Glad to hear that you made satisfactory arrangements to get the corned beef withdrawn. Sure we were right to insist on this and grateful to you for carrying it out.'[148]

The 8 January editions of the trade press were highly critical of the government. The *Grocers' Gazette* expressed sympathy for the 1819 stockholders, who faced either financial loss, and in some cases bankruptcy, or being pilloried if they ignored the standstill. They also expressed support for traders at all levels, who 'through the muddled incompetence of Whitehall find themselves in a serious predicament'.[149] The *Grocer* declared that corned beef was now a 'broken market'. The blame did not lie with the retailers and wholesalers, and it was understandable that the importers and distributors would want some compensation if they were unable to get rid of their 1819 corned beef. Meanwhile, the ministries were 'passing the buck'. But the *Grocer* did not only blame the government – they also criticised the large meat packers for not facilitating the return of the 1819 material to Argentina, and bemoaned the fact that 'a whole industry' had 'fallen into disrepute'.[150] The Conservative opposition attempted to capitalise on the situation. The shadow Minister of Agriculture was highly critical, asserting that there was no justification for, on the one hand, saying that the meat was fit for sale, and, on the other, to 'bully and coerce' the stockholders into not releasing it. He observed that there seemed to be a 'lack of liaison between departments' and that 'the Prime Minister has publicly humiliated two of his Ministers by taking care to let it be known that he himself had made them eat their own words and adopt an entirely different policy in regard to this matter'.[151] The *British Food Journal* reflected that the affair had been characterised by 'a profusion of statements . . . and what seemed like a fight between factions in the trade', with the positions of the ministries 'none too clear'. And all of this had been

---

[147] J. A. Anderson to Mr Hensley, 10 January 1966, PRO MAF 282/114.
[148] H. Wilson to F. Peart, 7 January 1966, PRO PREM 13/891.
[149] 'Who is fooling whom?', *Grocers' Gazette*, 8 January 1966, PRO MH 148/99.
[150] 'Corned beef hash!', *Grocer*, 8 January 1966, p. 35.
[151] 'Beef? "Unsavoury muddle"–Tory', *Grocers' Gazette*, 15 January 1966, pp. 7, 67.

'thrown into a thorough ferment by the political intervention by the Prime Minister'.[152]

Promises and frustration

MAFF lost no time in following up their commitments. Peart saw the Argentine *Chargé d'Affaires* and argued that it would be good for both countries if the episode could be resolved quickly. He arranged for the Foreign Office to write to the Ambassador in Buenos Aires, asking him to take up the issue.[153] But the Embassy reported that Argentine officials thought the British government should have maintained the position that reprocessed corned beef was safe in the face of adverse propaganda. They claimed that the 'propaganda' had been inspired by Argentina's competitors, and by stockholders who were seeking compensation. They thought it dangerous for the Argentine government to become involved in 'questions of commercial risks', and beyond their powers to 'sponsor a deal'. They would have no objection to private interests arranging a deal, but customs regulations would allow only temporary import for subsequent re-export.[154]

When Peart told Foley of the disappointing response, Foley did not seem unduly distressed. Peart agreed to clarify whether Argentina would agree to temporary import for reprocessing free of exchange, currency or other controls.[155] He also undertook to enquire of the Ministry of Health what documentation they would expect to provide in connection with exports of 1819 stock. The Ministry's response represented a partial retreat from earlier positions. First, the exporters were not bound to tell the Ministry what their intentions were. Second, if the Ministry was aware that suspect meat was being transported to a particular country, they would tell the health authorities what they knew, 'in the mildest possible terms'. Third, they did not feel obliged to provide information about reprocessed meat, but if the exporter wanted a certificate, the MOH who had supervised the reprocessing could provide one.[156]

At the beginning of March, Foley reported that he had approached the major packers for assistance with reprocessing, repackaging and marketing, but found them 'unhelpful if not hostile'. He was considering the possibility of the work being done by Establishment 1819, which had resumed exports to North

---

[152] 'The corned beef tangle', *British Food Journal*, 1966, vol. 68, p. 15.

[153] 'Note of a meeting held between the Minister of Agriculture, Fisheries and Food and Senor Horacio Marco on 10th January 1966'; Foreign Office to Buenos Aires, 11 January 1966, PRO MAF 282/114.

[154] Buenos Aires to Foreign Office, 26 January 1966, PRO FO 371/184663.

[155] W. S. Foley to J. Winnifrith, 2 March 1966, PRO MH 148/203; N. J. P. Hutchison to J. A. Hauff, 23 February 1966, PRO MH 148/205; Foreign Office to Buenos Aires, 17 February 1966, PRO FO 371/184663.

[156] M. A. J. Pearson to Mrs Hauff, 17 February 1966, PRO MH 148/207.

America for products other than canned meat. He suggested that the company might open its cannery and undertake the reprocessing if, as an inducement, the UK placed it on the approved list. He was also considering other destinations for the stock, having shipped some overseas in January. However, the buyers met with difficulties, 'possibly due to the adverse Publicity of December/January, or the follow-up advice given by the Ministry of Health', and there had been no repeat business. He was considering reprocessing or repackaging in fresh cans prior to export,[157] but officials opposed this as it would lead to a further round of publicity.[158]

MAFF agreed to take 'preliminary soundings' in any country that Foley considered exporting to. If required, a certificate could be provided, stating that reprocessing had taken place according to an approved method. But MAFF pointed out that exporting to most countries would present difficulties, because the authorities would require positive identification that the meat had originated from animals which had undergone ante- and post-mortem inspection.[159] Foley seemed unconcerned about this, and was more worried that the certificate envisaged might mention *Salmonella typhimurium*. He asked whether it could be simply stated that reprocessing 'ensures complete sterility'.[160]

Foley attended a further meeting at MAFF on 13 April 1966. He now felt that the ideal solution was to return the stock to the original plant. However, he understood that the Argentine authorities were obstructing the plant's application for 'approved' status following pressure from the major packers. The officials undertook to investigate and to continue enquiries about the exchange controls. As for the certificate covering reprocessed stock, there was some further softening of the previous line: it might be possible to avoid mentioning salmonella, and to refer to reprocessing ensuring 'commercial sterility of the product'. But prevarication continued on these points, and officials now also thought it pointless to use British government representatives in making enquiries overseas, as they would alert foreign officials to suspect consignments which they otherwise would not query.[161] Later MAFF provided a list of countries that did not require certificates, mostly in Africa and the Middle and Far East,[162] but Foley had already explored such outlets, finding the distributors hostile, as agents of the big packers.[163]

None of MAFF's activities were of any help by the time of Foley's next visit to the Ministry, accompanied by representatives of another company. They

---

[157] W. S. Foley to J. Winnifrith, 2 March 1966, PRO MH 148/203.

[158] N. J. P. Hutchison, 14 April 1966, PRO MAF 282/115.

[159] A. J. D. Winnifrith to W. S. Foley, 21 March 1966, PRO MAF 282/115.

[160] W. S. Foley to J. Winnifrith, 25 March 1966, PRO MH 282/115.

[161] N. J. P. Hutchison, 14 April 1966, PRO MAF 282/115.

[162] K. A. Bird to W. S. Foley, 24 May 1966, PRO MAF 282/115.

[163] 'Note for record', PRO MAF 282/115.

were 'clearly unhappy with the situation and felt that they were not being given all the assistance that might be possible'. Once again, little positive transpired. MAFF only undertook to consider whether their agents for the disposal of stockpile stock, Wallin & Thompson Ltd, might be permitted to help. Some clarification of the Argentine exchange control problems had been achieved, but there was no sign of the 1819 cannery reopening. Foley mentioned that 3500 cases of unreprocessed material had been disposed of in Europe using the original certificate but that 1000 were 'now not being moved', suggesting that MAFF may have passed on adverse information. This was denied by officials.[164] One official later recorded that the Ministry of Health also knew nothing of the matter. It was more likely that trade competitors were sabotaging Foley's efforts. As for the exports of the unreprocessed stock to date:

> So far as this Department is concerned we do not seek to influence either way the view a foreign administration may take . . . but if asked questions of fact, e.g. whether establishment 1819 is or is not on our approved list, we must answer truthfully. So far as the Ministry of Health is concerned they would feel obliged to mention the circumstances to the health authorities of the country concerned if it came to their notice that stocks were going to a particular country.[165]

There was an element of, if possible, 'turning a blind eye', and the dangers of this were recognised by another official. MAFF would be criticised if it became known that they had knowingly allowed 'material which was considered unsuitable for sale on the UK market, for health reasons, to be foisted on other countries'. But if MAFF did pass on information, the possible outlet would probably be closed and the 1819 stockholders would regard this as 'a stab in the back'.[166]

MAFF now took a harder line. If asked to supply a certificate, they would have to detail 'the whole of the facts in relation to the goods as set out in the Milne report plus the trade considerations which had prevented the sale of the material after reprocessing'. Foley regarded this as 'useless' and 'unduly obstructive'.[167] But it emerged that Foley had found an alternative method of certification for unreprocessed stock, avoiding contact with central government. Customarily, port health authorities provided a certificate for re-exported goods, which stated simply that goods in a particular bill of landing had arrived bearing an official certificate from another country, which was then quoted. According to the Ministry of Health, this was 'not covered by statute or under any specific control by the Health Departments'. There were therefore 'no grounds on which the Ministry of Health could or would wish to

---

[164] Ibid.
[165] N. J. P. Hutchison to Mr Payne, 14 July 1966, PRO MAF 282/115.
[166] K. A. Bird to Mr Hensley, 19 July 1966, PRO MAF 282/115.
[167] K. A. Bird to P. Humphreys-Davies, 2 August 1966, PRO MAF 282/115.

intervene'.[168] This was certainly drawing back from earlier positions, and when a MOH reported movements of stock in August, the Ministry decided that it did not need to know.[169] After one MOH interfered with the movement of stock and looked for support, discussion took place on how to avoid such incidents. It was decided not to circulate MOsH for fear of publicity, but to suggest to Foley that stockholders might send a courtesy letter to the local MOH whenever movement of 1819 stock was imminent, assuring them that it was within the terms of the agreement with the government.[170]

This method of certification proved only a small breakthrough, because the sales in question did not generate repeat orders and Foley again asserted that 'someone was damaging his interests in some clandestine way'.[171] Soon the 1819 stockholders were again 'restive',[172] and one declared his intentions to sell his stock for any purpose to the highest bidder. He asked for details of the legal penalty he might incur to help him decide whether he could offset the fine or gaol sentence against the commercial benefit.[173] It was now agreed to let Wallin & Thompson help. They were confident that they could find a market, and were soon introducing buyers and sellers. At around the same time, there was finally some progress on the question of the 1819 cannery. The veterinary attaché had visited the factory, which had been given a new code number, and he had specified the improvements which would have to be made for approval to be granted.[174]

The disposal of the 1819 produce proceeded slowly and Foley again became upset when MAFF refused to facilitate a barter of corned beef for butter. The stock he had disposed of had been 'consumed happily', but 'slanderous accusations' had obstructed repeat business and had even 'encouraged less reputable elements to what must plainly be regarded as Blackmail'.[175] In December, he complained that 'some sort of advice emanating from the UK Government' had resulted in the closure of one European market, with the goods returned. Such success as the stockholders had achieved, he declared, was entirely due to their own efforts, but their problems were due to 'Government Intervention twelve months ago, which gave substance to the combination of emotional hysteria and trade competitors' opposition'. They were now 'half way through the problem' but would face further difficulties if the 'intervention' continued.[176] From this point onward, Foley kept his distance from the ministries.

---

[168] N. J. P. Hutchison to Mr Skilling, 10 August 1966, PRO MAF 282/115.

[169] J. Ross to Mrs Pearson, 2 August 1966, PRO MH 148/99.

[170] Middleton to Mr Hutchison, 21 November 1966, PRO MH 148/99.

[171] J. P. Hutchison to Mr Middleton, 11 October 1966, PRO MAF 282/115.

[172] N. J. P. Hutchison to Mr Payne, 19 September 1966, PRO MAF 282/115.

[173] Middleton to Mr Payne, 19 October 1966, PRO MH 148/99.

[174] K. A. Bird to W. S. Foley, 26 August 1966; R. G. R. Wall to Mr Payne, 26 September 1966; N. J. P. Hutchison to Mr Middleton, 11 October 1966, PRO MAF 282/115.

[175] W. S. Foley to J. Winnifrith, 7 November 1966, PRO MAF 282/115.

[176] W. S. Foley to J. Winnifrith, 5 December 1966, PRO MAF 282/115.

And despite all the difficulties, when Bird wrote in September 1967 to tell him that the old Establishment 1819 had been accepted on to the approved list, Foley replied that he had already managed to dispose of the rest of his stock.[177] The problem had been solved but, largely in view of political considerations which precluded the reprocessing operation that the Milne Committee envisaged, the bulk of the 1819 stock had been shipped abroad and consumed in its original state.

Disposal of the suspect stockpile corned beef

During 1968, in view of changes in stockpile policy, the disposal of the stockpile suspect stock began to be reconsidered. There was a long-established policy of running down the amount of canned meat in the stockpile, as purchases were financed from sales, and some of the proceeds were diverted into purchases of other foods.[178] From 104,950 tons in 1956, the total corned beef stock dropped to 49,000 tons by 1964.[179] And in February 1965, as an economy measure, the Defence and Overseas Policy Committee decided to divert the £2 million that it was expected to raise from sales during 1965 and 1966, away from new purchases and towards maintenance costs.[180]

Corned beef was originally considered good for the stockpile because it was ready to eat, useful for maintaining morale, and protected against nuclear fall-out. But its nutrition to weight ratio was low, and it was the most expensive food in the stockpile.[181] It was also expensive to maintain, since it was kept in humidity-controlled cold stores.[182] In view of the expense, the future of the stockpile came under the investigation of the Home Defence Review from 1965,[183] and by 1967, canned meat was deemed no longer an essential component. All stocks were to be disposed of by August 1970.[184] It was estimated that by 1 April 1968 there would be 25,000 tons of canned beef left (including 2300 tons of stewed steak), 8100 of which were suspect.[185]

---

[177] K. A. Bird to C. M. Firth, 15 September 1967, PRO MAF 282/115.

[178] R. J. E. Taylor, 'Stockpile programme, 1963/64', PRO MAF 246/44.

[179] Meat and Livestock division, 'Stock-pile policy canned meat paper for meeting on 10th May 1961', April 1961; A. R. Parselle, 'Canned meat stockpile Brief for meeting April 2nd 1964', April 1964, PRO 246/44.

[180] J. R. Renolds to A. R. Parselle, 10 February 1965; N. J. P. Hutchison to R. J. E. Taylor, 15 February 1964, PRO MAF 246/178.

[181] R. J. E. Taylor to S. T. Charles, 'Strategic food stockpile programme, 1963/64', 15 March 1963, PRO MAF 246/44.

[182] B. H. Woollacott to J. Graham, March 1958, PRO MAF 246/73; Meat and Livestock division, 'Stock-pile policy canned meat paper for meeting on 10th May 1961', April 1961, PRO 246/44.

[183] R. J. E. Taylor to Mr Jotcham, 10 September 1965, PRO MAF 282/113.

[184] A. R. Parselle to G. H. B. King, 7 December 1967, PRO MAF 246/178.

[185] E. A. Townsend, 28 December 1967, PRO MAF 246/178.

In November 1968 it was decided to turn off the humidity controls from 1 December, in the expectation that despite increased deterioration, the cans would remain saleable until August 1970.[186]

By December 1968, £20,000 had been recovered by the sale of 500 tons of pre-1955 suspect meat for pet food manufacture in Italy, on conditions that precluded its return. This left about 600 tons of this material, which it was hoped to dispose of in the same way. As for the 5200 tons of post-1958 typhoid-suspect production, MAFF's Meat division officials sought permission for this to be sold to South America.[187] With ministerial permission obtained, MAFF's Meat division asked the Ministry of Health whether they had any objections to the proposed course of action,[188] and MAFF's Animal Health division II, which had not been party to the decision making so far, also became aware of the proposals.[189] In view of their public health responsibility for overseas meat inspection, Animal Health division II regarded themselves as the proper channel for communication with the Ministry of Health. They believed that the CMO would oppose the plan, and so it was arranged for Ministry of Health officials not to put it to him in the meantime, in case MAFF became 'landed with a ruling' that would be 'difficult to get round'.[190] Animal Health division II opposed the export of the suspect meat, because they thought it contrary to statements made to the press and in Parliament since October 1965. If it became known that disposal of the suspect stock was proceeding in spite of these statements, they thought that the 'political result' might be 'extremely serious'.[191] At an exchange of views between the divisions, Animal Health division II argued against the export of suspect stock in case it should lead to a typhoid outbreak, for which the British government would be responsible. They were especially opposed to the stock being sent to countries whose meat plants were approved by the UK. They had been trying to persuade the authorities of various countries to improve their hygiene standards, and the sale would cast doubt on their good faith. This position was supported by the External Relations division, and it was agreed, after all, that it was inadvisable to export the stock to either South America or Italy. Instead, export to Indonesia, Thailand and the Philippines, where there were no UK-approved establishments, would be explored. And disposal for animal food in the UK would also be considered.[192]

---

[186] O. R. Appleby to J. L. Cope, 14 November 1968; J. L. Cope to R. C. Evans, 25 November 1968, PRO MAF 246/178.

[187] 'Food stockpile – stocks of suspect canned corned beef Submission to the Minister'; O. R. Appleby to L. Hurst, 18 December 1968, PRO MAF 282/115.

[188] G. B. H. King to J. M. Firth, 6 December 1968, PRO MAF 282/115.

[189] O. R. Appleby to L. Hurst, 18 December 1968, PRO MAF 282/115.

[190] J. G. Carnochan to Mr Crump, 2 January 1969, PRO MAF 282/115.

[191] G. O. Lace to G. H. B. King, 18 and 24 December 1968, PRO MAF 282/115.

[192] 'Food stockpile – disposal of stocks of "typhoid suspect" canned corned meat Note of meeting held in Mr Carnochan's room at 3p.m. on 8th January 1969', PRO MAF 282/115.

With a view to possible sales in the Far East, MAFF consulted the FCO. They were alarmed at the idea that ministers should be involved in selling goods that could not be disposed of at home because of a possible health hazard to underdeveloped countries. They thought that if the transaction became known, ministers would be vulnerable to attack, and the only defence would be the need to save public funds. But there could be repercussions which would be detrimental to trade, and informal soundings with the Treasury and Board of Trade suggested that there would be further opposition to the proposal.[193]

Fortunately, Wallin & Thompson Ltd came up with an alternative proposal, namely for the material to be sold to a firm for reprocessing in Gibraltar at a cannery that could be leased for the purpose, with the product sold outside of the UK. The cannery's official certificate would be withdrawn temporarily to reduce the risk of the product returning to the UK, and the process would be supervised by Perfect Lambert Ltd and the Gibraltar health authorities. MAFF estimated that at 9d per pound this would provide a return of £450,000 for the 5860 tons of suspect corned beef.[194] The price was attractive, compared with a possible sale at 4d per pound for pet food manufacture. The potential proceeds also compared with an estimated cost of £150,000 for storage to destruction.[195] Animal Health division II again drew attention to possible problems. The minister would have to be told that undertakings had been given not only that the suspect meat would not be released for consumption in the UK, but also that it would not be released at all. The likelihood of 'political trouble' was reckoned to be small, but 'if it happened the trouble could be serious'. It would also become known in trade circles what the ministry was doing, which would damage Britain's reputation.[196]

The Meat division disagreed with the Animal Health division II's interpretation of the previous commitments, arguing that the emphasis had been directed:

> firstly to the potential risk to consumers in the U.K., and secondly to the possibility of damage to public confidence to canned meat markets generally in the UK which might ensue from releasing the meat on to the *home market* in any form.[197]

Selling the meat for supervised reprocessing abroad and sale outside the UK would hardly conflict with these undertakings. This position was based on a

---

[193] D. Evans to G. W. Jewkes, 13 February 1969; G. W. Jewkes to Mr Preston, 26 February 1969; G. W. Jewkes to D. Evans, 4 March 1967, PRO FCO/91.

[194] O. R. Appleby to L. Hurst, 'Food stockpile – stocks of "suspect" canned corned beef', 26 March 1969; O. R. Appleby to L. Hurst, 11 April 1969, PRO MAF 282/116.

[195] O. R. Appleby to A. G. Robinson, 1 April 1969, PRO MAF 282/116.

[196] L. Hurst to O. R. Appleby, April 1969, PRO MAF 282/116.

[197] O. R. Appleby to L. Hurst, 16 April 1969, PRO MAF 282/116.

press notice of 1965,[198] while Animal Health division II's was based on an answer to a parliamentary question on 22 December 1966.[199]

External Relations division advised that before putting the proposal to the Minister, the FCO should be consulted.[200] The FCO again found the plan distasteful, but were prepared to assist.[201] With the approval of the Ministry of Health obtained, a submission was put to the Minister of Agriculture in July. This was Cledwyn Hughes, who had succeeded Fred Peart in the post. The submission followed the lines of the original proposal, and named two potential purchasers of the meat, who would be asked to bid for the contract. The past policy statements were put to the Minister, but the document claimed that it was unlikely that 'disposal abroad under adequate health safeguards would be challenged'. As for possible accusations that Britain might be accused of 'double standards and thus might embarrass our veterinary staff in their efforts to raise standards among our less satisfactory suppliers', it was suggested that solving the problem of the suspect stock would be worth the risk.[202] The Minister gave his approval. By mid-August, arrangements for the supervision of the process had been agreed with the MOH for Gibraltar,[203] and the contract had been awarded.[204]

Implementing the scheme fell to the Emergency Services and Defence division, which devoted much thought and planning to potential public relations problems. Nevertheless, one official began to worry that the submission to the Minister had been too 'sanguine' in suggesting that there was little risk of adverse publicity. He suggested that certain journalists 'could work up quite a dramatic knocking story about our disposing of this meat in this way'.[205] He thought that the fact that the reprocessed product would not be allowed back into the UK should 'not be regarded as sufficient safeguard against the possibility of critical comment'. In the event, however, the operation proceeded unnoticed, until its existence was admitted after a theft of suspect stock from a store in South Wales, which came to light in December 1970. About 12cwt of the 500 tons of corned beef at the store, which was all destined for Gibraltar, was stolen by a workman involved in alterations, and sold to cafés and shared among friends.[206] The police who investigated proposed that

---

[198] Ibid.

[199] L. Hurst to O. R. Appleby, 22 April 1969, PRO MAF 282/116.

[200] D. Evans to O. R. Appleby, 22 April 1969, PRO MAF 282/116.

[201] D. Evans to G. W. Jewkes, 14 May 1969; G. W. Jewkes to D. Evans, 30 May 1969, PRO FCO/91.

[202] Meat division, 'Food stockpile – stocks of suspect canned corned beef Submission to the Minister', July 1969, PRO MAF 282/116.

[203] O. R. Appleby to R. J. Blake, 20 August 1969, PRO MAF 282/116.

[204] W. E. Crump to Mr Keeling, 17 September 1971, PRO MAF 282/116.

[205] J. G. Carnochan to Mr Crump, 12 February 1970, PRO MAF 282/116.

[206] Defence, Emergencies and Crop Improvement, 'Theft of suspect canned corned meat from Llantarnum buffer depot', PRO MAF 282/116.

a warning be issued through the local media. Animal Health division II advised the Permanent Secretary that although most of the stolen meat had probably been consumed, they would be 'very vulnerable if we did not exhaust every possibility of warning people generally. The meat is not more than suspect, but were a typhoid outbreak to result we would be gravely culpable if we had failed to issue warnings.' But against this it could be argued that it would be a mistake to worry the public unnecessarily, and the corned meat trade would be very critical of any action which might damage sales. The objective would be for publicity to be kept as local as possible, but the statement would probably be picked up by the national media and lead to a 'spate of Parliamentary Questions'.[207]

The warning issued did not mention typhoid but stated that the stolen meat was 'not suitable for human consumption'. It gave information about how to identify the cans, and advised anyone in possession of them to take them to their local public health department.[208] The following day MAFF issued a press notice which emphasised that it was extremely unlikely that anyone eating the corned beef would become ill, and expressed concern that the public should not become alarmed about the safety of corned beef in general. This notice explained that the meat had been withheld as a precautionary measure following the enquiry into the Aberdeen typhoid outbreak. A footnote added that the enquiry recommended that the suspect material could be made fit for consumption by reprocessing. The Ministry had arranged 'some time ago' for this to be 'carried out abroad under strict and approved conditions after which the meat is being disposed of for consumption outside the United Kingdom'.[209]

There is no evidence that this episode caused any significant political problems.[210] Some anxiety occurred, however, when, in December 1970, Dutch officials asked MAFF for details of why a consignment of corned beef that had arrived in the Netherlands from Gibraltar had needed reprocessing, and why Britain did not want it. While they were apparently satisfied with the explanation, this incident was thought unfortunate because the Dutch official certificate had been removed in September 1969 due to the laxity of their controls.[211] Some further worries occurred in August 1971 when the UK Managing Director of CAP claimed that one of his customers had been offered a supply of reprocessed corned beef via Belgium. The possibility of alerting customs and port health authorities was discussed, but as only a single sample

<hr />

207 R. P. Fraser to Secretary, 16 December 1970, PRO MAF 282/116.

208 W. E. Crump to Mr Fraser, 16 December 1970, PRO MAF 282/116.

209 Press notice, 'Canned corned meat', 17 December 1972, PRO MAF 282/116.

210 This statement is based on lack of evidence for this in file PRO MAF 282/116, the absence of questions related to the episode in *PD(C)* and *PD(L)*, and the lack of any report of the matter in *The Times*, revealed through the inspection of the indexes.

211 'Corned beef, Note for Mr Doling', PRO MAF 282/116.

tin was involved, this action was not taken, because it was thought likely that an 'unwarranted scare' would result.[212]

The successful disposal of the suspect corned beef, and the fading of public, press and parliamentary interest in the issue, effectively solved the last of the problems that arose for the government from the typhoid outbreaks of 1963 to 1964. But in view of political considerations, the solution had been very different to that imagined by the Milne Committee.

Conclusions

This chapter has provided a clear example of political factors taking priority over advice based on scientific assessments of health risks in food safety policy. It was the possible political implications of reprocessing of the suspect corned beef in accord with the Milne Committee's recommendation that proved decisive. As we have seen, the level of press, parliamentary and commercial attention the matter received in August and December 1965, and fear of further political repercussions, provoked the intervention of the Prime Minister, who dictated the line to be taken. The Minister of Agriculture was told the result to be achieved, and it was achieved within the confines of existing legislation by the application of threats of bad publicity and moral pressure upon the trade. The deal struck by the Ministry, whereby suspect stockpile stock would be permanently withheld in return for the permanent withholding of the commercial suspect stock, was accepted by the larger firms. They could potentially increase their sales if less stockpiled corned beef could be returned to the market. But this solution had no attraction for the smaller firms who held Establishment 1819 stock, who had no connection with the producers in Argentina, and therefore had no easy means of disposing of their suspect stock.

Ultimately, in the absence of any offer of compensation in view of a ruling by the Treasury, the result of the Prime Minister's intervention was that most of the Establishment 1819 stock was shipped abroad and consumed in its original state rather than after reprocessing as the Milne Committee had envisaged. However, this seemed acceptable to civil servants and politicians, so long as it only put at risk the populations of foreign countries. There is no evidence, however, at least in the Ministry of Health and MAFF files examined in the course of preparing this book, that any harm resulted.

In this chapter there has been some evidence of conflict within ministries over decision making, as well as the involvement of other ministries, especially

---

[212] W. E. Crump to Mr Bassett, 13 August 1971, PRO MAF 282/116; W. E. Crump to E. H. Doling, 16 August 1961; W. E. Crump to Mr Cope, 20 August 1971; L. Hurst to W. E. Crump, 20 August 1971, PRO MAF 282/116.

the Treasury and the Foreign Office. These additional layers in food policy making will be developed further in the next chapter, which considers one further decision-making process arising from the Aberdeen typhoid outbreak and the report of the Milne Committee.

9

British action to encourage improvements in Argentine meat hygiene, 1964 to 1969

Introduction

The visit to South America in early 1964 of Leo Grace, MAFF's chief technical adviser on meat inspection, not only showed that two plants were using untreated water. Grace was also shocked by the run-down and unhygienic state of most meat plants, and the disorganisation of the inspection service. Attempts by the British to apply pressure upon the South American governments to remedy this situation were not underway by the time of the Aberdeen outbreak, but the matter was pursued soon afterwards. The Milne Committee recommended that 'the hygienic requirements to be observed by establishments exporting meat and meat products to this country should be set out in as clear and detailed a manner as possible',[1] but upon publication of the report, the Secretary of State for Scotland was able to announce that it was already being attended to. He did not admit, however, that the responses of several countries, including Argentina, had not been satisfactory.

This chapter will follow the efforts to persuade the Argentine government to clean up their meat industry and to improve their meat inspection service. Similar problems occurred with other South American countries, but we will focus on Argentina since it produced the corned beef that was associated with the 1963 to 1964 typhoid outbreaks. Policy debate revolved around the 'official certificate procedure' which was the responsibility of one of MAFF's divisions, and which aimed to safeguard public health by regulation of overseas meat industries. It was this division which played a leading role, but, as we will see, its proposals were sometimes resisted by other MAFF divisions and other ministries. Eventually the meat plants were improved, largely for commercial reasons, but eight years after the Aberdeen typhoid outbreak, the control of Argentine meat plant hygiene was still unsatisfactory.

The 'official certificate' system for public health approval was described in Chapter 2.[2] As for animal health approval, the regulations applying to most countries were embodied in the Diseases of Animals Act, 1950, and the

---

[1] Scottish Home and Health Department, *The Aberdeen Typhoid Outbreak*, Edinburgh, 1964 (Milne report), p. 7.
[2] See pp. 43–4.

253

Importation of Carcasses and Animal Products Orders, 1954 and 1960, but the core regulations relating to South America dated to the Bledisloe agreement of 1928.[3] For some countries, the animal health risks were low and the meat inspection services efficient, so the government concerned was trusted with maintaining adequate standards. But there was a continuous risk of the importation of foot-and-mouth disease from South America, doubts about the effectiveness of inspection, and a history of problems with the meat arriving in the UK. A list of *frigoríficos* approved from the animal health perspective had therefore been prepared.

Adjustments to the animal health list, and exclusions of establishments from the public health certificate, were made in response to the advice of the veterinary attaché at the Embassy in Buenos Aires. Once a recommendation was made, and after the Ministry of Health was consulted in the case of public health matters, MAFF would inform the Foreign Office, the Foreign Office would inform the Embassy, and the Embassy would inform the Argentine government of the decision. But this simplifies the chain of communication, because it also involved inter-divisional exchanges, for example, between the Animal Health and External Relations divisions of MAFF. Decisions were published in the *London Gazette*, the British government newspaper, and conveyed to port health authorities, local authorities and MOsH.[4]

Action following the Aberdeen typhoid outbreak

Prior to the Aberdeen outbreak, while certain Argentine establishments had been excluded from the official certificate, there was no public health approved list. However, in mid-June 1964, after it was realised that the Argentine government had omitted Establishment 1819 from the list supplied to Grace, MAFF instructed the veterinary attaché, R. H. Ewart, to warn the Argentine veterinary authorities that, in future, produce would only be accepted from establishments approved by British inspections.[5] On 23 June, a list of acceptable South American canneries was published in the *London Gazette*.[6] This meant that, along with the list of establishments acceptable from the animal health standpoint, all Argentine establishments exporting to Britain had been identified.

These were 'emergency' measures, but the Aberdeen outbreak raised broader policy issues, discussed in a memorandum by Ken Bird, Chief Executive Officer of MAFF's Food Standards, Hygiene and Slaughterhouse Policy division. A long-term programme of visits to all supplying countries was planned, but

---

[3] See p. 39.
[4] 'Imported meat and meat products', 24 June 1964, PRO MAF 282/90.
[5] M. D. M. Franklin to Mr Lace, 16 June 1964, PRO MAF 282/90.
[6] G. O. Lace, 'Notice for insertion in the *London Gazette*', PRO MAF 282/90.

Bird suggested that the Minister needed to be able to provide reassurance about the safety of imported canned meat quickly. He proposed that a note be sent to all countries holding official certificates for meat products. This would stress that the certificate implied all necessary precautions had been taken to prevent dangers to public health, and seek assurances that the certificate would not be applied to canned meat cooled with non-potable water. A list of canneries meeting these standards would be requested and supplies from other canneries would then be rejected. This, Bird suggested, 'would produce results in the foreseeable future which would provide a reasonable safeguard'.[7]

Bird's strategy was adopted, and extended to all establishments (not only canneries) after high-level discussions. Selwyn Lloyd, Lord Privy Seal, prepared a note proposing an 'Independent all-Party enquiry into the system of importing canned food and food generally', but ministers concluded that 'it would be wrong to set up an outside enquiry, or . . . to refer to an "enquiry" of any kind, since this would arouse doubts about the adequacy of our arrangements which do not at present exist'. Instead, it was agreed to proceed along the lines of Bird's proposals, and to send supplying countries an *aide-mémoire* detailing the UK's 'specific requirements'. Within three or four months shipments would be accepted from approved establishments only, and more 'on-the-spot inspections' would be arranged. It was not proposed to publicise these moves, but the press would be given the gist of what was happening if they enquired.[8] The targeting of all relevant countries would help prevent offending the Argentinians' concerns about being singled out.

Anxieties about publicity were reinforced during preparation of the *aide-mémoire*, when Anthony Cowdy, who was writing on overseas meat inspection for the *Sunday Times*, asked for an interview. The MAFF officials 'batted as best we could against some well directed bowling', but warned that there were likely to be criticisms in the article. Cowdy might point to 'insufficient inspectors and hence insufficient overseas inspection'.[9] This was the thrust of the article, which appeared under the headline 'Britain's two-man tin check to get tougher'.[10] But this was not a sensational issue and it was not taken up by the rest of the press.

The *aide-mémoire* was cleared by the Foreign and Colonial Offices by 22 July,[11] and transmitted to fifty-four governments. The document began by mentioning the 1963 outbreaks 'which were associated with imported canned meat' and the recent outbreak in which the same connection had been

---

[7] K. A. Bird to G. O. Lace, 'Imported meat and meat products', 16 June 1964, PRO MAF 282/90.

[8] C. Soames to Lord Privy Seal, 25 June 1964, PRO MAF 282/90.

[9] K. A. Bird to Mr Hensley, 2 July 1964, PRO MAF 282/90.

[10] A. Cowdy, 'Britain's two-man tin check to get tougher', *Sunday Times*, 5 July 1964, cutting in PRO MAF 282/90.

[11] J. H. V. Davies to G. O. Lace, 22 July 1964, PRO MAF 282/90.

'publicly canvassed'. In view of these events, the British government had been considering 'arrangements for safeguarding human health in connection with imports of meat and meat products'.[12] The note asked for assurances that ante- and post-mortem inspections were carried out according to principles set out in appendices. As an indication of the minimum food hygiene standards, regulations pertaining to England and Wales were appended.[13] A further appendix declared that cooling water should be of a standard acceptable for public supplies, and specified the maximum number of organisms per millilitre, the treatment required for polluted sources, and the free chlorine content after treatment.[14] In conclusion, governments were asked to produce lists of establishments at which the principles indicated were being observed by the end of September.[15] The Embassy in Buenos Aires transmitted the *aide-mémoire* to the Argentine government on 14 August, and warned that a further communication in connection with Grace's visit would follow.[16]

Grace's report, dated 30 June 1964,[17] began with the immediate background to his trip – the 1963 outbreaks – but admitted that 'evidence of laxity in supervision of meat hygiene and meat inspection' had already accumulated from port health authorities. They had found a high incidence of meat infected with *Salmonellae*, and diseased offal. Grace reported that the Argentine meat inspection organisation consisted of a headquarters staff, with veterinary inspectors at each plant. Auxiliaries supplied by the plants carried out routine incisions of organs. On paper, the organisation was good, but in practice it was poor. Ante-mortem inspection was often inadequate. Frequently 'animals in an advanced state of disease' were mixed with healthy ones. Grace described the post-mortem inspection as often 'perfunctory . . . without any serious veterinary supervision'. He was alarmed by the serious deterioration of the buildings. Broken floors and walls, defective lighting, cracked wooden equipment, no facilities for sterilising implements, and primitive toilets, were all common. Because of 'filthy and impossible conditions' he recommended that

---

[12] 'Public Health (Imported Food) Regulations, 1937 and 1948 Official Certificate for Meat and Meat Products', PRO MAF 282/9.

[13] These were the Slaughterhouse (Hygiene) Regulations, 1958, the Food Hygiene (General) Regulations, 1960, and the Food Hygiene (Docks and Carriers, etc) Regulations, 1960. They were made under Sections 13 and 123 of the Food and Drugs Act, 1955. The equivalent Scottish regulations were the Food (Preparation and Distribution of Meat) (Scotland) Regulations, 1963, and 'Statutory provisions governing imported meat and meat products within Great Britain', MAF 282/90.

[14] 'Appendix VI: The standard of cooling water in canning factories', PRO MAF 282/9.

[15] Public Health (Imported Food) Regulations, 1937 and 1948 Official Certificate for Meat and Meat Products', PRO MAF 282/9.

[16] *Aide-mémoire*, 4 March 1965, PRO MAF 276/260; 'Additional paragraph: Government of Argentina', PRO MAF 282/90.

[17] L. B. A. Grace, 'Inspection of meat producing establishments in Argentina, Uruguay and Paraguay concerned with exports to the United Kingdom, 16th January to 11th April, 1964', 30 June 1964, PRO MAF 282/130.

two establishments be immediately excluded from the official certificate. He added, however, that he and Ewart had been embarrassed by the length of time this had taken, and that in future a faster procedure was needed. Four establishments 'on the fringe' were warned to make improvements quickly.

Grace sometimes found that diseased meat was sent to canneries and that veterinary officers thought this acceptable because the meat was sterilised during canning. They disclaimed knowledge of the UK's regulations that precluded this practice. Defects were found at all the canneries and only a few came close to the required standards. He paid special attention to the cooling water and checked the level of chlorine, making sure that there was now 'complete awareness of the essential need to chlorinate adequately'.[18]

When Grace and Ewart met the Director-General of Animal Health, they provided a copy of the British legislation covering imported meat and meat products. Grace expressed his disappointment about the 'lack of veterinary control' in most *frigorificos* and referred to specific inadequacies. As for enforcement, there was disagreement about procedures and the role of the veterinary attaché. Grace commented that had the Argentine authorities been doing their job, his visit would have been unnecessary. In response, the Director-General argued that since the British government maintained a veterinary representative in the country, it was impossible for the Argentines to withdraw approval from establishments. Grace rejected this, and reported that the 'Argentine authorities are now in no doubt that, from the pure public health angle, they are the responsible party'.[19]

At the end of July, A. J. D. Winnifrith, Permanent Secretary at MAFF, suggested that the Minister ought to glance through Grace's report, commenting that quite apart from the 'risk of typhoid as a result of using bad water . . . the general picture . . . is appalling'. He was concerned that there seemed to be evidence of this state of affairs even prior to the 1963 outbreaks, and that the Argentine authorities appeared to disclaim responsibility. A note on Grace's findings was submitted to the Argentine authorities towards the end of August.[20]

The fate of the *aide-mémoire*

It was envisaged that once the Argentine government had responded to the *aide-mémoire*, a list of acceptable *frigorificos* would be published in the *London Gazette*, and MAFF was anxious to proceed. During August, Ewart reported that he had visited an unsatisfactory establishment which he thought should be excluded from trade with the UK, but it was agreed that

---

[18] Ibid.
[19] Ibid.
[20] A. J. D. Winnifrith to Mr Franklin, 28 July 1964, PRO MAF 282/9.

action would have to wait until the Argentine government responded. However, Argentina, like some other countries, was in no hurry to reply. By 7 October only twenty-two replies had been received, and reminders were sent to thirty-two countries. It emerged that the Argentine authorities had lost the appendices to the *aide-mémoire*, which Bird regarded as a 'complete lack of realisation . . . of the importance of the matter'.[21] During discussion of the Milne report on 23 November, he disclosed that nineteen replies were outstanding, and that the defaulters still included Argentina. Winnifrith and the Minister, Fred Peart, now proposed that strong action be taken. A few days later, Bird told Assistant Secretary G. O. Lace, who was responsible for Animal Health division II (formerly Food Standards, Hygiene and Slaughterhouse Policy), that the only threat available was withdrawal of the official certificate. However, to execute this threat would be 'very serious', and Meat and Livestock division, whose brief was to advise on supply, might argue that market conditions precluded such a step. In this case, a new reminder would have to be issued 'in the strongest possible terms', but without a threat it would probably be ineffective.[22]

Meat and Livestock division expected Argentine chilled beef supplies to fall from 2300 tons a week to less than 2000 in 1965,[23] and as Assistant Secretary N. J. P. Hutchison saw it, the main point was the 'vital need of Argentine chilled beef in setting the whole tone of the market'. There were concerns 'lest high prices for beef . . . once again hit the headlines', and in these circumstances 'even a little Argentine chilled beef is better than none at all – which would really scare the market'. The health risks, he thought, 'would have to be very obvious indeed before public opinion would accept "famine" prices'.[24] Hutchison later reported that Argentina was diverting supplies to Italy, where prices were higher, but that they regarded 2000 tons per week as the minimum needed to keep an effective place in the British market. He was considering an appeal for an increase in the quota, but was not optimistic.[25]

Bird concluded that revoking the official certificate would have a serious effect upon prices. The only course, if the Argentine government failed to provide the reassurances, would be for MAFF to draw up its own list of acceptable *frigoríficos*. Lace commented to John Hensley, the Under-secretary responsible for the Animal Health divisions, that this would effectively put the slaughterhouses 'on the same footing' as the canneries.[26] There would be

---

[21] K. A. Bird to Mr Lace, 2 December 1964, PRO MAF 276/260.

[22] Ibid.

[23] S. Relton to C. R. Wrigley, 8 December 1964, PRO MAF 246/222.

[24] N. J. P. Hutchison to Mr Small, 10 December 1964, PRO MAF 246/222.

[25] N. J. P. Hutchison, 'Conversation with Mr Viceconte, Deputy Head of the European Office of the Argentine Meat Board on 15th December, 1964', PRO 246/222.

[26] G. O. Lace to J. Hensley, 31 December 1964, PRO MAF 246/222.

no practical change in terms of supplies, in view of the list of canneries and the existing animal health approved list. In Hensley's view, the right course was for the Foreign Office to have the Embassy take up the issue in stronger terms, 'putting the matter as one of courtesy and efficiency in international relations'.[27]

A note for the Minister, dated 4 January 1965, advised that since Argentine establishments were named by the Milne Committee, 'pressure must be put on them for a reply' and that this was 'presentationally necessary even though the risk . . . is slight'.[28] On the possibility of MAFF producing its own list, this 'would leave matters in an unsatisfactory condition from both sides', since the Argentine government would be on record as having 'shown themselves unable to give elementary assurances'.[29] In addition, Britain would have been 'unable to obtain any response' from the Argentine government and would have been 'compelled to do their work for them'. But Ewart had at least reported that Argentina had reorganised their veterinary service, in view of MAFF's complaints and the adverse publicity caused by the Aberdeen outbreak. The CVO had been demoted and a new chief instated, who would hopefully 'wish to make a show of efficiency'. In conclusion, the note recommended that the Ambassador should be instructed to make strong and urgent representations about the 'deplorable impression which will be presented by any delay' and the unsatisfactory situation that would arise if Britain was forced to draw up its own list.[30]

With their strategy approved, MAFF officials set about preparing documents for the Foreign Office, but inter-divisional differences soon emerged. F. M. Kearns, Under-secretary responsible for External Relations, commented to Winnifrith that the Foreign Office should be informed that if an early reply was not forthcoming, moves would be made towards removal of the official certificate. He thought that the Argentine government could not be allowed to ignore the *aide-mémoire*, or else Peart would be unable to maintain that 'everything had been done to meet the recommendations of the Milne Committee'.[31]

Hensley advised caution, suggesting that it was not 'necessary to talk in terms of a threat of action so damaging to trade and international relations'. He further remarked that 'Damp patches in walls can be cured without setting fire to the house'. In his view, the threat of drawing up a list would be sufficient.[32] Kearns replied that his main point had been the need to 'ginger up the Foreign Office'. Winnifrith agreed with the harder line, and asked Hensley

[27] J. Hensley to Mr Kearns, 4 January 1964, PRO MAF 246/222.
[28] Animal Health division II, 4 January 1964 [*sic*], PRO MAF 246/222.
[29] Ibid.
[30] Ibid.
[31] F. M. Kearns to Secretary, 7 January 1965, PRO MAF 246/222.
[32] J. Hensley to Secretary, 8 January 1965, PRO MAF 246/222.

to prepare a letter to the Foreign Office showing that 'we intend to thrust this through'.[33]

A few days later, however, Hutchison re-emphasised the supply considerations. He thought it might be necessary to go to South American governments 'at a high level to see what they could do to improve their deliveries', and asked, 'Would there not . . . be some danger of the right hand appearing not to know what the left hand was doing? Would we not risk inviting the comment that beggars cannot be choosers?'[34] Hutchison's immediate superior also cautioned against allowing the Ambassador to think that 'we have up our sleeve a weapon that we should not be prepared to use'.[35]

After a further exchange of views, Hensley's position prevailed. The letter to the Foreign Office merely remarked that MAFF could not 'stress too strongly' that Peart 'must have these reassurances quickly', and spoke vaguely about 'consequences which could have serious repercussions on trading relationships'.[36] The telegram sent to the Embassy noted:

> In the event of further delay we may be compelled to make some reference to the matter, and in doing so to explain that in default of a response to our request we had to draw up our own list of establishments in respect of which we were prepared in future to recognize the Official Certificate.[37]

The Ambassador was asked to make 'urgent representations'.

In sum, it seems that the Minister and Permanent Secretary initially favoured strong action to encourage a response to the *aide-mémoire*. However, the strength of the threat the Ambassador was encouraged to make depended upon interactions between various MAFF divisions. External Relations division, which was responsible for dealings with the Foreign Office, favoured strong threats. But the Meat and Livestock division, cognisant of supply questions, favoured a softer approach, and Animal Health division II accepted their point of view. We will see, however, that as time went on and the reform of Argentine meat plant hygiene and meat inspection proved elusive, the positions of the divisions changed. Animal Health division II became frustrated by lack of progress, since the action they advocated was obstructed by other issues taking priority, and the concerns that the External Relations division shared with the Foreign Office.

---

[33] A. J. D. Winnifrith to J. Hensley, 8 January 1965, MAF 246/222.
[34] N. J. P. Hutchison to Mr Payne, 12 January 1965, PRO MAF 246/222.
[35] J. A. Payne to Mr Kearns, 13 January 1965, PRO MAF 276/260.
[36] F. M. Kearns to J. G. Rennie, 21 January 1965, PRO MAF 276/260.
[37] Foreign Office to Buenos Aires, 25 January 1965, PRO MAF 276/260.

Britain draws up a list of approved establishments

Winnifrith complained that without the phrase 'urgent *personal* representations' in the telegram sent to the Embassy in Buenos Aires, the Ambassador would merely 'send the third secretary', and so a further communication stressed this point.[38] The Embassy reported that the Ambassador had submitted a note to Argentine officials and verbal assurances of immediate action were given.[39] On 19 February, MAFF learned that Ewart, the veterinary attaché, had received what was presumed to be a response from the Assistant Director of the Argentine Directorate General of Animal Health. But there were inaccuracies and errors. The Embassy asked the Foreign Office's opinion as to whether the 'channel and form' of communication was acceptable, but advised that 'it may be wise . . . not to concern ourselves unduly' with such matters.[40] Ewart commented: 'At least, we can be satisfied that the subject is not being ignored.'[41]

The document gave assurances about the meat inspection arrangements and stated that the British regulations had been circulated. Orders had been issued regarding the quality of water.[42] As for the errors, the main problem was the list of establishments and details of what they were producing.[43] A few days later, Ewart reported that a more satisfactory list had been received, and a formal communication from the Ministry of Foreign Affairs and Worship was expected.[44] Hensley commented that 'the Argentine Government machine is beginning to grind out an answer',[45] while Bird remarked: 'It looks as though the penny has dropped.'[46] However, this optimism proved misplaced, since the formal communication repeated the earlier errors (including the wrong list), and the reassurances were not clearly addressed to either the British government or the Embassy. The Embassy requested a correction.[47]

At the end of March, the Ministry of Foreign Affairs and Worship sent a satisfactory statement, but an accurate list of establishments had yet to materialise.[48] By mid-April, MAFF officials were becoming anxious to publish

---

[38] J. Winnifrith to F. M. Kearns, 29 January 1965; Foreign Office to Buenos Aires, 29 January 1965, PRO MAF 276/260.

[39] British Embassy Buenos Aires, 2 February 1965; Buenos Aires to Foreign Office, 3 February 1965, PRO MAF 276/260.

[40] Buenos Aires to Foreign Office, 19 February 1965, PRO MAF 276/260.

[41] Ewart to A. Gwyn Benyon, 19 February 1965, PRO MAF 276/260.

[42] Ramiro García, 'Reference Note No 261 of the British Embassy', 11 February 1965, PRO MAF 276/260.

[43] R. H. Ewart, 18 February 1965, PRO MAF 276/260.

[44] R. H. Ewart to K. Bird, 22 February 1965, PRO MAF 276/260.

[45] J. Hensley to P. Humphreys-Davies, 26 February 1965, PRO MAF 276/260.

[46] K. Bird to R. H. Ewart, 1 March 1965, PRO MAF 276/260.

[47] *Aide-mémoire*, 4 March 1965, PRO MAF 276/260.

[48] Ministry of Foreign Affairs and Worship, 31 March 1965; Buenos Aires to Foreign Office, 9 April 1965, PRO MAF 276/260.

the list, as Ewart wished to remove another establishment that he found inadequate,[49] but two months later Ewart reported that the list was still not forthcoming. He explained: 'This dilatoriness is typical of the frustration involved in dealing with the Argentine government.' The Embassy had sent repeated reminders, and made many representations, without success.[50] It was finally agreed that MAFF would draw up its own list. This was finalised in July, and transmitted to the Argentine authorities, published in the *London Gazette*, and circulated to port health and local authorities in August.[51] The two unsatisfactory establishments were omitted.[52] On 31 August, the Embassy reported that the Argentines had finally produced another list. It still contained errors but was, in any case, too late.[53]

Over the next eighteen months approvals of several establishments were removed on Ewart's recommendations. Examples included a plant where standards deteriorated after rebuilding was suspended because of labour problems, a CAP establishment taken over by a workers' co-operative, and a plant suspected of financial irregularities.[54] The process of adjusting the animal and public health approved lists and disseminating information about them was complex and laborious, and involved much duplication of effort, prompting one MAFF official to comment on the matter in early 1967. When dealing with an adjustment to the animal health list she asked a colleague: 'Can't we tie up the Public Health ends at the same time? It does seem idiotic to me that this sort of thing is done piece-meal.'[55] This point was taken up quickly because a few days later, when transmitting a decision to the Foreign Office, MAFF commented that they would in future send papers concerning animal and public health approvals, or disapprovals, together.[56] This, however, was a very small step towards integrated policy making, and, as we will see, during 1967 and 1968, the separation of public health and animal health considerations caused significant problems.

Besides Ewart's advice, other information about the state of Argentine meat plants also reached MAFF, including reports of contaminated meat arriving in Britain. Furthermore, in December 1966, Grace's opposite number in Germany informed him that his government had stopped imports from one

[49] T. J. B. Dawes to A. C. Richardson, 15 April 1965, PRO MAF 276/260.

[50] R. H. Ewart to K. A. Bird, 10 June 1965, PRO MAF 276/260.

[51] K. A. Bird to R. H. Ewart, 16 June 1965; G. O. Lace to K. A. Bird, 7 July 1965; S. Relton to MacInnes, 12 August 1965; G. O. Lace to Port Health Authorities, Certain Local Authorities, 31 August 1965, PRO MAF 276/260.

[52] Draft note to Government of Argentina, PRO MAF 276/260.

[53] S. Relton to MacInnes, 31 August 1965, PRO MAF 276/260.

[54] A. E. Griffiths to G. E. Clark, 25 August 1966; N. W. Wright to K. Adams, 1 September 1966; N. W. Taylor to A. C. Richardson, 16 May 1966; R. H. Ewart to J. R. Kerr, 25 November 1966, PRO MAF 276/260.

[55] Kate to Alan, 3 January 1967, PRO MAF 276/260.

[56] M. E. Beckworth to Wilcock, 13 January 1967, PRO MAF 276/260.

establishment that was still exporting to Britain. In transmitting this information to Ewart, Grace commented that he thought it was time for the South American meat plants to be re-inspected, proposing that his deputy, Roger Blamire, should make the trip.[57]

A new report on Argentine meat hygiene, and animal health complications

In view of the recommendation of the Milne report for medical participation, and the agreement between the ministries, MAFF realised that the Ministry of Health would have to be informed about the plan for a visit to South America during 1967.[58] Bird proposed, however, to send the Ministry of Health the provisional programme for the year and to suggest that other visits might be more appropriate. Even if they wanted to be involved in the South American visit, he doubted whether a medical officer would have the time to spare.[59] This strategy achieved the hoped-for result. The Ministry gave little thought to the South American trip and declined to join the other visits since the volume of imports involved was so low.[60]

Blamire spent from 11 April until 19 May in South America, and visited fifteen Argentine establishments. He found conditions little changed from the time of Grace's visit. In the slaughterhalls, floors and walls were seldom constructed of impervious material, ceilings were generally unlined, lighting was poor, and facilities for washing knives and hands were inadequate. In some offal rooms there was no separation between areas handling 'red offals' and those for cleaning intestines. Some cutting and boning rooms used wooden surfaces and lacked sterilisers for knives. In general, Blamire commented that 'the standards of hygienic practice are dictated largely by commercial needs', rather than any attempt to comply with regulations. He gave an example of the rejection of a consignment at Smithfield because of mould on the carcasses, after which new hygiene procedures were introduced at the establishment concerned.

Blamire reserved his strongest criticism for the meat inspection service, which had deteriorated further. The benefits of appointing a new CVO had not materialised. Senior veterinarians received low salaries and often held other jobs. Many should have retired but were unable to because of inadequate pensions. Their time in the factories was spent mostly on paperwork, and they were looked down upon by the management and had little authority. The auxiliaries exhibited 'varying degrees of skill' and were subject to 'varying

[57] L. Grace to R. H. Ewart, 13 December 1966, PRO MAF 276/260.
[58] T. J. B. Dawes to Mr Bird, 30 December 1966, PRO MAF 282/9.
[59] K. A. Bird to Mr Lace, 2 January 1967, PRO MAF 282/9.
[60] J. E. King to G. O. Lace, 15 February 1967, PRO MAF 282/9.

degrees of supervision'. As for water supplies, Blamire reported that 'the lesson had been learnt'. He found no dangerous water supplies, although the meat inspection service seemed to have no role in monitoring.

According to Blamire's account of his meeting with the Argentine CVO, after referring to past events and continuing problems, he emphasised that the 'root of the trouble seemed to be the extremely poor standard of the meat inspection service'. According to the CVO, a levy on slaughtering to pay for the service had been appropriated for other purposes. Later, the Minister of Agriculture explained the difficulties of persuading his government, 'which was dedicated to reducing bureaucracy' that 'many more bureaucrats should be employed at very much higher salaries'. To this, Blamire responded that other countries were prepared to maintain the services necessary to enjoy access to British markets and that 'the United Kingdom could not tolerate a state of affairs which left them open to unnecessary health risks'.

Blamire concluded his report by noting that standards in Argentina fell far below those outside South America, and did not reach the level required of new suppliers. He recommended that the Argentine government be told that any establishment which did not take immediate steps to ensure compliance with the UK's requirements within a stated time would be removed from the approved list. He suggested twelve months for major items such as the replacement of floors and three months for the provision of washing facilities and sterilisers, the replacement of wooden equipment and so on. As for the meat inspection service, it would take years to reform, but Blamire suggested that they insist that a start be made immediately. If no changes became evident, the entire official certificate should be revoked.[61]

Blamire's report was dated 4 July, a few weeks before Peart was due to make a goodwill visit to Argentina, and MAFF officials became engaged in preparing briefing documents. They suggested that Peart might express approval of Blamire's findings on water supplies, before indicating that in view of his other findings, the Argentine government would soon receive a note indicating that the future of their meat exports to Britain would be at stake unless further improvements were made.[62] But Peart was also advised to raise another question, namely the control of foot-and-mouth disease. The desire of officials to take up this issue complicated matters and delayed concerted action over public health problems.

By 1967, endemic foot-and-mouth had long been eliminated in Britain by slaughter and movement restrictions arrangements during outbreaks, and the same standards were required of most countries exporting meat to Britain. However, as mentioned in Chapter 2, during the late 1950s and early 1960s

---

[61] R. V. Blamire, 'Visit to South America – Argentina', 4 July 1967, copy supplied to the project by R. V. Blamire.
[62] 'Minister's visit to South America Public Health (Imported Food) Regulations Meat and Meat Products', PRO MAF 246/328.

the disease continued to cause problems.[63] But in Argentina the disease remained endemic. In 1966, for example, there were some 5000 outbreaks. But as officials explained to Peart, South American imports were allowed to continue, to enable Britain to obtain 'supplies of high quality chilled beef at relatively low prices'.[64]

In 1960, the unusually high level of 298 outbreaks in Britain arose from twenty-six primary outbreaks, half of which were attributed to imported meat, bones or swill. In Argentina, a vaccination campaign had been applied to cattle but not to pigs, because suitable vaccines were not available. South American pork imports were therefore prohibited from 1 February 1961, a decision seemingly vindicated when the number of outbreaks dropped rapidly. In 1962 there were only five outbreaks, none in 1963 and 1964, and only one in 1965. In 1966 there were thirty-four outbreaks, while in January 1967 there were twenty-nine. The relative freedom of Britain from foot-and-mouth since 1962 was also attributed to regulations requiring the sterilisation of waste food used for feeding animals, and improved controls in continental countries. But the majority of the remaining cases were either firmly or tentatively attributed to South American produce.[65]

Against this background, the MAFF division responsible for animal health, Animal Health division I, sought to use Peart's visit to Argentina to raise the question of strengthening Britain's defences against foot-and-mouth disease. They suggested that subjecting South America to similar controls as applied to other countries should be considered.[66] The Minister's speaking notes proposed that he might pay tribute to Argentina's vaccination campaign before explaining that soon a revision of the UK's animal health requirements was likely. A visit to Argentina for discussions by MAFF's CVO might be suggested.[67]

Peart, however, apparently failed to say anything about foot-and-mouth, which made it more difficult for officials to decide how to raise the matter in the light of the urgent need to press demands on the public health issues.[68] As officials began to prepare a draft note to the Argentine government, two camps

[63] See pp. 39–40.

[64] 'Minister's visit to South America UK import regulations: animal health', PRO MAF 246/328.

[65] Ministry of Agriculture, Fisheries and Food Department of Agriculture and Fisheries for Scotland, *RAHSGB 1960*, p. 23; *RAHSGB 1961 and 1962*, pp. 10, 12; *RAHSGB 1965*, p. 9; *RAHSGB 1966*, pp. 11, 16. *RAHSGB 1967*, p. 11; Ministry of Agriculture, Fisheries and Food, *Report of the Committee of Inquiry on Foot-and-Mouth Disease 1968, part one*, London, 1968.

[66] 'Minister's visit to South America UK import regulations: animal health', PRO MAF 246/328.

[67] 'Minister's visit to South America July/August, 1967, meat trade: human and animal health aspects Speaking Note', 20 July 1967, PRO MAF 246/328.

[68] E. H. Bott, 23 August 1967, PRO MAF 246/328.

emerged as to the best strategy, and it was eventually left to the Minister to decide on the way forward. According to one line of reasoning, expressed by the Meat division, it was essential to include a warning about projected changes in the foot-and-mouth regulations in the note about the public health problems. This view held that it would be wrong to 'persuade the Argentine Government to insist on a lot of work being done' for public health reasons, and then to refuse the meat on other grounds.[69] The other perspective, articulated by Hensley, pointed to the difficulties of raising the animal health issues after Peart's goodwill visit, and of explaining why action was necessary when the vaccination campaign was apparently having some success.[70] The discussion had reached this point when a food poisoning outbreak occurred, apparently linked with Argentine meat. This provides an opportunity for exploring the practical difference, if any, that the typhoid outbreaks had made to the handling of such incidents.

The *Salmonella typhimurium* incident

On Friday, 25 August, the chief meat inspector of the London Borough of Islington invited MAFF to examine some frozen mutton carcasses from Argentine Establishment 1408. These showed evidence of ineffective inspection and poor hygiene; in some cases there were faeces in the abdominal cavity.[71] Later that day, further news precipitated action. Dr Anderson of the PHLS informed MAFF that over recent weeks there had been several *Salmonella typhimurium* poisoning cases, including one death, in Manchester. The phage type, U244, had not been recorded in Britain before, except in a sample of Establishment 1408 mutton recently supplied by the Port of London health authority.[72]

Establishment 1408 had already been under investigation. When Blamire visited the plant he indicated the improvements that were needed, but since his return to Britain, eight out of ten samples from one consignment, and fourteen out of twenty samples from another consignment of Establishment 1408 produce tested positive for various *Salmonellae*.[73] Some further consignments were admitted without testing. Blamire asked Ewart to re-inspect Establishment 1408, suggesting that if conditions had not improved, the plant might be removed from the approved list. No remedial action was evident, but Ewart recommended that twenty days be allowed for improvements. This

---

[69] Ibid.

[70] J. Hensley to Mr Bott, 24 August 1967, PRO MAF 246/328.

[71] K. A. Bird to G. O. Lace, 30 August 1967, PRO MAF 276/260.

[72] Ibid.

[73] K. A. Bird to G. O. Lace, 30 August 1967; K. A. Bird to G. O. Lace, 5 September 1967, PRO MAF 276/260.

warning was issued and appeared to produce the desired response: on 24 July Ewart advised that the plant was now satisfactory.[74]

After hearing from the PHLS, MAFF officials seemed much more anxious to act quickly than in the early days of the 1963 to 1964 typhoid outbreaks. Instead of relying upon the Ministry of Health for immediate policy, they agreed that everything should be done to stop the entry of further Establishment 1408 supplies *before* seeking the views of Dr Ross at the Ministry of Health.[75] A cable was despatched to Ewart asking him to inform the Argentine authorities that no further exports from Establishment 1408 would be accepted, pending investigations.[76] Port inspection staff were asked to detain Establishment 1408 produce,[77] and it emerged that a further consignment was being unloaded in London.[78] The remaining material was detained while that which had already passed through the port was stopped at Wrexham and elsewhere.[79] Once MAFF had protected their position, however, the resolution of the situation relied heavily upon Ministry of Health advice.

On 31 August, Lace explained to Winnifrith that Ministry of Health enquiries had not confirmed the connection between Argentine mutton and the incident. Only one patient died, and 'this could have happened with other strains of Salmonella'. It was not even certain that *Salmonella* poisoning was 'the cause, or the only cause, of death', and it was now unlikely that the Ministry of Health would take 'dramatic action' against Establishment 1408 meat in circulation. In conclusion, he noted that one matter illuminated by the incident was that the Port of London had not been as forthcoming as they could have been over the laboratory findings.[80]

Winnifrith felt the action taken safeguarded MAFF's position, but was surprised that despite adverse findings on Establishment 1408 produce, the Port of London health authority had 'calmly released' batches of this material. He suggested that there was a case for writing to the Ministry of Health, 'telling them of our feelings about these incidents and requesting them to take steps to prevent any recurrence'. As for the Establishment 1408 stock produced before Ewart's visit which was still in circulation, he observed that it was up to the Ministry of Health to decide whether to withdraw it, commenting 'If they like to take this risk that is their business.'[81]

Bird subsequently reported a discussion with the chief inspector at the Port of London health authority. The latest information was that the U244 *Salmonella typhimurium* had not been found in a sample of mutton as had been

---

[74] K. A. Bird to G. O. Lace, 30 August 1967, PRO MAF 276/260.
[75] Ibid.
[76] G. O. Lace to R. H. Ewart, 25 August 1967, MAF 276/260.
[77] K. A. Bird to G. O. Lace, 30 August 1967, PRO MAF 276/260.
[78] PD(C), vol. 760, cols 365–6 (14 March 1968).
[79] K. A. Bird to G. O. Lace, 5 September 1967, PRO MAF 276/260.
[80] G. O. Lace to Secretary, 31 August 1967, PRO MAF 276/260.
[81] A. J. D. Winnifrith to G. O. Lace, 4 September 1967, PRO MAF 276/260.

assumed, but in a sample of the frozen hearts.[82] The closest they were to proof of a connection between Establishment 1408 and the food poisoning incident was a 'recollection of a meal of roast mutton' but there was no information as to whether the meat was home-produced or imported. The isolation of U244 from offal rather than meat did not strengthen the position. Nevertheless, Lace recorded, 'we can justify what we did as a precaution'.[83] Subsequently, Blamire and Lace met Ross and the port medical officer for London on 12 September, and they decided that there was no justification for holding stock, or for holding up further shipments. As for the question of the communication of test results by the ports, a meeting between MAFF and medical officers of the main ports was planned.[84]

Communication and relationships between port health authorities and the central authorities were matters that had been considered by the Milne Committee. As mentioned in Chapter 7, the Milne report argued that the responsibility for imported meat hygiene should pass from MAFF to the Ministry of Health immediately upon unloading rather than after inspection, as previously, and agreement on this was easily achieved.[85] However, in 1967, there was clearly still scope for communication problems, and even Winnifrith was not clear what the relationships and responsibilities were supposed to be. But he clearly thought that what mattered most was that MAFF could justify their actions. Once the emergency had passed, he was unconcerned as long as any continuing risk to health was demonstrably the responsibility of the Ministry of Health.

On the whole, there is little evidence that the experiences of 1963 to 1964 made significant changes as to how the civil servants managed these problems. There was certainly no breakdown in 'departmentalism' and some signs that greater concern among officials to safeguard their positions had reinforced 'departmentalism'. The episode concluded with a cable on 13 September from Lace to Ewart asking him to advise the Argentine authorities that shipments from Establishment 1408 could resume.[86]

Policy prevarication and the foot-and-mouth outbreak

In mid-September, as the *Salmonella typhimurium* 'emergency' passed, debate about longer term problems concerning South American meat recommenced. Consensus emerged on the importance of the public health issues, and on the

---

[82] K. A. Bird to G. O. Lace, 5 and 6 September 1967, PRO MAF 276/260.

[83] G. O. Lace to Secretary, 13 September 1967, PRO MAF 276/260.

[84] Ibid.

[85] See pp. 199–200.

[86] Ministry of Agriculture, Fisheries and Food to Ewart, 13 September 1967, PRO MAF 276/260.

suggestion that the CVO should visit South America for animal health discussions. However, there were still disagreements over whether to raise both matters simultaneously, or to deal with public health first. Now Hensley favoured the former approach, while F. M. Kearns and J. A. Payne, of the External Relations, and the Meat and Livestock and Fatstock Marketing divisions, favoured the second.[87] In mid-October, the Minister was consulted.[88] He was advised that a decision was urgent in view of an impending visit from the Argentine Minister of Economy, Dr Krieger Vasena, and because the longer action on Blamire's report was left, the less impact it would make.

The submission explained the two schools of thought. According to one, combining the public health ultimatum with the animal health warning would 'give the South Americans the impression we are seeking a pretext to stop the carcass meat trade'. They would therefore 'hesitate to incur the expenditure required on the public health side'. Since the public health matter was urgent, it was reasonable to deal with it first. According to the second view, raising the two issues consecutively would create an impression of 'double dealing', and once the public health requirements had been met, Peart would be under pressure from colleagues to 'let well alone'.[89]

Imposing safeguards on South America similar to those imposed on continental countries would stop South American carcass beef imports for the foreseeable future, but this trade now represented only 10 per cent of Britain's beef supplies. No problems would arise in good supply situations, but at other times prices might rise. The Minister was advised that if the South Americans could not meet the public health requirements:

> we should have good grounds for stopping the imports in spite of the likely opposition of the Board of Trade on the grounds of foreign policy, trade, and loss of British investments in South American meat plants and in shipping. If, on the other hand, the public health requirements were met, the animal health reasons for stopping the trade would be unlikely to prevail by themselves against these wider considerations.[90]

A draft note summarised Blamire's findings and referred to the requirements that had been notified to Argentina following the Aberdeen typhoid outbreak. A deadline of 1 June 1968 was envisaged for upgrading the meat plants, and 1 January 1969 for structural alterations and major repairs. After these dates, plants failing to comply would be removed from the approved list, and unless improvements in the meat inspection service became evident, Argentina's

---

[87] J. Hensley to Mr Tame, 18 October 1967, PRO MAF 246/328.

[88] 'Imports of meat from South America. Foot-and-mouth disease risk. Submission to the Minister', 18 October 1967, PRO MAF 246/328.

[89] *RAHSGB 1967*, p. 10.

[90] 'Imports of meat from South America. Foot-and-mouth disease risk. Submission to the Minister', 18 October 1967, PRO MAF 246/328.

official certificate would be withdrawn.[91] A further draft note suggested a visit by the CVO to discuss improving notification of foot-and-mouth outbreaks, a more intensive vaccination policy, and the certification of farms and areas as foot-and-mouth disease-free.[92]

The submission attracted further comment by Deputy Secretary W. C. Tame, who favoured raising both issues simultaneously, suggesting that if the animal health questions were delayed, it would be 1969 before any improvements could be made. He explained that the proposals were 'tough on public health' but 'tender on animal health' because otherwise Argentine carcass meat imports would be precluded, and added:

> We do not think that we could get away with this in Whitehall even though . . . we could do without the meat. To fight this battle in Whitehall now would cause further delays with the probability of an unsatisfactory outcome: to suggest it after the Argentinians have gone to the trouble and expense of tightening up on the public health side . . . would be bound to fail.[93]

Tame hoped that without demanding the impossible, they could 'persuade or bully' Argentina into adopting the best possible safeguards. Winnifrith added:

> the present arrangements are quite illogical. We insist on the carrying out of our code on the Continent . . . [but in] . . . the case of the Argentine, we have deliberately pulled our punches, partly because up to now we have needed their meat, and partly because of our industrialists' investments in abattoirs, refrigerated ships etc. There is no doubt that this kid glove policy increases the incidence of foot-and-mouth disease in this country, and that the compensation we have to pay, and the losses our farmers suffer, is the price for getting 10 per cent of our beef imported from the Argentine.[94]

The outcome of the consultation was that officials were instructed to prepare a firm note on the public health issues for the Ambassador to deliver, with the animal health trip by the CVO to follow in due course. The note was still under consideration at the Foreign Office at the end of October when Vasena arrived in Britain.

Over recent months, prospects for trade with Argentina, especially in armaments, had strengthened. In July it was reported that Argentina might buy British HS748 aircraft, and in October Argentina ordered some British missiles. The British government were anxious to develop the relationship,

91 'Appendix I Note by Her Majesty's Government to the Government of Argentina', PRO MAF 246/328.
92 'Carcass meat imports animal health safeguards', PRO MAF 246/328.
93 W. C. Tame to Secretary, 18 October 1967, PRO MAF 246/328.
94 A. J. D. Winnifrith to Minister, 19 October 1967, PRO MAF 246/328.

and offered assistance to firms selling capital equipment to Argentina.[95] Vasena's visit was expected to further stimulate trade, and he met Peart to promote the meat trade.[96]

Officials again produced briefing documents. These stated that the Argentine veterinary service had 'no grip on the vital functions of meat inspection' and that supervision was 'virtually lacking', but the Aberdeen typhoid outbreak demonstrated the 'magnitude of the consequences which can stem from laxness'. Assurances provided by Argentina needed to be 'given foundation in fact'.[97] The papers suggested that when mentioning the forthcoming note on meat hygiene, Peart should assure Vasena that the last thing wanted was disruption of the meat trade. However, he was also advised to say that unless public health improvements were made, not only would British consumers be exposed to 'indefensible risks', but the 'continuance of the trade' would also be jeopardised. The proposed visit by the CVO could then be mentioned and advances in foot-and-mouth control presented as in the interests of both countries, removing 'possible impediments' to the continuation of trade.[98] Peart adopted the approach suggested and Vasena assured him that the new Argentine Minister of Agriculture was anxious to deal with the problems. But they swiftly moved on to other issues, such as price problems.[99]

The British Ambassador warned the Argentine Minister of Agriculture about the forthcoming note on 20 November, and he claimed to have already ordered an overhaul of the veterinary service. The Ambassador then urged that the delivery of the note be postponed for four reasons. The first was the repercussions of a foot-and-mouth outbreak that had begun in Shropshire on 25 October. The Argentines were 'sensitive' about accusations in the British press that their meat had caused the outbreak. Second, the Argentines were concerned about the effect of the devaluation of sterling on the meat trade. Third, there was a 'great opportunity' to increase exports to Argentina as a consequence of the devaluation and Vasena's visit. Finally, Britain was seeking Argentine support in the United Nations over Middle East issues. In view of these factors the Ambassador suggested that the 'peremptory admonitions against the Argentine' be delayed until the veterinary attaché had held discussions with the new head of the Argentine veterinary service.[100]

---

[95] 'Argentina possible purchase of HS 248 aircraft from Britain', *The Times*, 21 July 1967, p. 17d; Kenneth Owen, '£5m missile order for Belfast firm', *The Times*, 10 October 1967, p. 20g; Jorge Rocka, 'Boost for Argentina by Britain', *The Times*, 7 October 1967, p. 17d.
[96] J. E. Dixon to Mr Williamson, 27 October 1967, MAF PRO 246/328.
[97] 'Visit of the Argentine Minister of Economy 29th October to 1st November meat – public health and animal health questions', PRO MAF 246/328.
[98] Ibid.
[99] 'Minister's meeting with Dr. Krieger Vasena', PRO MAF 246/328.
[100] Buenos Aires to Foreign Office, 20 November 1967, PRO MAF 246/328; Ambassador, British Embassy, Buenos Aires to M. Stewart, 3 May 1968, PRO MAF 246/329.

Despite his pleas, the Ambassador was instructed to proceed. The note, delivered on 24 November, called for an assurance that remedial measures had been put in hand by the end of 1967, and gave the deadlines for improvements mentioned above.[101] But the diplomatic problems were compounded by reports that MAFF was considering banning Argentine meat imports in view of the foot-and-mouth epidemic. The Argentine Foreign Minister warned the Ambassador of serious consequences if a ban was imposed. On 30 November, a deputation representing Argentine trade, industrial and agricultural interests warned that a ban would 'deeply and negatively' affect purchases of British goods by Argentine companies. Without success, the Ambassador attempted to persuade the Argentine government to voluntarily withhold shipments.[102] On 4 December Peart announced a temporary ban on carcass meat and offal imports, covering all countries apart from nine with a history of freedom from foot-and-mouth disease.[103]

The Argentine government seemed reassured that the ban was not permanent, but faced agitation for retaliatory action. On 8 December they informed the British Ambassador that Argentina might be obliged to 'orientate its trade by preference to those countries which were ready to trade in a positive way in accordance with reciprocity'. The armed services and state enterprises had already been ordered not to enter into contracts with British suppliers.[104] Peart, however, faced pressure to extend the ban, but he and his junior ministers consistently reiterated that it was subject to review.[105] On 22 December, when the Argentine Ambassador asked when the ban would be lifted, emphasising Argentina's anxiety about being singled out, Peart reminded him of his wish for a senior veterinary officer to visit Argentina, which he hoped would take place soon. A British note offered further reassurance that the ban was temporary, but an Argentine response claimed that the measure was 'not only lacking justification but causing grave damage to the international reputation of Argentine products'.[106] In mid-January 1968, two Argentine veterinary officials visited Britain to collect evidence about the source of the epidemic, and on return to Argentina announced that they had found no connection with Argentine meat.[107] This was accepted by the

---

[101] Foreign Office to Buenos Aires, 30 May 1968, PRO MAF 246/329.

[102] Ambassador, British Embassy, Buenos Aires, to M. Stewart, 3 May 1968, PRO MAF 246/329.

[103] *PD(C)*, vol. 755, cols 997–9 (4 December 1967).

[104] Ambassador, British Embassy, Buenos Aires, to M. Stewart, 3 May 1968, PRO MAF 246/329.

[105] *PD(C)*, vol. 756, cols *1485–6* (21 December 1967); ibid., vol. 757, col. *383* (24 January 1968); ibid., vol. 757, cols *228–9* (29 January 1968); ibid., vol. 759, col. *197* (23 February 1968).

[106] Ambassador, British Embassy, Buenos Aires, to M. Stewart, 3 May 1968, PRO MAF 246/329.

[107] Ibid.; M. Cresswell to Foreign Office, 1 February 1968, PRO MAF 246/329.

Argentine Minister of Agriculture, who the British Ambassador found 'defensive and generally hostile' throughout the affair, an attitude supported by the powerful Argentine Rural Society.[108]

In mid-January Peart announced that he would appoint a committee to examine foot-and-mouth policy,[109] and by the end of February the chair, the Duke of Northumberland, and members had been named.[110] On 15 February he told the House of Commons that he was examining the results of an investigation into the source of the outbreak.[111] The government faced further calls for the extension of the ban,[112] but some MPs echoed the anxieties of the Latin-American Export Council. One quoted a figure of £180 million-worth of trade at stake with Argentina alone, and suggested a compromise of allowing boned meat to be imported from foot-and-mouth areas, as bones were often implicated as the source of imported infections.[113]

With interest focused upon foot-and-mouth disease, Animal Health division II became concerned that the public health issues might be sidelined. The Argentine government had not provided the initial assurance requested. Lace told Bird that 'The essential thing is that we never let the Foreign Office, the Embassy, or the Argentine Government forget that . . . the requirements of our public health note . . . have got to be met in full'.[114] However, Bird was persuaded by the External Relations division that the South American ministers took the situation sufficiently seriously to make a formal note pressing for reassurances unnecessary. This would avoid an approach at a time when Britain's relations with Argentina were 'not at their best'.[115]

It emerged that the Ambassador *had* been active on the public health issues and had sent a reminder to the Argentine Ministry of Foreign Affairs. The Ministry replied that the note had been 'passed to the relevant organizations capable of finding a quick solution', but the Ambassador thought this unsatisfactory. However, Ewart met the Argentine CVO, who declared that once the President had signed a new set of regulations he would reorganise the meat inspection service, making it full time, increasing salaries, recruiting new staff, and sacking the incompetent workers. On 9 February the Ambassador reported that the regulations were not yet signed, but commented that such delay was not unusual. There was no evidence of disputes about the regulations, but there were 'no visible steps' by the veterinary service to improve *frigorífico* hygiene. However, the press had reported a meeting on sanitary controls involving

---

[108] Ambassador, British Embassy, Buenos Aires, to M. Stewart, 3 May 1968, PRO MAF 246/329.

[109] *PD(C)*, vol. 756, col. 589 (17 January 1968).

[110] Ibid., vol. 759, cols 1393–4 (28 February 1968).

[111] Ibid., vol. 758, cols 1589–90 (15 February 1968).

[112] Ibid., vol. 759, col. 643 (22 February 1968).

[113] Ibid., vol. 758, col. 1594 (15 February 1968).

[114] G. O. Lace to K. A. Bird, 23 January 1968, PRO MAF 260/261.

[115] M. E. Beckwith to Mr McCall, PRO MAF 276/261.

officials, the National Meat Board and the firms. The Ambassador felt that something was happening at last.[116]

Later in February, Ewart reported that there was still no evidence of increased control by the veterinary service,[117] and Bird told Blamire that he did not like the way things were developing:

> it seems to me that we may be up against a technique which we have seen before. It appears that the Argentine Government are going to make new regulations which on the face of it will ensure that our requirements are met. Unfortunately, however, we know only too well that what is required on paper is a very different thing from what may happen in practice.[118]

On 4 March 1968, Peart told the House of Commons that the report into the origins of the epidemic prepared by MAFF's CVO (now John Reid) was about to be published. The report contained circumstantial evidence that a consignment of South American lamb and offal had been the cause of the first and some of the subsequent primary outbreaks. On 15 April, the ban on beef imports would be lifted, but the ban on sheep meat and offal would continue. The Argentine government had invited a British veterinary mission for talks, which would leave for Argentina shortly.[119] MAFF officials realised that the briefing telegrams to the Ambassador would allow them to follow up the public health issue.[120] They arranged for him to be instructed by the Foreign Office to remind the Argentine authorities of the 'importance we attach to an early and effective response to our representations on public health standards and our wish to see this separate question quickly cleared so as to avoid any possible further interruption of trade'.[121]

Press interest in the public health issue and action on the 1 June deadline

Reid's report brought to light an unfortunate coincidence, leading to intense press interest and questioning of ministers. Reid concluded that the source of the foot-and-mouth epidemic was probably Argentine Establishment 1408 lamb that had reached the Fatstock Marketing Corporation of Wrexham on 25 August 1967. The meat was supplied to a butcher, who sold some to a farm,

---

[116] M. Cresswell to J. G. S. Beith, 9 February 1968, PRO MAF 276/261.

[117] Ewart to Foreign Office, 19 February 1968, PRO MAF 276/261.

[118] K. A. Bird to R. V. Blamire, 21 February 1968, PRO MAF 276/261.

[119] PD(C), vol. 760, col. 39 (4 March 1968).

[120] J. E. Dixon to Evans, 1 March 1968, PRO MAF 276/261.

[121] Foreign Office to Buenos Aires, 4 March 1968, PRO MAF 276/261.

including bones for the farm dogs.[122] The consignment in question had been held up temporarily during the *Salmonella typhimurium* incident.

On 6 March the Chairman of Wrexham Health Committee revealed that the lamb implicated in the foot-and-mouth epidemic had been impounded on the instructions of the Port of London health authority. Bacteriological tests were arranged, but before they were carried out the Ministry of Health ruled that the carcasses could be released.[123] Emlyn Hooson, MP for Montgomery, then took up the matter,[124] and his intention to table a series of parliamentary questions was reported under the front-page headline, 'Health warning on Argentine imports "before epidemic"'.[125] A *Times* editorial concluded that while the 'type of salmonella was less serious than the variety which brought about the Aberdeen typhoid epidemic', it was 'luck rather than good management' that prevented a serious incident.[126]

Hooson's questions generated a series of clarifications on the identity, movements and testing of the lamb destined for Wrexham.[127] The *Salmonella typhimurium* affair also featured in a House of Commons debate on 13 March on an opposition motion deploring the lifting of the beef import ban. Peart emphasised the mechanisms for a 'continual watch on any possible hazards to human health' and declared that 'meat plants . . . are inspected by officers of my Ministry and we do not import from any plant which is not satisfactory'. In view of this, he could not accept 'that the Government's decision . . . should be linked to public health considerations. If we become aware of any real risk to public health, we take action immediately.'[128] Hooson continued to probe the *Salmonella typhimurium* incident in early April and at the end of May,[129] but by this time press interest had passed.

In retaliation for the four months' lost business, and in the hope of pressurising Britain to guarantee that the market would remain open, the meat-packing companies resolved not to immediately resume exports to Britain.[130] This position was supported by the Argentine government, which also introduced a new 'freight-on-board prices agreed' system to prevent prices from depending upon the volatile Smithfield market, which resulted in frequent

[122] J. Reid, *Origin of the 1967–68 Foot-and-Mouth Disease Epidemic*, London, 1968, p. 3.

[123] '"Suspected" meat was released', *The Times*, 7 March 1968, p. 2f.

[124] *PD(C)*, vol. 760, col. 1424 (13 March 1968).

[125] G. Clark, 'Health warning on Argentine imports "before epidemic"', *The Times*, 7 March 1968, p. 1g.

[126] 'Wrexham's double jeopardy', *The Times*, 8 March 1968, p. 9a.

[127] *PD(C)*, vol. 760, col. 365–6 (14 March 1968).

[128] Ibid., col. 1413 (13 March 1968).

[129] Ibid., vol. 762, col. 360 (3 April 1968); ibid., 1967–8, vol. 762, col. 214 (9 April 1968); Ibid., vol. 765, col. 246 (29 May 1968).

[130] 'Ban on meat to Britain', *The Times*, 25 March 1968, p. 16f; R. Wigg, 'Beef guarantee sought', *The Times*, 8 March 1968, p. 1e.

losses.[131] Two months later, however, in the face of severe drought, they urged exporters to sell as much as they could to Britain. However, the aim of avoiding Smithfield market prices remained, which inhibited the resumption of trade at the pre-ban level.[132]

The British veterinary mission successfully restored relations at a technical level and carried through a renegotiation of the Bledisloe agreement, subject to the approval of both governments.[133] A ten-day visit to Britain by a team of Argentine veterinary officers followed, led by the Nobel Laureate, Bernado Houssay.[134] In London, Houssay commented that the British ban had been justified, but on returning to Argentina he claimed that foot-and-mouth disease was endemic in Britain, and that the attribution of outbreaks to imported meat was erroneous. In spite of this, the British Ambassador hoped that the Houssay mission had opened the way for eventual agreement between the veterinary authorities.[135]

Besides the veterinary missions, press and parliamentary interest during March and April focused on the progress of the Northumberland Committee, the recrudescence of the epidemic, and the impact of the epidemic on trade. The question of permitting only boned meat to be imported from foot-and-mouth endemic countries was raised several times, and this was the policy eventually recommended by the Northumberland Committee.[136] However, by early May 1968 the number of news items and parliamentary questions had declined, and the British Ambassador wrote that the 'most difficult and complicated' situation created by the ban had now 'to a greater degree been resolved'.[137]

In the light of the amount of unfinished business, this assessment was optimistic. It had been envisaged that an officer would be sent to check progress after the 1 June deadline, and that in early 1969 a senior officer would

---

[131] 'Argentine meat terms', *The Times*, 16 March 1968, p. 3d.

[132] Latin American correspondent, 'Beef export campaign by Argentina', *The Times*, 27 May 1968, p. 4f.

[133] Ambassador, British Embassy, Buenos Aires, to M. Stewart, 3 May 1968, PRO MAF 246/329.

[134] A. Kenworthy, 'Now Britain gets blame for farm plague', *Daily Express*, 22 April 1968, p. 11; T. J. B. Dawes to Mr Carnochan, 22 April 1968, PRO MAF 246/329; Agricultural Correspondent, 'Wind blamed for foot-and-mouth', *The Times*, 23 March 1968, p. 4g.

[135] Ambassador, British Embassy, Buenos Aires, to M. Stewart, 3 May 1968, PRO MAF 246/329.

[136] *PD(C)*, vol. 767, col. 81 (26 June 1968); 'Fear of new Shropshire outbreak', *The Times*, 20 March 1968, p. 2c; 'Support for lifting of the beef ban', *The Times*, 6 March 1968, p. 2g; R. Wigg, 'Argentine links damaged', *The Times*, 7 March 1968, p. 5a; 'Meat ban loses air order by Argentina', *The Times*, 22 April 1968, p. 2g; R. Wigg, 'Argentine links damaged', *The Times*, 7 March 1968, p. 5a; *PD(C)*, vol. 760, col. 106–7 (6 March 1968); 'Boneless beef imports to beat farm virus', *The Times*, 2 May 1969, p. 2a.

[137] Ambassador, British Embassy, Buenos Aires, to M. Stewart, 3 May 1968, PRO MAF 246/329.

investigate establishments where extensions had been given, and the meat inspection service. Blamire pointed out that unless action was taken in connection with the first deadline, there was no prospect of the second being taken seriously. An office meeting concluded that the establishments should be inspected, and that the most unsatisfactory would have to be struck off the approved list.[138] Deputy Secretary Tame commented that 'we cannot take risks in the field of public health . . . however much we may wish to avoid additional irritation to Argentina'.[139]

Under-secretary Kearns, who was now responsible for the Meat and Livestock division, advised that if individual establishments were proscribed, this would have minimal effect upon meat supplies, but he thought that the matter should be kept as routine as possible. Although 'after Aberdeen we cannot take any new risks in the field of public health', it would be unrealistic, he thought, 'not to take any account of the circumstances of the last few months'. He therefore suggested that they should not send officers as a 'specialist mission' but as help for the staff already in the country. He concluded: 'we should not wish to give Argentina any basis . . . on which to argue that we were determined to wreck her meat trade.'[140] Under-secretary Payne, who was now responsible for the External Relations division, remarked: 'I do not think we can pursue this public health question in isolation from the other matters we still have under consideration', alluding to the new animal health precautions which were being finalised.[141]

The outcome of this exchange of views was a letter to the Ambassador in Buenos Aires stating that the deadline would have to be followed up because of the risks to public health, press awareness of the issue, and the possible need for ministers to answer questions. This was 'entirely separate' from the animal health questions, although there were 'dangers of misunderstanding and misrepresentation'.[142] But the Ambassador warned that the public and animal health issues were 'closely connected in the minds of the Argentinians who are very sensitive to both'.[143] The results of the inspection were not encouraging. The veterinary officers sent as 'temporary reinforcements for local staff' were greatly concerned about the conditions they found, and recommended that four establishments, which had accounted for half of Britain's pre-ban supplies from Argentina, be removed from the approved list. Three were American-owned, including Swift Rosario, which had been implicated in the Aberdeen typhoid outbreak, while the fourth was owned by CAP. The recommendation was included in a submission to the Minister (now

[138] G. O. Lace to Mr Tame, 15 May 1968, PRO MAF 276/261.
[139] W. C. Tame to Mr Payne, 16 May 1968, PRO MAF 276/261.
[140] F. M. Kearns to Mr Tame, 17 May 1968, PRO MAF 276/261.
[141] J. A. Payne to Mr Tame, 20 May 1968, PRO MAF 276/261.
[142] Foreign Office to Buenos Aires, 30 May 1968, PRO MAF 276/261.
[143] M. Cresswell to Foreign Office, 31 May 1968, PRO MAF 246/329.

Cledwyn Hughes). The submission, presented to Hughes on 31 July, started by reminding him of the background:

> In recent years standards have generally risen, but in some South American countries they have fallen. Although, for political reasons and considerations of commercial policy, we have continued to accept their meat, we have, especially since the typhoid outbreak of 1964, made strenuous efforts to persuade particularly the Argentine Government to both bring their meat inspection service to a satisfactory standard, and to get the frigorificos and canneries brought up to our standards.[144]

Despite these efforts, only three out of seventeen Argentine plants passed the recent inspection without qualification. Ten were making efforts to comply with British requirements. Of the latter, it was suggested, five should be allowed three months to complete their improvements and five should be allowed six. The remaining four plants had made no attempt to correct shortcomings. It was recommended that a note be prepared removing approval from these plants. Leaving them on the approved list would subject British consumers to risks of typhoid, paratyphoid, botulism and staphylococcal toxin, and would 'remove all credibility from our pressure on the Argentine Government'. On the meat inspection service, Hughes was informed that the new law remained unsigned and that 'minimal progress' had been made.

During subsequent discussions, the question of withdrawing approval from the unsatisfactory establishments lost out in the process of deciding the order of priority of issues to be taken up with the Argentine government. The other matters, concerning animal health, included completion of a 'Record of Understanding', the implementation of amendments to the Bledisloe agreement, and arrangements for the Northumberland Committee to visit Argentina. J. G. Carnochan and members of the External Relations division talked these matters over with the Foreign Office before a meeting with an Argentine Embassy representative. Carnochan reported that their strategy was to 'avoid any unnecessary precipitation of a crisis', while the Argentine negotiator 'seemed anxious to get as much as he could without reaching breaking point'. Discussion proceeded satisfactorily on the animal health issues, but as for the public health issues, Carnochan remarked:

> Although it goes against the grain, External Relations and I are agreed that we should let some weeks elapse before we push on. . . . There is some risk that meantime we might be harried in our in-activity by certain newspapers but I think we can handle this. . . . During our meeting the Argentinians dropped some hints

---

[144] 'Imports of Meat from Argentina and Uruguay, Submission to the Minister', 31 July 1968, PRO MAF 276/261.

on this subject but they clearly do not expect any good news; by mutual consent we avoided direct discussion.[145]

Lace expressed his division's disappointment, commenting that they were concerned 'not only with the physical danger of illness which would not have come in had we moved earlier . . . but also by the weakening of the impact made by visits from our officers'.[146] Once again, public health policy implementation was delayed in the pursuit of other objectives, which were prioritised for diplomatic and economic reasons.

Rather than being able to 'push on' within weeks, the Animal Health division II experienced further frustration over another problem – the risks of Argentine frozen cooked beef. There was a small trade in this product,[147] but it was unaffected by the December 1967 ban because it was safe from the animal health perspective. The question arose of whether larger quantities could be shipped, and Ewart was asked to investigate, because of concerns about the adequacy of cooking and the risk of contamination after cooking.[148] MAFF and the Ministry of Health met to consider the matter in August 1968. Dr Howie, Director of the PHLS and member of the Milne Committee, had advised that under Argentine manufacturing conditions the product presented risks of 'botulism, *Clostridium welchii* food poisoning and staphylococcal food poisoning', and it was the view of the CMO that the trade should be stopped. But MAFF officials thought that removing the official certificate for frozen cooked beef only would be problematic. Five establishments were exporting the product to Britain, two of which were among the four most unsatisfactory plants, and it was envisaged that supplies from the latter would cease shortly. As for the other establishments, it was agreed that they should be approached informally, with a view to stopping the trade voluntarily. The situation would then be reviewed in early 1969.[149]

About a week after the withdrawal of approval from the four establishments was suspended, Lace returned to the frozen cooked beef problem. To 'keep to the spirit of understanding with the Ministry of Health', it would be necessary to speak to the importers. However, Lace still expected action against the four establishments after the January 1969 deadline, and it would be awkward asking two of them to suspend shipments of one commodity a few months

---

[145] J. G. Carnochan to Mr Tame, 5 August 1968, PRO MAF 276/261.

[146] G. O. Lace to J. G. Carnochan, 8 August 1968, PRO MAF 276/261.

[147] R. V. Blamire, 'Visit to South America – Argentina', 4 July 1967.

[148] K.A. Bird to Mr Lace, 15 December 1967, PRO MAF 276/260; K. A. Bird to E. H. Ewart, 3 January 1968, PRO MAF 276/260.

[149] G. O. Lace to Mr Tame, 16 August 1968; 'Note of a meeting on Friday August 2nd to discuss the importation of Argentinian frozen cooked beef', PRO MAF 246/329; J. W. Howie to J. M. Ross, 16 July 1968; J. M. Firth to L. Hurst, 8 August 1968, PRO MAF 276/261.

earlier. Alternatively, Argentine frozen cooked beef could be formally banned, but this would involve 'an unpleasant communication' which would be difficult without evidence of illness associated with the product. One option was to 'live with the risk', but Lace warned that if 'anything went wrong the blame would be entirely ours, since the two senior medical officials in the country have warned us'. Alternatively, they might attempt to alter the priority of the animal health over the public health issues, but he thought that 'the machinery' had already 'reached an irreversible point'.[150]

By the time a meeting was convened to explore the options, Ewart had suggested that the four unsatisfactory plants could now be given a deadline for improvements, because remedial work had started.[151] CAP was spending £200,000, while Swift was spending £1,000,000.[152] It was therefore agreed that the Argentine government would be told of the June inspection results, but that rather than removing approval from any establishment, deadlines would be set on the understanding that 'in view of the special risk involved' the cooked frozen beef trade would cease immediately.[153] The Animal Health division II prepared a submission along these lines for Hughes,[154] but it was criticised by Mr Dixon of the External Relations division. He pointed out that there was no detail of how long Britain had been importing frozen cooked beef, and whether there had been a recent deterioration in standards. There was nothing on how it was proposed to approach Argentina, or on the next step if they rejected voluntary action. Dixon appreciated that the CMO's statement presented a problem, but declared that more attention to the 'External Relations implications' was needed.[155] Hughes, however, was satisfied with the submission.[156]

It was only after Hughes had approved the proposals that Dixon's points were considered,[157] and the External Relation division's caution eventually prevailed. By early October it was agreed that because there was little time before the final deadline, 'it would be counter-productive to ask the Argentinians at this point to undertake voluntary restraint on frozen cooked meat'. It might 'undermine the will they at present seemed to be showing to improve standards'.[158] The acceptance by the Argentine government of changes to the Bledisloe agreement, including compulsory vaccination against

<hr>

[150] G. O. Lace to Mr Tame, 16 August 1968, PRO MAF 245/329.

[151] R. J. Blake to Mr Lace, 22 August 1968, PRO MAF 246/329.

[152] Animal Health II, 'Submission to the Minister imports of meat from Argentina – public health', 29 August 1968, PRO MAF 246/329.

[153] R. J. Blake to Mr Lace, 22 August 1968, PRO MAF 246/329.

[154] Animal Health II, 'Submission to the Minister imports of meat from Argentina – public health', 29 August 1968, PRO MAF 246/329.

[155] Dixon to M. D. M. Franklin, 12 September 1968, PRO MAF 246/329.

[156] D. F. Williamson to Mr Lace, 12 September 1968, PRO MAF 246/329.

[157] M. D. M. Franklin to Mr Carnochan, 12 September 1968, PRO MAF 246/329.

[158] J. E. Dixon to Mr Richardson, 1 October 1968, PRO MAF 276/261.

foot-and-mouth disease, was announced on 22 October.[159] This potentially cleared the way for the application of some pressure on public health issues, but no question was raised of revising the agreed approach. By the end of the month, MAFF had persuaded the Ministry of Health to withdraw their insistence that the frozen cooked beef imports be stopped.[160]

A note was delivered to the Argentine government on 27 November explaining that the June inspection had found only three meat plants to be satisfactory and that upgrading of the others was required by 1 January 1969. The new legislation on restructuring the veterinary service had now been published and was welcomed, but the note warned that the British inspectors would expect to see signs of improvement by January.[161] The Argentine official who received the note said he would endeavour to ensure that all the meat plants were either up to standard or 'at least, well advanced in the necessary work' by January.[162] These remarks had an 'ominous ring' about them, commented Lace, and increased the 'pessimism' he had 'always felt about the outcome of the efforts which we have been told the Argentine establishments have been making'.[163]

After Blamire, accompanied by Ross of the Ministry of Health, left for South America on 26 January, Carnochan attempted to prepare the ground for action on adverse reports. He wrote a memorandum observing that recommendations to remove plants from the approved list would be accompanied by 'loud squealing' from the Argentine government. While MAFF might be 'tempted to listen sympathetically', he declared that they should not allow themselves to be persuaded in any way. Anticipating the recommendations of the Northumberland Committee, he added that the preparation of boneless beef presented new opportunities for bacterial contamination, making it all the more important to achieve satisfactory standards.[164]

Inspections of Argentine meat plants 1969 to 1972

The news from Argentina was again worrying. On 19 February, Blamire reported that he had already seen four unsatisfactory plants, and that the meat inspection services were little improved.[165] The Ambassador also sent an anxious cable to the FCO. In the context of Argentine forebodings about the

---

[159] 'Safer meat rules accepted', *The Times*, 23 October 1968, p. 4b.

[160] G. O. Lace, 'Imports of meat from South America: public health control Submission to the Minister', 31 October 1968; G. O. Lace to Mr Carnochan, 31 October 1968; J. G. Carnochan to Mr Williamson, 1 November 1968, PRO MAF 276/261.

[161] British Embassy, Buenos Aires, 27 November 1968, PRO MAF 276/261.

[162] M. Gale to C. W. Wallace, 29 November 1968, PRO MAF 276/261.

[163] G. O. Lace to Mr Hurst, 9 December 1968, PRO MAF 276/261.

[164] J. G. Carnochan to Mr Tame, 7 February 1969, PRO MAF 276/261.

[165] R. V. Blamire to G. O. Lace, 19 February 1969, PRO MAF 276/261.

Northumberland report, any decision to strike plants off the approved list was likely to 'cause considerable disruption in the trade here and there are bound to be complaints'. It would 'keep the temperature down' if it could be made clear that approvals could be swiftly restored following improvements. In a further telegram he reported representations from the Argentine Under-secretary for International Affairs, who claimed that at one plant, Swift La Plata, which made 'a very important contribution to Argentine meat exports to the U. K. market', the remedial work had been completed after the inspection. Blamire was adamant, however, that there was no time for re-inspection. The following day the Ambassador was relieved that Blamire had had a satisfactory final meeting with the Argentine CVO. The CVO appreciated the line taken with Swift La Plata, but the Ambassador hoped that approval could be retained on the basis of an inspection by Ewart.[166] According to the record of a telephone conversation between MAFF's External Relations division and the Embassy, it was subsequently agreed that re-inspection by Ewart would take place three weeks after Blamire's departure. This was welcomed by the FCO, which had been preparing a strong letter to MAFF 'expressing disquiet' about developments and 'emphasising the need for due attention to be paid to the political factors'.[167]

The softer line, however, was not in accordance with the full record of Blamire's conversation with the CVO. According to this, there were internal political issues involved: over lunch the CVO revealed that his minister wanted him to resist pressure for him to encourage re-inspection of Swift La Plata. Blamire still recommended the removal of approval from this plant, and four others.[168] Three of the five were among the four candidates for removal from the approved list that had been identified after the June 1968 inspection. The Swift Rosario plant was now satisfactory, while the two new unacceptable plants were both owned by the British firm Bovril.[169] Blamire observed that there were signs of improvements in meat hygiene, but in order to give these a chance to develop, it was important to 'give full support' to the CVO who had shown that he was prepared to take a strong line. If the approvals were not removed immediately, Blamire thought, 'we shall lose the confidence' of the CVO and 'weaken the effort he is making to control the hygiene standards and inspection services'.[170]

Kearns, of the Meat division, approved of Blamire's recommendations, and told Carnochan of Animal Health that it was important to deal with them

---

[166] Buenos Aires to Foreign and Commonwealth Office, 21, 26 and 27 February 1969, PRO MAF 276/261.

[167] J. E. Dixon to Mr Evans, 28 February 1969, PRO MAF 276/261.

[168] R. V. Blamire to Mr Lace, 4 March 1969, PRO MAF 276/261.

[169] J. M. Ross and R. V. Blamire, 'Visit to Argentina – Jan/Feb 1969', 8 April 1969, supplied by R. Blamire to the project.

[170] R. V. Blamire to Mr Lace, 4 March 1969, PRO MAF 276/261.

quickly 'before we are caught up in the further problems on the animal health side arising out of the Northumberland Committee's report'.[171] The External Relations division and the FCO now seemed to support Blamire's recommendations, in the light of his report of his encounter with the Argentine CVO. MAFF was also under pressure to act from the DHSS (formerly the Ministry of Health). Lace reported that the DHSS were considering 'elevating the matter "to the highest level" apparently on a basis highly critical of this Ministry [MAFF]'.[172] The Embassy, however, continued to lobby against the removal of approval of the Swift plant, and to warn of the possible loss of export contracts to Argentina at a time when Britain was 'at last making headway' and looking forward to a trade fair during 1970.[173] Instructions were issued to Ewart to carry out an inspection, and the plant received a reprieve. Four plants were therefore removed from the approved list by means of a notice placed in the *London Gazette* on 1 April.[174]

Apart from the faults of the plants proposed for removal from the approved list, the full report by Blamire and Ross was remarkably positive. It began as follows:

> In a period of less than two years there has been a remarkable transformation in most of the premises on the U.K. approved list. Modern systems of slaughtering have been installed, the fabric of the buildings and internal surfaces of slaughterhalls and workrooms have been greatly improved, wooden equipment has been eliminated and equipment in general has been brought up-to-date.[175]

As regard hygiene standards, these were generally greatly improved. Metal or plastic scabbards, sterilisers and hand-washing facilities were now commonly in use. As for frozen cooked beef, in view of the improvements, and the fact that only 'very small supplies' of this product were 'occasionally exported to the UK', the report concluded that this was no longer 'an urgent health risk requiring immediate action'.[176] A report on this matter followed, leading to the issue of a memorandum recommending the necessary hygiene precautions.[177]

When turning to the meat inspection service, the tone changed. The standard of meat inspection was far below that normally expected and the

---

[171] F. M. Kearns to Mr Carnochan, 6 March 1969, PRO MAF 276/261.

[172] G. O. Lace to Mr Carnochan, 20 March 1969, PRO MAF 276/261.

[173] Buenos Aires to Foreign Office, 17, 21 March 1969; G. O. Lace to Mr Carnochan, 20 March 1969, PRO MAF 276/261.

[174] Animal Health Division II, 'Draft note to Argentine Government', 16 April 1969, PRO MAF 276/261.

[175] J. M. Ross and R. V. Blamire, 'Visit to Argentina – Jan/Feb 1969', 8 April 1969, copy supplied by R. V. Blamire to the project.

[176] Ibid.

[177] R. H. Goodhand, 'Visit to Argentina 1972', 14 September 1972, PRO MAF 282/133.

degree of supervision was 'still nominal'. At one slaughterhouse any animal capable of walking to the stunning pen passed ante-mortem inspection. In addition, Blamire and Ross saw carcasses being passed as fit which would be rejected in the UK for fever, emaciation or oedema.

Apart from these observations, the report observed that the law restructuring the meat inspection service was finally being implemented. The Argentine Ministry of Agriculture had the power to employ veterinarians at enhanced salaries, and allowed them to absorb, as government servants, the assistants employed by the factories. It was expected that by mid-February about 200 veterinarians and 250 assistants would be employed on the new basis. Finally, the current CVO seemed to be 'a strong man capable of resisting the enormous pressures which can be exerted upon one in his position'. If he were to remain in post, a steady improvement of the inspection service might materialise.[178]

In view of the failure to rigorously follow up the June 1968 inspection, an alternative explanation is required of the stimulus to the improvements in place by the time of the Blamire/Ross visit. An indication of such an explanation is provided by an article published in *The Economist* in January 1969 which claimed that since the end of the beef ban, changes in market conditions were leading to a boom in the Argentine beef trade. As a result of the Argentine government's attempts to find a new way of trading, the trade in consignments of chilled sides of beef at Smithfield Market had declined. However, an alternative trade had arisen in selected chilled or frozen cuts direct to supermarkets, hotels and restaurants on a fixed-price basis. This avoided price fluctuations, and the cuts fetched much higher prices.[179] The investment in plant seen by Blamire and Ross was therefore probably a result of economic buoyancy, and the need for improved hygiene to allow the reliable preparation of cuts of beef. Furthermore, the article makes it clear that it was already widely expected that the Northumberland Committee would recommend that South American meat imports be limited to boneless meat. Satisfactory boneless meat production certainly needed hygienic facilities. It therefore appears that commercial considerations, as much as direct pressure applied by the British or Argentine government, were responsible for the improvements seen in February 1969.

The Northumberland report was published on 1 May, and three days earlier an *aide-mémoire* to the Argentine government confirmed the predicted recommendations. The document referred to the hygiene standards needed for boneless beef production, and to the recent improvements in the *frigoríficos* and continuing deficiencies of the meat inspection service. On the latter matter it was stated that 'Her Majesty's Government trusts that the plans . . .

---

[178] Ross and Blamire, 'Visit . . . Jan/Feb 1969'.

[179] 'Argentina: the ban which became a boon', *The Economist*, 25 January 1969, cutting in PRO MAF 276/261.

for improvements will be vigorously prosecuted'.[180] As usual, the Argentine government complained of discrimination against them and threatened trade retaliation. But Hughes presented the policies as discrimination in Argentina's favour, since meat imports were normally banned altogether from foot-and-mouth endemic countries.[181]

Eight months later, Ewart reviewed the state of the meat inspection service. He recorded that in a few establishments there was 'semi-effective control in all departments or at least . . . veterinarians taking an active and intelligent interest'. In others there was some veterinary control in the killing halls, while the rest remained unimproved. Some of the *frigorifico* veterinarians, he felt, had taken the job as 'a lucrative sinecure'. Out of twenty establishments, he rated 'meat inspection' as 'good' at two and 'poor' or 'bad' at four. As for 'general veterinary control', only one establishment was 'good' and ten were 'poor' or 'bad'. Ewart commented that:

> The Argentines now have sufficient numbers of veterinarians and auxiliary personnel . . . but progress in increasing veterinary control is increasingly slow. Nevertheless, the basic structure is there and compared to the situation a year ago there had been improvement but they have . . . a long way to go before the veterinary service . . . can be regarded as satisfactory and dependable.[182]

The senior staff were of varying quality. There was no case of suspension of exports in view of hygiene defects without British prompting. Ewart was also beginning to lose faith in the CVO because he had recommended several plants for approval which Ewart deemed unsatisfactory.

A further visit by a MAFF inspector, which took place from May to July 1972, reported very favourably on all but a few establishments:

> Regarding the general standard of hygiene one could not fail but be impressed on entering the majority of the plants. It was abundantly clear that the operatives had been fully trained in the use of sterilising and hand-washing facilities.[183]

Equipment was routinely sterilised between carcasses, rooms were well lit, air-conditioned and ventilated, separate rooms were provided for different operations, and the freedom from rust, and routine cleaning of trolleys and overhead rails was impressive. But in some plants the requirements of the British memorandum on the preparation of frozen cooked meats were not fully observed.

---

[180] 'Aide-mémoire', 26 April 1969, PRO MAF 276/261.
[181] C. Hughes to E. F. McLoughlin, 8 May 1969, PRO MAF 276/261.
[182] R. H. Ewart, 'Conditions in the Frigorificos and assessment of the Argentine Frigorifico Veterinary Service – January 1970', 16 January 1970, PRO MAF 246/330.
[183] R. H. Goodhand, 'Visit to Argentina 1972', 14 September 1972, PRO MAF 282/133.

The veterinary service also continued to give cause for concern. The CVO whose appointment had held such promise had vacated the post, and the inspection service was controlled by a temporary replacement. The report stated that the service should 'play a greater part in the general supervision of the plants', and expressed concern about its lack of involvement in 'canning techniques, and the control of water supplies'. It recommended that an assurance be sought in connection with these matters, and that one plant should be removed from the approved list until the water supply was improved.

Evidently, since the typhoid outbreaks, Argentine meat hygiene had finally much improved, but the connection between this improvement and the pressure applied by the British government is unclear. Questions of domestic and international politics and trade, and action on animal health regulations frequently delayed and blunted such pressure. In the years immediately following the typhoid outbreaks, the publicity given to the problems with the water supplies seems to have stimulated cannery managers to make sure that cooling water was adequately treated. Eight years after the Aberdeen outbreak, however, in the absence of the rigorous control of canning by government inspectors, there were some signs that one of the most important lesson of the typhoid outbreaks (the danger of contaminated cannery cooling water) was beginning to be forgotten.

10

Summary and conclusions, and food safety since 1964

After the historical introduction to typhoid and food poisoning in Chapter 1, we began the examination of government policy making in connection with the typhoid outbreaks in Chapter 2, which continued in chapters 5 to 9. The first observation we may make from these chapters is that the process of constructing and implementing policy was often very complicated. Several ministries, several divisions within ministries, and a variety of other actors were often involved. Rarely, if ever, did action follow directly and unproblematically from scientific or technical principles, or suppositions concerning risk, or even evidence of actual food-related disease. Decisions on risks deemed theoretical were particularly subject to long drawn-out prevarication, although when there was concrete evidence of food poisoning cases, decision making and action on the basis of technical advice was sometimes achieved relatively quickly. In 1963, three typhoid outbreaks in rapid succession were necessary before a theoretical risk was deemed sufficiently real to justify action. At all times, however, the decision-making process was invariably conditioned, to a greater or lesser extent, by such considerations as the need to protect reputations, the likelihood or otherwise of damaging press publicity, and wider political and economic interests.

In the case of the 1963 typhoid outbreaks, Chapter 2 argued that sensitivity to broader economic and political factors, connected with the recent problems caused by the glut of Argentine chilled beef imports, influenced the way that the civil servants handled the situation. These factors, and the traditional civil service preference for making decisions and acting secretly or quietly, meant that when action was deemed necessary, publicity was avoided as far as possible. Had this not been the case, it might be suggested that the reactions of the public, and the managements of the South American meat plants, may have been such that the Aberdeen typhoid outbreak would not have happened. This notion is reinforced when it is considered that, no matter what other defects British inspectors found in the Argentine meat plants and meat inspection service after 1964, the quality of the cooling water employed in the manufacture of canned meat was almost invariably satisfactory (apart from at one plant in 1972).

Despite the concerns of the civil servants to avoid publicity, the connection made between typhoid and corned beef was mentioned in the public and professional press in 1963, although the matter had apparently not come to

287

the attention of Ian MacQueen and his colleagues in Aberdeen. Again, had MAFF and the Ministry of Health been more open about the action taken after the Bedford outbreak, had there been effective communication between the English and Scottish central health departments about the issue, and had the central health departments kept MOsH informed, the action taken in the early days of the Aberdeen outbreak may have been more decisive. The source of the outbreak, for example, may have been revealed to the public more quickly, avoiding one cause of some of the tension between the MOH and the local public during the first week.

The actions of MacQueen were an important feature of the Aberdeen outbreak, were controversial at the time, and are particularly well remembered by many of our interviewees, due to the media coverage and the critical comment in the Milne report. However, Chapter 3 also sought to provide an account of the activities of the other sectors of the health service, and other personnel within MacQueen's department, and to provide some insights into patient experiences. It was the GPs, the hospital doctors and the laboratory workers whose activities were, as much as MacQueen and his staff, responsible for bringing the outbreak under control. But in view of the criticisms of the Milne report, it is incumbent upon us to provide, in this conclusion, some further comments on MacQueen's performance.

MacQueen claimed in his evidence to the Milne Committee that his handling of the press during the Aberdeen typhoid outbreak was strategic. In Chapter 4, however, we argued that although MacQueen had previously been interested in the use of the press for health education, his relationship with the press during the outbreak was partly the result of his responses to the criticisms of the local public and press during the first week. The media provided a means by which MacQueen communicated with the population, but also provided a channel of communication between the population and MacQueen. MacQueen was faced with a situation outwith his previous experience and the typhoid outbreak was as much a learning experience for him as it was for many others.

But whether or not MacQueen's use of the press was based on a preconceived strategy, he was condemned for it, and the various control measures that he instituted, by the Milne Committee. The rationale of the committee's position was that, they claimed, MacQueen overestimated the infectivity of typhoid. However, as shown in the first section of Chapter 5, MacQueen's concern with the likelihood of 'waves' of infection was shared with key personnel at the SHHD – which was not acknowledged in the Milne report. The same personnel were also sympathetic towards MacQueen during the outbreak, in view of the pressure he was under from the press.

Chapter 6 discussed how the general 'shape' of the Milne report was arrived at – the censure of MacQueen and the lenient treatment of the ministries and the firms. While the general thrust of the report certainly suited the ministries there is no indication that they contributed to the critical treatment of MacQueen – rather this originated from local and professional opinion. On the other hand, in view of the contrast between the sometimes verbal flamboyance of MacQueen, and the habitual reserve of civil servants, it is not surprising that there are signs that some of them approved of the Milne report's criticisms of MacQueen. In addition, the criticism of MacQueen could also distract attention from such mild criticisms of the ministries as were included in the report. Some of the positions taken by local actors were no doubt conditioned by longer term problems relating to the relationships between the sectors of the NHS, and MacQueen's strategy for public health. For example, his enthusiasm for expanding the roles of health visitors maintained tensions between public health and GPs which had existed since the emergence of the MOH in the nineteenth century.[1] However, the judgement of James Howie, Director of the PHLS and key expert member of the committee, was also important, and his professional agenda was reflected in several of the committee's recommendations. Wider economic and political influences, and the avoidance of publicity in connection with the 1963 outbreaks, as discussed in Chapter 2, were not covered in the ministries' evidence. Such matters would not have been considered as suitable areas for investigation by the ex-civil servant and civil servant who acted as chair and secretary of the committee, and who did much to influence the agenda.

The evidence presented to the Milne Committee by the London-based ministries sought to establish that their actions in connection with and following the 1963 outbreaks had been reasonable, in the light of current knowledge and experience. And as far as can be judged without the full record of the Milne Committee's proceedings, the committee seems to have accepted the ministries' evidence at face value. Besides the neglect of broader dimensions of the handling of the 1963 outbreaks, there appears to have been no detailed consideration of the adequacy of the ministries' responses to the earlier Pickering incident in 1955. The veterinary attaché in Buenos Aires may have been expected to be aware of the potential problems of using unchlorinated river water for cooling purposes in canneries, but in mid-1963 he seems to have been oblivious to the issue. Likewise, the Milne Committee seems to have given no consideration to the evidence of hygienic failures at specific canning plants that had accumulated by the early 1960s. Since, as mentioned in Chapter 1, such evidence was in the hands of W. C. Cockburn, Director of the epidemiological research laboratory of the PHLS, this issue would have raised questions about the role of the PHLS, as well as the ministries. As it

---

[1] L. Diack and D. F. Smith, 'Professional strategies of Medical Officers of Health in the post war period (1): 'innovative traditionalism': the case of Dr Ian MacQueen, MOH for Aberdeen 1952–1974', *Journal of Public Health Medicine*, 2002, vol. 24, pp. 123–9; L. Diack and D. F. Smith, 'The media and the management of a food crisis: Aberdeen's typhoid outbreak in 1964', in V. Berridge and K. Loughlin, *Medicine, the market and the Mass Media*, London, forthcoming, 2005.

was, the PHLS was held up as a model of good practice, against which the deficiencies of the Scottish laboratory service could be compared.

Uncritical acceptance of the evidence of the ministries, leaving the aforementioned issues unexplored, would make anything other than a lenient approach towards the firms linked with the 1963 and Aberdeen outbreaks difficult to sustain. Little was made by the committee of the points that the chlorination of canning plant cooling water had apparently become standard practice in South America after 1955, but that Establishment 25 neglected the lesson. Likewise, there was only brief mention of the point that Establishment 1A, which was linked with both the Pickering and Aberdeen outbreaks, apparently learned but then overlooked the lesson. In view of the rejection by the firms of the possibility that typhoid germs could enter cans undetected, the committee's sessions with their witnesses concentrated upon persuading them that such an event was indeed possible.

Chapter 5 continued the examination of food safety policy making begun in Chapter 2, in the context of the Aberdeen outbreak. Whereas the decisions during 1963 were all handled by civil servants, during the emergency situation created by the Aberdeen typhoid outbreak, besides the ministers of the departments directly concerned, other senior Conservative politicians became involved in managing the affair. The outbreak was an emergency at more than one level. In view of the widespread publicity it was a political as well as a food safety emergency, especially in the context of the impending general election, and the threat posed by the Labour Party led by Harold Wilson. The appointment of the Committee of Enquiry, proposed by senior civil servants and approved by the politicians, was part of the strategy for political management of the outbreak, arising from the allegation that stockpile corned beef was involved. During the emergency, the expert advice of the CMO resulted in swift action involving the withdrawal, publicly, of several batches of canned meat. As we saw in Chapter 8, however, as the emergency passed, the predominant view in MAFF resisted the CMO's advice against releasing any stockpile corned beef until after the publication of the Milne report. And after MAFF's position was endorsed by ministers, the CMO proved willing to modify his advice.

As became apparent in Chapter 7, the CMO's advice, as a rule, was taken seriously. If the CMO favoured the Milne Committee's recommendation that a medical officer should accompany a veterinary officer on overseas meat inspection trips, MAFF would find the recommendation difficult to resist. Even without the Ministry of Health's and the CMO's enthusiasm, resisting the recommendation was risky, in view of the criticism that would result in the event of further mishap. However, besides fear of publicity, Chapter 7 also demonstrated the roles of pre-existing policy agendas, and interdepartmental and inter-professional rivalry in conditioning food safety policy making. MAFF's veterinarians who were responsible for overseas meat plant hygiene were very anxious to protect the small niche in veterinary public health that they occupied on behalf of the British veterinary profession. In consequence, while the recommendation on medical involvement in overseas meat inspection was implemented, the method of implementation smacked very much of tokenism.

The implementation of some of the other recommendations, including those concerning the powers of MOsH, and hygiene in cold meat retailing, was discussed briefly at the end of Chapter 6. Here it seemed that officials were very willing to take account of the views of industry bodies and to disregard the views of professional bodies such as the Public Health Inspectors' Association, which significantly softened the impact of the Milne Committee's proposals. But there was no evidence of any conflict in this connection between MAFF and the Ministry of Health. As in the decision making over the 1963 typhoid outbreaks, Ministry of Health officials seemed no less willing than their colleagues at MAFF to take into account the interests of the food trade, and they were no more willing to substitute voluntary agreements and informal methods of operating with legal regulations.

We have observed that politicians became involved in the decision making during the Aberdeen typhoid outbreak. In Chapter 8 we discussed a further episode concerning the fate of the suspect corned beef, which during 1965 also entailed political intervention at the highest level – from Harold Wilson who was now Prime Minister. In this case, the effect was to prevent the application of the advice of the Milne Committee that the suspect corned beef could be made safe by reprocessing. For all his apparent enthusiasm for science,[2] for Wilson public sentiment and political instinct were better guides to action than scientific advice. The Labour Party won the October 1964 general election with a majority of only five, and it would not be until March 1966 that they achieved a comfortable majority.[3] In these circumstances Wilson was bound to take a keen interest in such issues of public and press concern, and to seek to present the government as the protector of the people. Ironically, however, the Prime Minister's intervention eventually led to the ministries effectively turning a blind eye to the bulk of one batch of suspect corned beef (from Establishment 1819) being exported abroad for consumption without reprocessing.

The involvement or intervention of government politicians in food safety policy making was only occasional, but civil servants routinely included political and economic calculations in their decision making. The role of those in the Foreign Office (or FCO), and the External Relations and Meat divisions of MAFF, and the Treasury, were precisely to take such matters into account. But those whose remit was public health, such as the staff of MAFF's Animal Health division II, were also frequently willing to adjust their recommendation

---

[2] H. Rose and S. P. R. Rose, *Science and Society*, London, 1969, p. 93.
[3] For the election results see Richard Kimber, 'Political science resources British governments and elections since 1945', internet: http://www.psr.keele.ac.uk/area/uk/uktable.htm, accessed 6 April 2004.

in the light of such matters as supply and prices. Chapter 9, which related the tortuous story of the efforts to encourage improvements in Argentine meat plant hygiene and the Argentine meat inspection service which followed the typhoid outbreaks, highlights the interdivisional as well as the interdepartmental interactions involved in policy making. There is little indication of food safety being accorded any higher priority than before the typhoid outbreaks. Furthermore, the brief account of the 1967 *Salmonella typhimurium* incident suggested that any more vigorous activity in a possible emergency situation was aimed mainly at protecting departments from criticism.

The long 'drag' on policy on Argentine meat hygiene was exacerbated by the foot-and-mouth outbreak of late 1967, when animal health priorities took precedence over public health. Even the clear advice of the CMO and James Howie on the hazards of frozen cooked beef were effectively ignored in the summer and autumn of 1968, due to the priority taken by animal health and wider economic and political matters. When the improvement in the hygiene of the Argentine meat plants eventually came, it appears to have been as much or more the result of commercial considerations rather than any attempt to adhere to regulations.

While the advice of the CMO may have been occasionally frustrated, MAFF officials normally felt constrained by the CMO's advice, and would sometimes strategically delay or avoid seeking it. As we saw in Chapter 9, this occurred at one point during the discussion about the disposal of the suspect corned beef in the stockpile. In contrast, the advice of MAFF's veterinary advisers on overseas meat inspection was of lower status, especially within the wider policy-making arena. In this connection it is worth referring to some additional primary material. Some unusually candid remarks by C. D. Wiggin, a member of the FCO's American Department, appear in a letter that he wrote to the ambassadors in South America in April 1970, and illustrate external perceptions of MAFF veterinarians, and the interdivisional dimensions of MAFF policy making.

Wiggin's letter was prepared in the context of a difficult situation that arose in Brazil, after MAFF recommended removal of their official certificate as a result of shortcomings in the hygiene of their meat plants, and animal health risks. For those concerned with foreign affairs, Wiggin said, it was a 'long and painful business to get helpful decisions out of MAFF; and all too often one is reduced to trying to prevent really disastrous decisions being taken'. He intimated that he had been 'worried by the attitude of our veterinary experts in Latin America, not to speak of the technical side of MAFF'. The technical experts did not seem to realise that in technical decisions, judgements involving 'diplomacy, timing, tactics and so on' could be of 'the greatest importance'. From Wiggin's perspective, the approach of MAFF's experts seemed not to be how to ensure that meat was exported to the UK under proper conditions and to make adverse decisions as 'palatable as possible to the Latin Americans', but rather 'Let's teach these somethings a lesson'. However, in concluding, he added that it was unfair to speak of MAFF as a 'monolithic hostile force'. There were also 'a lot of people in MAFF who realise that meat is a politically explosive subject and that action on the meat front can have the most damaging repercussions on major British interests'. It was the 'custodians of animal and human health in MAFF' who were 'not so foreign affairs minded'.[4] A few months later Wiggin told a colleague: 'We have just emerged from a potentially awkward brush with the Brazilians over meat exports which in our view, shared by other Whitehall departments, was in part brought about by the over purist (and tactless) line taken by MAFF veterinarians.'[5]

This incident also provides a further example of high-level political involvement in decision making. The question of whether Brazilian meat and meat products should be banned immediately in view of the unhygienic state of the country's meat plants came before a ministerial committee on agricultural policy, after which the Minister without Portfolio, Peter Shore, wrote to Harold Wilson. Shore, pointing out that:

> conditions at the Brazilian meat-processing plants from which come the products exported to Britain appear to have become worse over the last few years, since the Aberdeen typhoid outbreak in 1964 (attributed to similar conditions in an Argentine meat cannery), despite our own pressure to maintain and improve them.[6]

Brazil also appeared not to be applying the revised animal health precautions agreed after the 1967 to 1968 foot-and-mouth outbreak. However, Shore remarked that while the volume of meat imports from Brazil was small, a ban would arouse resentment and 'cause damage to our exports to that country, currently running at over £40M per year'. The Agricultural Policy Committee had agreed that rather than an immediate ban, 'there should be representations at a high level to the Brazilian Government expressing our serious concern at standards of hygiene in their meat industry . . . and stating that within months . . . there must be substantial improvement'. Wilson signalled his agreement with this strategy, annotating the letter: 'I think the conclusion to put them on notice is the right one at this stage.'[7] The association made between the state of the Brazilian meat industry and the Aberdeen typhoid outbreak did not seem to alarm Wilson in the same way that he had been alarmed in 1965, when he intervened to prevent the reprocessing and distribution of suspect corned beef. This may reinforce the suggestion made at the end of Chapter 9, namely that some of the lessons of the Aberdeen typhoid outbreak were beginning to fade by 1970. Yet it may also reflect the difference between intense press interest in the 'reprocessing' issue during a difficult political situation in 1965 and minimal interest in the hygiene of the Brazilian meat

---

[4] C. D. Wiggin to D. Hunt, 27 April 1970, PRO FCO 7/146.
[5] C. D Wiggin to Mr Mills, 7 October 1970, PRO FCO 7/1491.
[6] P. Shore to Prime Minister, 21 May 1970, PRO PREM 13/3036.
[7] Ibid.

industry in May 1970, and the unimportance of the issue in the context of the 1970 general election a few weeks later.

Whether or not the press was interested and knowledgeable about particular issues certainly influenced the positions of politicians, and among the civil servants, whatever the other differences between them, there was an almost universally shared preference for making decisions in private. However, there is one example of some dissent from the usual civil service ethos of secrecy, articulated in August 1968, when action on the latest shocking report on the state of the Argentine meat industry was under discussion, in the difficult political circumstances of the aftermath of the foot-and-mouth outbreak. One MAFF official argued that the likely reaction to and impact of removing the approval of the most unsatisfactory establishments could be mitigated if the Minister was armed with a 'good plain tale' about the hazards of not taking action. The Minister could use this to persuade the trade, the public and his colleagues that the possible price rises and political consequences involved would have to be faced. This suggested both a more open and a more strategic conception of press relations, but the idea was rejected by a more senior official, who feared that the plan would backfire and call into question their whole past strategy on the safety of Argentine meat imports. He favoured the traditional preference for making decisions quietly and assuring the public that all was well.[8] In Chapter 8, however, we saw that there were occasions when the policy makers were willing to use the press as a weapon in the pursuit of policy objectives, when the effect of the publicity would cast the actions of others in a negative light (holders of Establishment 1819 suspect stock) and encourage them to tow the government line.

The early 1960s was a period when a new, more vigorous style of investigative journalism was developing, and when there were more specialist reporters and competition within the media, and a less reverential attitude towards ministers, senior officials and others in authority, including scientists.[9] This may account for some of the intense media activity surrounding the Aberdeen typhoid outbreak, but it should also be remembered that earlier outbreaks, dating at least as far back as the 1897 asylum outbreak near Maidstone, mentioned in Chapter 1, had received much publicity which had influenced events. But the 1960s did also see the beginning of press interest in new environmental concerns such as the impact of the use of the insecticide DDT, and a high-profile and shocking medical scandal, the thalidomide affair.[10] However, in this book we have seen no evidence of the development,

---

[8] Mr Kearns to J. G. Carnochan, 31 July 1968; J. G. Carnochan to Mr Kearns, 1 August 1968, PRO MAF 276/261.

[9] K. Loughlin, 'Networks of mass communication: reporting science, health and medicine from the 1950s to the 1970s', in V. Berridge (ed.), *Making Health Policy: Networks in Research and Policy after 1945*, Amsterdam, forthcoming, ch. 11.

[10] R. Carson, *Silent Spring*, London 1963; P. I. Folb, *The Thalidomide Disaster, and its Impact on Modern Medicine*, Cape Town, 1977.

in response to such trends, of any new, more sophisticated press or other strategies by the civil servants and ministries involved in such issues. There was nothing new in the way that a committee of enquiry was appointed to defuse the political situation, and dramatic headlines created in early June 1964 by the Aberdeen typhoid outbreak and Ian MacQueen's accusations about the possible involvement of stockpile corned beef. And there was nothing new about the way civil servants constantly factored calculations as to the possibility of press and political interest into their decision making – as, for example, when deciding on the implementation or non-implementation of the Milne Committee's recommendations.[11] Analysis of the early days of the bovine spongiform encephalopathy (BSE) affair suggest that by the late 1980s the ministries were attempting even tighter control of information.[12] And it would not be until a decade later, with the formation of the Food Standards Agency, that there would be a decisive shift towards a policy of openness in policy making and press relations, as will be mentioned at the end of this chapter.

Having outlined some of the key points made in previous chapters of this book, we will now attempt to put together some of the insights gained, in order to outline some of the key features of the food safety policy-making system of the 1960s. This will build on our analysis of the process of implementation of the Milne Committee's recommendation for medical involvement in overseas meat inspection, which appeared in a previous publication,[13] and which was expanded in Chapter 7. The conceptual scheme is illustrated schematically in Figure 10.1 (note that the original generation of the recommendation is not covered). The essential features are the *context* (the most important aspects of which were existing policy agendas and the possible political and press comment in the case of non-implementation of the recommendation), and the *interplay of interests* within the policy-making machinery (the ministries and their technical advisers). Figure 10.2 attempts to expand this diagram in

---

[11] For examples of policy making in the field of nutrition, and officials' strategies in connection with official or quasi-official expert committees appointed following adverse press publicity, see D. F. Smith, 'The rise and fall of the Scientific Food Committee during the Second World War', in D. F. Smith and J. Phillips (eds), *Food, Science, Policy and Regulation in the Twentieth Century: International and Comparative Perspectives*, London, 2000, pp. 101–16; and D. F. Smith, 'The social construction of dietary standards: the British Medical Association – Ministry of Health Advisory Committee on Nutrition Report of 1934', in D. Maurer and J. Sobal (eds), *Eating Agenda: Food and Nutrition as Social Problems*, New York, 1995, pp. 279–304.

[12] D. Miller, 'Risk, science and policy: definitions, struggles, information management, the media and BSE', *Social Science and Medicine*, 1999, vol. 49, pp. 1239–55.

[13] L. Diack, T. H. Pennington, E. Russell and D. F. Smith, 'Departmental and professional agendas in the implementation of the recommendations of a food crisis enquiry: the Milne report and inspection of overseas meat plants', in D. F. Smith and J. Phillips (eds), *Food, Science, Policy and Regulation in the Twentieth Century: International and Comparative Perspectives*, London, 2000, pp. 189–206.

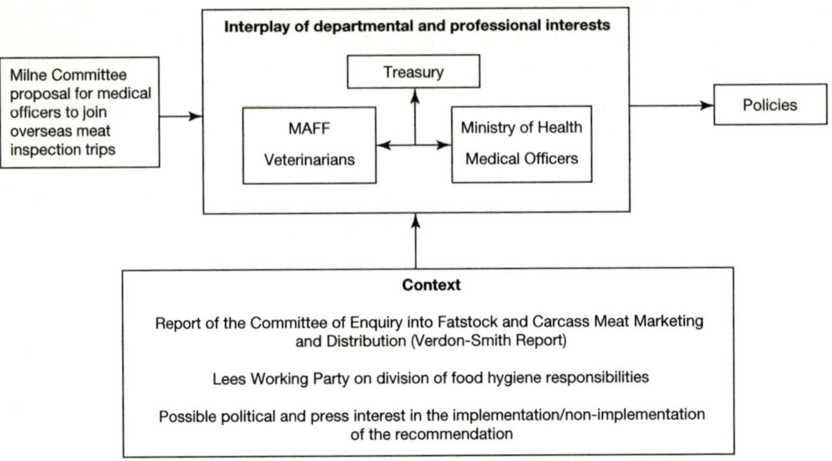

Figure 10.1 Decision making on the Milne Committee recommendation for medical involvement in overseas meat inspection

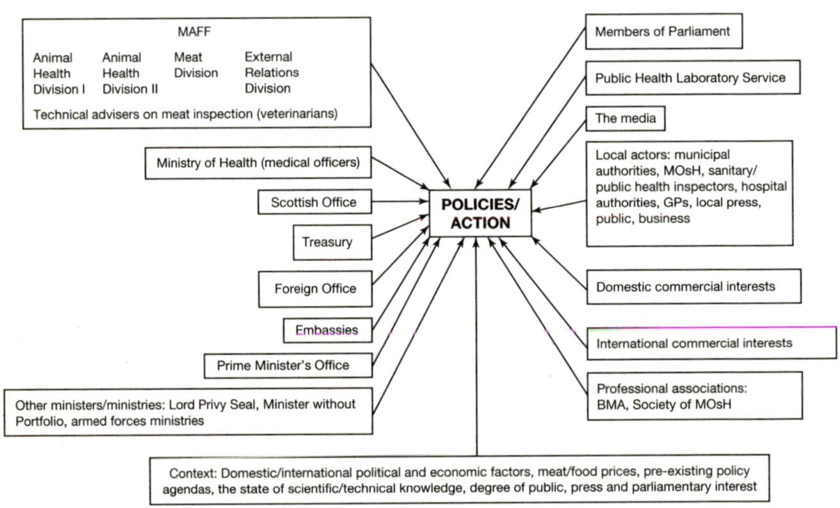

Figure 10.2 Simplified schematic representation of food safety policy making in the 1960s

order to take in the more complex and varied policy-making processes covered in other chapters of this book. This brings in a wider variety of actors both within and outside the machinery of government, and expands and generalises the relevant aspects of the context. Within each department of government there are, of course, specialised divisions, but no attempt has been made to represent these, except in the case of MAFF – as interdivisional differences within MAFF formed an especially important feature of the action discussed in Chapter 9. All the actual and potential interactions between the actors involved in different specific examples of policy making would be difficult to represent, and so this has not been attempted. Clearly, the importance of different actors, and different aspects of the context, varied from issue to issue. The relative importance of different actors and contextual factors varied, for example, according to whether an emergency or chronic problem was under consideration.

Figure 10.2, and the above discussion of food policy making, may be compared with Erik Millstone's four 'models' of food policy making, and the interaction of science and ethics, as put forward by actors and analysts.[14] The first, which he labels 'positivisitic extremism', involves policy flowing directly from science, and is plainly a non-starter in the world revealed by archival research. The second supposes that science and ethics both contribute to policy, but separately. To generalise, we might substitute economics, politics and culture for 'ethics'. This is also clearly inapplicable in our examples where the science was uncertain, and both scientific/technical and lay policy makers took account of scientific and extra-scientific factors. Millstone's third and fourth models are that scientific debate is 'nothing but a form of social conflict', and that 'science and ethics are richly interconnected but nonetheless distinguishable'. The former position Millstone attributes to M. Schwartz and M. Thompson, who take the view that it is impossible to separate 'politics, technology and social choice' and that they are, rather, 'an entanglement: an inchoate mass'.[15] The latter position implies that the scientific and extra-scientific considerations are 'analytically distinct' but 'can and do reciprocally influence each other', but that the extent to which they 'can be distinguished and separated in practice' is a 'matter for specific investigation in particular cases'.[16] This is a similar stance to that taken by the media analyst David Miller, who remarks that 'the generation, communication and promotion of expert advice is itself an integral part of the policy process. Expert assessments are not simply political, but neither are they straightforwardly neutral and factual.'[17]

---

[14] E. Millstone, 'Food safety: the ethical dimensions', in B. Mepham (ed.), *Food Ethics*, London, 1996, pp. 84–100.

[15] M. Schwartz and M. Thompson, *Divided we Stand: Redefining Politics, Technology and Social Choice*, London, 1990, p. 1.

[16] Millstone, 'Food safety', pp. 88–9.

[17] Miller, 'Risk, science and policy', p. 1241.

Millstone explains the approach to food policy analysis that he favours further in a joint paper with Patrick van Zwanenberg. The authors describe their stance as a 'constructivist approach grounded in epistemological realism' which they illustrate with a case study comparing US and UK pesticide regulation. They regard the US regulatory regime as more effective, greater openness being one important contributing factor. They also claim that using their approach, the analyst can point to risk assessments that are likely to be more or less robust, and can therefore make a contribution to policy making.[18] It is not necessary here to consider the philosophical dimensions of van Zwanenberg and Millstone's framework, but it should be clear that we sympathise with their approach. We have already discussed such themes as when policy has/has not followed more or less directly from scientific advice and, like them, we also consider that analysts can identify pathogenic aspects of regulatory regimes. Like van Zwanenberg and Millstone, and Miller, we consider that secrecy is one such characteristic – without which the Aberdeen outbreak may have been avoided.

The detailed history of food poisoning in Britain since the 1963 to 1964 typhoid outbreaks has yet to be written, but we will conclude this chapter with a brief account that will indicate some of the features, episodes and themes of that period. First, it should be noted that while the typhoid outbreaks had some impact on the history of food safety, they certainly did not occasion any thoroughgoing changes in approach. The 'Drive for clean food' that the *Municipal Journal* hoped would follow the Aberdeen typhoid outbreak[19] was not sustained for long and fundamental reforms did not take place until three decades later.

The confidence of the early 1960s that food poisoning was being brought under control by the food hygiene regulations, mentioned in Chapter 1, did not last. During the late 1960s and 1970s, in passages concerning food poisoning in the SHHD annual reports, optimism soon gave way to circumspection. In 1968, one particularly disappointing *Salmonella* outbreak in Glasgow was mentioned, which involved more than 450 cases and seven deaths. Later, there was little or no comment about the trend in food poisoning notifications.[20] The reports of the CMO of the Ministry of Health (later DHSS, later Department of Health) ventured few remarks on food poisoning trends. In the late 1960s the CMO (George Godber) emphasised the poor quality of the data,

---

[18] P. van Zwanenberg and E. Millstone, 'Beyond skeptical relativism: evaluating the social constructions of expert risk assessment', *Science, Technology and Human Values*, 2000, vol. 25, pp. 259–82.

[19] 'Drive for clean food may follow Aberdeen typhoid', *Municipal Journal*, 1964, vol. 72, p. 2044.

[20] *RSHHD 1965*, p. 15; *RSHHD 1966*, pp. 9, 99; *RSHHD 1967*, pp. 12, 110; *RSHHD 1968*, p. 105; *RSHHD 1969*, p. 18; *RSHHD 1970*, pp. 21, 70; 'Food poisoning in West Scotland', *British Medical Journal*, 1968, vol. iii, p. 750.

and linked one rise in notifications to a 'warm summer and autumn'. In his report for 1973 he drew attention to a drop in food poisoning in England for the second year running.[21] But the resumption of the overall upward trend passed without comment, except in the CMO's report for 1984, when the total number of cases stood at 19,744 (compared to 8088 in 1970[22]). The CMO (Henry Yellowlees) remarked simply that 'there are many factors which influence these statistics and no particular inference should be drawn from apparent trends'.[23]

Food poisoning was of low priority for the central government health departments in the 1970s, despite the upward trend in notifications, some local initiatives and the efforts of certain organisations. The latter included the professional associations of the public health inspectors (later environmental health officers) which attempted to intensify a long-standing campaign to raise the profile of food poisoning (pre-dating the Aberdeen typhoid outbreak). The British Association for the Advancement of Science also produced a report on *Salmonella*.[24] The lack of interest within the central health departments may be illustrated by the almost total absence of any mention of food poisoning and microbiological food safety in the high-profile public health policy document, *Prevention and Health, Everybody's Business: A Reassessment of Public and Personal Health*, which appeared in 1976.[25] And in a paper given at a symposium to celebrate the centenary of the Sale of Food and Drugs Act, 1875, the CMO (Henry Yellowlees) acknowledged that there had been a rise in food poisoning since 1964, but declared that it did not indicate a fault with the legislation. Rather, he stated that there was a need for stricter enforcement,

---

[21] *RCMO 1967*, p. 37; *RCMO 1969*, p. 34; *RCMO 1973*, p. 62.

[22] *RCMO 1970*, p. 195.

[23] *RCMO 1984*, p. 47. For a graph showing food poisoning notifications in England between 1948 and 1988, see the Committee on the Microbiological Safety of Food, *The Microbiological Safety of Food Part I* (Richmond report), London, 1990, p. 11. For food poisoning notifications per 100,000 population for England and Wales, Scotland and Northern Ireland between 1975 and 1989, see the Committee on the Microbiological Safety of Food, *The Microbiological Safety of Food Part II* (Richmond report), London, 1991, p. 42.

[24] 'London boroughs favour food shops registration', *Municipal Engineering*, 1963, vol. 140, p. 970; 'Food hygiene regulations have not reached expectations', *Municipal Engineering*, 1964, vol. 141, p. 794; 'Food hygiene and the public', *Municipal Journal*, 1964, vol. 72, p. 1477; 'Working party on food hygiene', *Environmental Health*, 1971, vol. 79, p. 275; 'Towards cleaner food', *Environmental Health*, 1972, vol. 80, pp. 175, 177; 'New hygiene campaign by restaurant inspectors', *The Times*, 15 May 1972, p. 4f; 'Health inspectors urge complaints on dirty food shops', *The Times*, 2 June 1972, p. 4d; 'No complacency by Scottish health officers', *Municipal and Public Services Journal*, 1973, vol. 81, p. 902; British Association for the Advancement of Science, *Salmonella the Food Poisoner: A Report by a Study Group*, London, 1978.

[25] Department of Health and Social Security, *Prevention and Health, Everybody's Business: A Reassessment of Public and Personal Health*, London, 1976.

a problem caused by the failure of local authorities to train enough environmental health officers.[26]

There were only occasional parliamentary questions about food poisoning during the 1970s. These usually asked for data on trends in food poisoning or whether ministers were satisfied with the food safety hygiene regulations.[27] There were also sporadic questions about *Salmonella* poisoning caused by the consumption of poultry, which had been identified as an increasing problem in the late 1960s.[28] But food poisoning remained of little interest to politicians until 1984 to 1989 when there was a series of food safety incidents and problems, and when food poisoning notifications were increasing dramatically, reaching 52,557 in 1989.[29]

One factor accounting for part of the increase in the food poisoning notifications during the 1980s was the identification of a new food poisoning organism, *Campylobacter*, in 1977. By 1984, *Campylobacter* was described as 'second only to salmonellosis as a cause of gastro-enteritis' in Scotland.[30] Improved surveillance was also certainly part of the explanation for the increase. Scotland became a founder participant in the WHO Programme for the Control of Foodborne Infections and Intoxications in Europe, and the SHHD report for 1981 suggested that part of the increase in *Salmonella* infections was due to better reporting to the CDSU, in view of the WHO scheme.[31] Thereafter, the number of laboratory isolations of *Salmonella* in Scotland remained roughly static, while in England and Wales, there was a rapid increase. The ratio of isolations of *Salmonella* in England and Wales compared to Scotland increased to the expected 10:1 by 1988, suggesting that improved recording in England and Wales was an important aspect of the increase in food poisoning during this period.[32] The latter phenomenon may be connected with a new system of collection of data by the Office of Population and Statistics, and the development of the work of the Communicable Disease Surveillance Centre (CDSC). Established at the PHLS in 1977 with a staff of

---

26 H. Yellowlees, 'Food safety: a century of progress', in Ministry of Agriculture, Fisheries and Food, *Food Quality and Safety a Century of Progress*, London, 1976, pp. 62–7, at p. 65.
27 *PD(C)*, vol. 821, cols 44–5 (13 July 1971); vol. 846, col. 69 (14 November 1972); vol. 850, col. 387 (15 February 1973); vol. 861, col. 450 (23 October 1973); vol. 872, cols 410–11 (30 April 1974); vol. 943, col. 179 (1 February 1978); vol. 965, cols 27–8 (26 March 1979).
28 *RCMO 1967*, p. 38; *RCMO 1968*, pp. 29–30, 129; *RSHHD 1971*, p. 9; *PD(C)*, 1970, vol. 798, col. 18 (16 March 1970); *PD(C)*, 1972, vol. 838, col. 451 (12 May 1972); *PD(C)*, 1976, vol. 905 col. 231 (11 February 1976); 1976, vol. 907, cols 298–9 (11 March 1976); 1976, vol. 914, col. 65 (28 June 1976).
29 *RCMO 1990*, p. 129.
30 *RCMO 1978*, p. 46; *RCMO 1981*, p. 47; *RSHHD 1981*, p. 25; *RSHHD 1984*, p. 30.
31 *RSHHD 1981*, p. 26; *RSHHD 1986*, pp. 41–2. The surveillance system for salmonellosis is described in *RSHHD 1988*, pp. 52–3.
32 *RSHHD 1988*, pp. 54–5.

three, the CDSC developed a network of regional epidemiologists during the 1980s and merged with the PHLS Epidemiological Research Laboratory.[33] However, the Committee on the Microbiological Safety of Food, appointed in 1989 to investigate and advise on the apparent increase in food poisoning, concluded that despite improved recording, there was a real increase in food poisoning during the 1980s, linked to changes in food technology, lifestyle and habits, hygiene awareness, and international travel and commerce.[34]

The first high-profile food poisoning incident was the Stanley Royd Hospital *Salmonella* outbreak of 1984, which was caused by cross-contamination in the hospital kitchen between raw chicken and cooked beef which was not properly refrigerated. This led to a public enquiry and a series of parliamentary questions about food poisoning, outbreaks in hospitals, and the question of removing Crown immunity from prosecution under the Food and Drugs Acts for NHS hospitals.[35] This had been the subject of a long-standing campaign by environmental health officers.[36] Although the report of the enquiry, published on 21 January 1986, did not favour removing Crown immunity, the government conceded the point. By this time, environmental health officers, MPs, trade unions, the National Association of Metropolitan Authorities, and the National Association of Health Authorities were all lobbying in favour of the change. A private member's bill was dropped in favour of government legislation, which came into effect from 7 February 1987.[37] The Stanley Royd report also contributed to a review of public health infrastructure, attempts to remedy weaknesses that had developed since the abolition of MOsH in 1974, and the further expansion of the CDSC.[38]

[33] *RCMO 1982*, p. 58; C. L. R. Bartlett, 'The Communicable Disease Surveillance Centre 1977–2003: an overview', *Communicable Disease and Public Health*, 2003, vol. 6, pp. 87–96.

[34] Richmond report, *Part I*, p. 103; Richmond report, *Part II*, pp. 22–3.

[35] Department of Health and Social Security, *Report of the Committee of Inquiry into an Outbreak of Food Poisoning at Stanley Royd Hospital*, London 1986, pp. 1, 10; T. H. Pennington, *When Food Kills, BSE, E. Coli and Disaster Science*, Oxford, 2003, pp. 45–54; PD(C), vol. 65, cols 520, 608, 807–8, 1084 (22, 24, 25, 31 October 1984); vol. 68, cols 228, 327, 356, 386, 424, 454, 470, 546, (22, 23, 26, 26, 27, 27, 27, 29 November 1984); vol. 69, col. 321 (7 December 1984); vol. 70, col. 49 (17 December 1984); vol. 72, col. 247 (31 January 1985); vol. 74, col. 621 (8 March 1985); vol. 75, col. 118 (12 March 1985); vol. 76, col. 16 (23 March 1985); vol. 77, cols 565–6 (26 April 1985); vol. 80, col. 737 (11 June 1985); vol. 84, col. 443; vol. 86, cols 415–16, 426 (12 November 1985); vol. 87, col. 507; cols 650–2 (28 November 1985).

[36] 'Hospital kitchens', *Environmental Health*, 1973, vol. 81, p. 130; 'Food hygiene in NHS kitchens', *Environmental Health*, 1975, vol. 83, p. 324; PD(C), vol. 855, col. 352 (3 May 1973); vol. 939, cols 328–9 (17 November 1977); vol. 91, col. 602 (7 February 1986).

[37] PD(C), vol. 81, cols 184–6 (18 June 1985); vol. 90, cols 190–202, 493 (21, 28 January 1986); vol. 91, cols 140–1, 211, 232–3, 601–610 (4, 6, 6, 7 February 1986); vol. 95, cols 795–828 (15 April 1986); vol. 99, cols 26–149 (9 June 1986).

[38] *Food Poisoning at Stanley Royd*, pp. 110–11; D. Acheson, Statement 251, 6 November 1998, BSE Inquiry, internet: http://www.bseinquiry.gov.uk/files/ws/s251.pdf., accessed

Microbiological food poisoning was by now firmly on the agenda of a growing network of pressure groups that Tim Lang has described as the 'new food movement', in which the London Food Commission, which he directed, played a leading role. The commission was founded in March 1985 with sufficient funds for five years from the Greater London Council. The commission took up a wide range of issues, including the microbiological hazards of cook-chill foods.[39] It also nurtured a campaign against the introduction of food irradiation, which had been put forward as a means of controlling food poisoning organisms in various foods, especially poultry.[40] With an increasingly sophisticated public relations and media strategy, the food movement was able to build a broad alliance of opposition to food irradiation. This included large sections of the food industry and women's and consumers' organisations, as well as professional opinion represented by, for example, the British Medical Association Board of Science and Education. In brief, the movement argued that hygienically produced food would not need to be irradiated.[41]

During 1987, a form of food poisoning caused by the contamination of foods by *Listeria monocytogenes* came to medical, public and political attention. There had been several high-mortality food-borne *Listeria* outbreaks abroad,[42] and in Switzerland there were forty cases with three deaths associated with *Vacherin Mont D'or* soft cheese. In response, the CMO of the Department of Health (Donald Acheson) issued a food hazard warning in November 1987, and the cheese was withdrawn from sale.[43] In August 1988 hygiene guidelines were issued to cheese manufacturers. By the end of 1988 only four cases of listeriosis had been linked to contaminated food in Britain, but surveys showed high levels of contamination not only of soft cheeses but also of raw and pre-cooked chicken, and cook-chill meals. The organism was of special public concern because of its ability to grow at temperatures as low as 4°C, and cause abortion, stillbirth and neonatal disease.[44]

In addition, in mid-1988 the problem of BSE came to the attention of politicians and the public. The possibility of the infective agent crossing the species barrier and causing a new form of Creutzfeldt-Jakob disease (CJD) in

25 March 2004; D. Acheson, *Public Health in England*, London 1988; Bartlett, 'Communicable Disease Surveillance Centre'; 'Stanley Royd: the epidemiological lesson', *British Medical Journal*, 1986, vol. 1, pp. 644–5.

[39] T. Lang, 'Going public: food campaigns during the 1980s and 1990s', in D. F. Smith, (ed.), *Nutrition in Britain: Science, Scientists and Politics in the Twentieth Century*, London, 1997, pp. 238–60; J. Sheppard, *The Big Chill: A Report on the Implications of Cook-chill Catering for the Public Services*, London, 1987.

[40] *RSHHD 1987*, p. 47.

[41] British Medical Association, Board of Science and Education, *Irradiation of Foodstuffs*, London, 1987; T. Webb, *Food Irradiation in Britain?*, London, 1985.

[42] *RCMO 1988*, p. 134.

[43] *RCMO 1987*, p. 109; *RCMO 1988*, p. 134; *PD (C)*, vol. 123, col. 763 (4 December 1987).

[44] *RCMO 1989*, p. 106.

humans was mentioned in the first parliamentary question on the matter in June.[45] The official line was that, like scrapie in sheep, BSE was unlikely to be transferable to humans. However, the measures introduced from 1988 onwards to remove from the food chain overtly infected cattle, and later certain tissues from all other cattle, emphasised that the extent of the risk was unknown, and that it was also worth taking seriously. A working party chaired by Sir Richard Southwood was appointed to consider the issue, which first met in June 1988 and reported in February 1989. Its report concluded that on the one hand, 'the risk of transmission of BSE to humans appears remote', but, on the other, that if the working party's assessment proved incorrect 'the implication would be extremely serious'.[46] But government policy was driven by the first of these conclusions until March 1996.

Finally, the problem of *Salmonella* in eggs, which had been the subject of several carefully worded warnings by the CMO, became sensational news in December 1988, following a statement by Edwina Currie, junior minister at the Department of Health. During an interview with Independent Television News, Currie remarked that 'most of the egg production in this country, sadly, is now infected with *Salmonella*'. The media, sensing newsworthy policy differences between MAFF and the Department of Health, gave wide publicity to the issue. A sudden drop in egg consumption and demands for compensation from the egg industry followed, as did Currie's resignation on 16 December. A £19 million rescue package was announced three days later, and a scheme of compensation for the slaughter of infected flocks and other control measures were introduced.[47]

The House of Commons Agriculture Committee mounted an investigation into *Salmonella* in eggs,[48] and press interest in food poisoning began to subside, but was revived in early February 1989, when mounting evidence of widespread contamination of foods by *Listeria* led to further food hazard warnings.[49] Food safety was by now a matter for mainstream politics. On 21 February 1989, the leader of the Labour Party, Neil Kinnock, opened a debate in the House of Commons condemning the Conservative government for 'its failure to fulfil its duty of care and safeguard the safety and quality of food and water in Britain'. The debate lasted for six hours and 488 MPs voted at 10 p.m.[50]

---

45 *PD(C)*, vol. 135, col. *511* (21 June 1988).

46 Ministry of Agriculture, Fisheries and Food, and Department of Health, *Report of the Working Party on Bovine Spongiform Encephalopathy*, London, 1989.

47 D. Miller and J. Reilly, 'Making an issue of food safety: the media, pressure groups and the public sphere', in D. Maurer and J. Sobal (eds), *Eating Agendas: Food and Nutrition as Social Problems*, New York, 1995, pp. 305–36; *RSHHD 1989*, p. 75; Ministry of Agriculture, Fisheries and Food, *Salmonella in Eggs – A Progress Report*, London, 1990.

48 House of Commons Agriculture Committee, *Salmonella in Eggs*, London, 1989.

49 'Anything to eat?', *Lancet* 1989, vol. 1, pp. 416–18; House of Commons Social Services Committee, *Listeria and Listeriosis*, London, 1989.

50 *PD(C)*, cols 852–938 (21 February 1989).

Ministers had announced reviews of food legislation in 1977 (despite the CMO's views), and 1983, and in 1984 a consultation document had been issued by all the central agricultural and health departments in England, Wales, Scotland and Northern Ireland.[51] But it was not until the spring of 1989, following the publicity given to *Salmonella* and *Listeria* and other food poisoning issues, that there was finally sufficient political will for a Cabinet-level decision to proceed with a bill. That this decision was taken by the Conservative government of Margaret Thatcher, which had been pursuing policies of deregulation of industry for ten years, emphasises the depth of the food safety crisis at this time.[52] In February 1989, the Committee on the Micro-biological Safety of Food, chaired by Sir Mark Richmond, was also established. The committee was asked to produce an interim report on the incidence of food-borne microbiological disease in time for its recommendations to be taken into account during the passage of the new legislation.[53] In addition, in May 1989 a leaflet providing food hygiene advice for the public was launched and 15 million copies were distributed.[54]

Following the release of a White Paper in July,[55] the Food Safety Bill was introduced in December 1989, received the royal assent on 29 June 1990 and came into effect on 1 January 1991. The new Act, unlike the legislation it was designed to replace, covered the whole of the UK. It relied greatly upon enabling powers to make it possible to introduce a wide range of food safety measures, and to implement European Community legislation. The Act finally addressed a number of issues relevant to the Aberdeen typhoid outbreak and the Milne Committee's recommendations. It allowed ministers to make emergency control orders so it would be no longer necessary to rely upon voluntary action by industry in order to remove suspect food from the market. In addition, local authorities would have the power to have whole batches of food condemned when any portion was proven dangerous. Ministers would also be able to set training requirements for food handlers. In addition, minis-ters could require food businesses to be licensed or registered. It was envisaged

---

[51] *PD(C)*, vol. 940, cols *420–1* (1 December 1977); *PD(C)*, vol. 49, col. *197* (22 November 1983); 'Review of food and drugs acts', *British Food Journal*, 1978, vol. 80, p. 36; Agricultural Departments in the United Kingdom, Department of Health and Social Security, Welsh Office, Scottish Home and Health Department, Department of Health and Social Services Northern Ireland, *Review of Food Legislation*, London, 1984.

[52] Pennington, *When Food Kills*, pp. 26–7; J. Reilly and D. Miller, 'Scaremonger or scapegoat? The role of the media in the emergence of food as a social issue', in P. Caplan (ed.), *Food, Identity and Health*, London, 1997, pp. 234–50; T. H. Pennington, 'Recent experiences in food poisoning', in D. F. Smith and J. Phillips (eds), *Food, Science, Policy and Regulation in the Twentieth Century: International and Comparative Perspectives*, London, 2000, pp. 223–38, at p. 235.

[53] Richmond report, *Part 1*, p. 1.

[54] *RCMO 1988*, pp. 132–3.

[55] HM Government, *Food Safety: Protecting the Consumer*, London, 1989.

that premises requiring tight control, such as dairies and food irradiation plants, would be licensed, while other premises would simply have to be registered with local authorities to facilitate inspections. The Act increased the penalties for food safety offences and removed Crown immunity entirely except with regard to premises with national security implications.[56] But these measures did not go far enough for some opposition members of both Houses of Parliament. In the debates on the Food Safety Bill, they argued for statutory licensing for all food premises, and quoted the views of the Richmond Committee on this point. Some also called for the creation of an independent 'food safety and standards agency'.[57] These were issues which became the subject of further debate later in the 1990s.

In accordance with the recommendations of the Richmond committee, the national microbiological surveillance system for food was strengthened by the creation of two new committees, the Steering Group on the Microbiological Safety of Food and the Advisory Committee on the Microbiological Safety of Food, which first met in 1991. The former consisted of officials with a number of experts, its role being to develop the surveillance system. The role of the latter, which was composed of independent experts, was to interpret the results of surveillance, to identify risks and to advise on food safety. The two committees later merged.[58]

The implementation of the Food Safety Act, and control measures such as those intended to clean up the national poultry flock, were slow to produce noticeable effects. When the total number of food poisoning notifications in England rose to 63,347 in 1992, the CMO (Kenneth Calman) could only remark: 'There is no obvious explanation for this increase, but the study of human infectious intestinal diseases in England will provide further information on the epidemiology of foodborne disease.'[59] This was a reference to the work of the Steering Group on the Microbiological Safety of Food. Despite all the enquiries and policy making since the late 1980s, arresting the growth in food poisoning notifications now seemed more complicated than ever, a problem only amenable to further scientific enquiry. One increasing problem of the 1990s was *E. coli* 0157 poisoning, which came to a head with the November 1996 outbreak in Wishaw, near Glasgow. This involved just over 500 cases and twenty-one deaths, and centred upon a church lunch for elderly people, the meat for which was supplied by a popular local butcher, John

---

[56] *PD(L)*, vol. 513, cols 743–50 (5 December 1989); C. Baylis, *Food Safety Law and Practice*, London, 1994.

[57] *PD(L)* vol. 513, cols 756–818 (5 December 1989); *PD(C)* vol. 168, cols 1023–94 (8 March 1990); vol. 173, cols 812–98 (7 June 1990); Richmond report, *Part I*, p. 113.

[58] *RCMO 1991*, pp. 154–5; *RCMO 1995*, p. 179.

[59] *RCMO 1992*, p. 175.

Barr. It was the subject of an enquiry by a working party chaired by Hugh Pennington, and a fatal accident enquiry.[60]

New general food hygiene regulations, implementing a European Council directive of June 1993, were embodied in the Food Safety (General Food Hygiene) Regulations, 1995, and came into force in September 1995. The measures introduced included new staff training requirements. Proprietors of food businesses were required to 'ensure that food handlers engaged in the food business are supervised and instructed and/or trained in food hygiene matters commensurate with their work activities'.[61] The regulations were also informed by the control strategy known as 'hazard analysis critical control point' (HACCP), which had been advocated by the Richmond Committee.[62] This system was promoted by the WHO in the 1980s,[63] and had been developed by the American food company Pillbury from 1959, for use in the preparation of foods for the manned space programme of the American National Aeronautics and Space Administration.[64] The Food Hygiene Regulations 1995 specified that a proprietor of a food business should 'identify any step in the activities of the food business which is critical to ensuring food safety and ensure that adequate safety procedures are identified, implemented, maintained and reviewed', and outlined the principles of HACCP.[65] The Wishaw outbreak demonstrated, however, that not only HACCP, but even some of the most basic points of good practice specified in legislation, regulations and codes of practice introduced since the 1950s Food and Drugs acts, had failed to penetrate and alter the practices of some food handlers. The essential cause of the outbreak at Wishaw was cross-contamination between raw and cooked food at the butcher's shop, a problem that had been well understood for decades.[66] The Pennington report revived the question of licensing of food businesses, and new regulations requiring the licensing of butchers' shops came into force in 2000. Licensing is now subject to satisfactory hygiene conditions being in place, including compliance with existing food hygiene legislation, the operation of documented food safety management

[60] Pennington Group, *Report on the Circumstances Leading to the 1996 Outbreak of Infection with E. coli 0157 in Central Scotland*, Edinburgh, 1997; Pennington, *When Food Kills*.

[61] RCMO 1995, p. 180; Statutory Instrument 1995, No. 1763, The Food Safety (General Food Hygiene) Regulations, 1995, internet: http://www.legislation.hmso.gov.uk/si/si1995/Uksi_19951763_en_1.htm#tcon, accessed 15 April 2004.

[62] Richmond report, *Part I*, pp. 64, 38–40, 72–81.

[63] International Commission on Microbiological Specifications for Foods, 'Prevention and control of food-borne salmonellosis through application of hazard analysis critical control point', *International Journal of Food Microbiology*, 1987, vol. 4, pp. 227–47.

[64] Committee on the Review of the Use of Scientific Criteria and Performance Standards for Safe Food, *Scientific Criteria to Ensure Safe Food*, Washington, 2003, pp. 20–1.

[65] Food Safety (General Food Hygiene) Regulations, 1995.

[66] Pennington, *When Food Kills*, p. 20.

controls in line with the principles of HACCP, and enhanced staff hygiene training.[67] The implementation of HACCP across a wide range of food businesses has intensified in recent years, but some commentators have begun to criticise overemphasis upon the bureaucratic rather then behavioural dimensions of the system.[68]

Before the Wishaw *E. coli* outbreak, the long-running BSE/new-variant CJD saga had reached a climax in March 1996. In a statement in the House of Commons, the Secretary of State for Health finally revised the official line since the late 1980s that 'British beef is safe', and declared that the two diseases might be linked. Intense scrutiny of the affair by the media and politicians followed, and several books on the subject were published during 1996 and 1997. Long before the announcement of the BSE enquiry in December 1977 and the publication of its exhaustive report in October 2000, it was widely acknowledged that MAFF's remit of promoting and protecting the agricultural industry played a role in the underestimation of the risks from BSE and delayed effective action.[69] Pennington also argues that the BSE/CJD crisis, and an impending general election, conditioned the decisions by the Secretary of State for Scotland Michael Forsyth to establish the Pennington working party, and to accept its recommendations. A right-wing conservative, who in the 1980s had objected to the compulsory pasteurisation of milk in Scotland because of its effects on small businesses and traditional cheese making, now endorsed the licensing of butchers.[70]

Food safety was an important issue in the 1997 general election. The Labour Party manifesto declared that 'Labour will establish an independent food standards agency. The £3.5 billion BSE crisis and the *E. coli* outbreak which resulted in serious loss of life, have made unanswerable the case for the independent agency we have proposed.'[71] The plan for the agency was based on a report by Phillip James, Director of the Rowett Research Institute, Aberdeen,

---

[67] Pennington Group, *Report*, ch. 7; Food Standards Agency, 'Licensing of butchers' shops in England Guidance Notes', internet: http://www.foodstandards.gov.uk/foodindustry/meat/meatplantsprems/butcherslicensing/, accessed 15 April 2004.

[68] C. Taylor, 'Moving on from bureaucracy to behaviour change in food business', *Communicable Disease and Public Health*, 2003, vol. 6, pp. 3–4.

[69] S. Dealler, *The Lethal Legacy: BSE Search for the Truth*, London, 1996; Brian J. Ford, *BSE: the Facts*, London, 1996; R. J. Maxwell, *An Unplayable Hand?: BSE, CJD and British Government*, London, 1997; 'The inquiry into BSE and variant CJD in the United Kingdom', internet: http://www.bseinquiry.gov.uk/index.htm, accessed 15 April 2004; M. McKee, T. Lang and J. A. Roberts, 'Deregulating health: policy lessons from the BSE affair', *Journal of the Royal Society of Medicine*, 1996, vol. 89, pp. 424–6.

[70] Pennington, 'Recent experiences', p. 225; Pennington, *When Food Kills*, p. 201; PD(C), vol. 69, cols 883–8 (10 December 1984).

[71] 'New Labour because Britain deserves better', internet: http://www.psr.keele.ac.uk/area/uk/man /lab97.htm, accessed 15 April 2004.

prepared shortly before the election at the request of Tony Blair, then leader of the opposition. James' proposal was to remove MAFF's involvement in food safety policy making and to make the Department of Health the responsible department, which would act on the advice of the new independent agency. A White Paper, *The Food Standards Agency – A Force for Change* was released in January 1998, and the Food Standards Bill introduced to Parliament in June 1999. The Act received the royal assent on 11 November 1999 and the Food Standards Agency (FSA) was launched on 1 April 2000, with a UK head-quarters in London, and national offices in Scotland, Wales and Northern Ireland.[72]

The FSA took over the responsibility for most food safety matters, but MAFF retained responsibility for a number of issues including on-farm strategy with regard to control of food-borne zoonoses. The Department for Environment, Food and Rural Affairs (DEFRA) retained these responsibilities when MAFF was abolished in June 2001, immediately after the general election, following MAFF's poor handling of the foot-and-mouth disease outbreak which began in February.[73] The Meat Hygiene Service, which was established in 1995 and finally centralised meat inspection under veterinary control, is now an executive agency of the FSA. However, the CVO, on the staff of DEFRA, is head of profession for the veterinarians employed by the service.[74] The Food Standards Agency itself not only has national offices, but also an internal structure consisting of a Food Safety Policy Group, Enforcement and Food Standards Group and Corporate Resources and Strategy Group. Local authorities retain the responsibility for the enforcement of food standards regulations.[75] While there have been important changes, the system for the making and application of food policy inevitably remains complex. There is certainly continuing potential for the kind of interdepartmental, interdivisional and inter-professional tensions and conflicts which sometimes made decision making and action so difficult during the 1960s. However, the principles of transparency and disclosure by which the FSA operates, which are facilitated by use of the internet, probably help to limit the influence of such factors. The BSE saga has been described as a 'paradigm of policy failure',

---

[72] 'The Food Standards Agency – a force for change', 1998; 'Food Standards Act, 1999', internet: http://www.foodlaw.rdg.ac.uk/index.htm, accessed 16 April 2004.

[73] D. Brown, 'Mixed rural welcome for Beckett super-ministry', 11 June 2001, internet: http://portal.telegraph.co.uk/news/, accessed 16 April 2004; 'The new son of MAFF', 18 June 2001, internet: http://www.guardian.co.uk/leaders/story/0,3604,508681,00.html, accessed 16 April 2004.

[74] 'Concordat between the Department for Environment, Food and Rural Affairs and the Food Standards Agency', internet: http://www.defra.gov.uk/corporate/fsaconcd/concord. pdf, accessed 16 April 2004; Food Standards Agency, 'Meat hygiene service', internet: http://www.food.gov.uk/enforcement/meathyg/mhservice/, accessed 16 April 2004.

[75] Food Standards Agency, 'Structure of the Agency', 5 October 2001, internet: http:// www.food.gov.uk/aboutus/how_we_work/agency_structure#h_3, accessed 15 April 2004.

the lessons of which can guide more effective future strategies.[76] It is the hope of the current authors, however, that as the work of the FSA develops and become more routine, the historical insights into food policy making and action provided by this book may also sensitise participants and commentators to the kind of problems which may re-emerge.[77]

[76] P. van Zwanenberg and E. Millstone, 'BSE: A paradigm of policy failure', *The Political Quarterly*, 2003, vol. 74, pp. 27–37.

[77] At the time of completing the final proof-reading of this book in March 2005, two issues concerning the safety and hazards of food and food products have recently arisen. The first involves processed foods contaminated with the carcinogenic Sudan I food dye, which was in chilli powder imported from India. The second concerns the possibility of importing the bird flu virus, which threatens the health of humans as well as poultry, in consignments of feathers from China. While it is dangerous for historians to make predictions, these two, or similar issues, may well give rise to problems of the kind explored in this book. As for the Sudan I episode, questions have already arisen about the effectiveness of the machinery for monitoring the safety of imported food constituents, but in the months ahead concerns may shift to the effectiveness of the identification, withdrawal and disposal of suspect food. On the feathers/bird flu issue, on 5 March 2005 there was an interesting discussion on the BBC's 'Farming Today' programme. Here the debate was on the efficacy of DEFRA's procedures and guidelines, and the value of veterinary inspectors' touch, smell and visual checks upon consignments of feathers at ports, as a means of assessing whether the feathers have been correctly processed. The trustworthiness of the Chinese government's supervisory system, and the validity of the 'official certificates' accompanying the goods were also debated. In the light of the West's ambitions to exploit the opportunities offered by the economic development of China, the possible parallels between this issue and the 1960s corned beef and typhoid affair are obvious. Food Standards Agency, 'Sudan Dyes' internet, http://www.food.gov.uk/safereating/sudani/, accessed 6 March 2005; BBC, 'Bird flu threat from feathers', internet http://news.bbc.co.uk/2/hi/health/4321059.stm, accessed 6 March 2005.

Appendix

Recommendations of the Milne Committee[1]

In the light of our findings we have felt it desirable to make a number of recommendations. Briefly these are as follows:

1 That the hygienic requirements to be observed by establishments exporting meat and meat products to this country should be set out in as clear and detailed a manner as possible and should contain a requirement that all water used in such an establishment which is likely to come into contact with the product should conform to a minimum bacteriological standard of purity. We understand that this recommendation is now being implemented.

2 That the personnel presently employed in the inspection of canning establishments abroad should be augmented and that any inspection team, particularly at the time of a first visit, should also include a medical officer.

3 That consideration should be given to suggesting to the Food and Agricultural Organisation of the United Nations the setting up, under the auspices of the International Codex Commission, of a system of inspection for all establishments engaged in the manufacture for export of meat and meat products.

4 That the present division of responsibility between the Ministry of Health and the Ministry of Agriculture, Fisheries and Food so far as meat and meat products are concerned should be revised with regard to the point at which responsibility passes from one department to the other.

5 That the powers available to medical officers of health to close premises in which infection may exist should be re-examined to consider whether strengthening of the present powers is desirable.

6 That there should be prepared in consultation with the trade a code of practice on the hygienic handling of cold cooked meats in retail establishments.

7 That the Food Hygiene Regulations should be amended as soon as may be considered practicable to ensure that where cold cooked meat is displayed for sale the temperature in such a display should not exceed 40°F.

[1] Scottish Home and Health Department, *The Aberdeen Typhoid Outbreak*, Edinburgh, 1964, pp. 7–8.

8 The law whereby a medical officer of health has power to examine a person whom he has reason to believe may be suffering from infectious disease should be extended to cover persons who may reasonably be suspected of carrying infectious disease.

9 A person engaged in food handling should be obliged to declare whether or not he or she has had typhoid fever, paratyphoid fever or any other serious gastro-intestinal infection.

10 Only detergents and sterilisers whose bactericidal properties have been proved should be used in food premises; the responsibility for approving such materials should rest with the central health departments.

11 The organisation of the bacteriological services in Scotland should be re-examined to establish whether the needs of the local authorities and central department in this respect are being adequately met. We are informed that this re-examination is concurrently being carried out.

12 The present method of educating all staff in the food trade in matters relating to food hygiene should be examined with a view to improvement.

13 A standing committee should be set up to advise ministers on the risk of infection which may arise from the consumption of any particular food.

14 It is for consideration whether powers to compel the withdrawal of stocks of suspect food already distributed by the trade should be sought.

Bibliography

Acheson, D., *Public Health in England*, London, 1988.

Agricultural Departments in the United Kingdom, Department of Health and Social Security, Welsh Office, Scottish Home and Health Department, Department of Health and Social Services Northern Ireland, *Review of Food Legislation*, London, 1984.

Andrews, C., 'James Craigie', *Biographical Memoirs of Fellows of the Royal Society*, 1979, vol. 25, pp. 233–40.

Ash, I., G. D. W. McKendrick, M. H. Robertson and H. L. Hughes, 'Outbreak of typhoid fever connected with corned beef', *British Medical Journal*, 1964, vol. 1, pp. 1474–8.

Atkins, P. J., 'The pasteurisation of England: the science, culture and health implications of food processing, 1900–1950', in D. F. Smith and J. Phillips (eds), *Food, Science, Policy and Regulation in the Twentieth Century: International and Comparative Perspectives*, London, 2000, pp. 37–52.

Bartlett, C. L. R., 'The Communicable Disease Surveillance Centre 1977–2003: an overview', *Communicable Disease and Public Health*, 2003, vol. 6, pp. 87–96.

Baylis, C., *Food Safety Law and Practice*, London, 1994.

Berridge, V., 'Public or policy understanding of history', *Social History of Medicine*, 2003, vol. 4, pp. 511–23.

Berridge, V. (ed.), *Making Health Policy: Networks in Research and Policy after 1945*, Amsterdam, forthcoming.

Berridge, V., and K. Loughlin (eds), *Medicine, the Mass Media and the Market*, London, forthcoming, 2005.

Berridge V. and J. Stanton, 'Science and policy: historical insights', *Social Science and Medicine*, 1999, vol. 49, pp. 1133–8.

Blackhall, S., 'The jam jar' in S. Blackhall, *Reets*, Aberdeen, 1990, pp. 58–61.

Blackhall, S., *Reets*, Aberdeen, 1990.

Blamire, R. V., 'Meat hygiene: the changing years', *Journal of the Royal Society of Health*, 1984, vol. 5, pp. 180–5.

Borough of Maidstone, *Epidemic of Typhoid Fever 1897*, London, 1898.

Bradley, W. H., 'An epidemiological study of Bact. Typhosum D4', *British Medical Journal*, 1943, vol. 1, pp. 438–41.

Bradley, W. H., 'The control of typhoid fever', *Public Health*, 1949, vol. 62, pp. 159–63.

British Association for the Advancement of Science, *Salmonella the Food Poisoner: A Report by a Study Group*, London, 1978.

British Medical Association, Board of Science and Education, *Irradiation of Foodstuffs*, London, 1987.

Brodie, J., 'Antibodies and the Aberdeen typhoid outbreak of 1964. I The Widal reaction', *Journal of Hygiene*, 1977, vol. 79, pp. 161–80.

Brodie, J., 'Antibodies and the Aberdeen typhoid outbreak of 1964. II Coombs', complement fixation and fimbrial agglutination tests', *Journal of Hygiene*, 1977, vol. 79, pp. 181–92.

Brodie, J., I. A. MacQueen and D. Livingstone, 'Effect of Trimethoprim-Suphamethoxazole on typhoid and Salmonella carriers', *British Medical Journal*, 1970, vol. 3, pp. 318–19.

Browning, C. H., *Chronic Enteric Carriers and their Treatment*, Medical Research Council Special Report Series No. 179, London, 1933.

Bynum, W. F. and R. Porter (eds), *Companion Encyclopaedia of the History of Medicine*, London, 1993.

Caplan, P. (ed.), *Food, Identity and Health*, London, 1997.

Carson, R., *Silent Spring*, London, 1963.

Christie, A. B., 'Treatment of typhoid carriers with ampicillin', *British Medical Journal*, 1964, vol. 1, pp. 1609–11.

Cockburn, W. C., 'Reporting and incidence of food poisoning', in W. C. Cockburn, J. Taylor, E. S. Anderson and B. C. Hobbs (eds), *Food Poisoning Symposium*, London, 1962, pp. 3–14.

Cockburn, W. C., J. Taylor, E. S. Anderson and B. C. Hobbs (eds), *Food Poisoning Symposium*, London, 1962.

Committee on the Microbiological Safety of Food, *The Microbiological Safety of Food Part I*, London, 1990.

Committee on the Microbiological Safety of Food, *The Microbiological Safety of Food Part II*, London, 1991.

Committee on the Review of the Use of Scientific Criteria and Performance Standards for Safe Food, *Scientific Criteria to Ensure Safe Food*, Washington, 2003.

Couper, W. R. M., K. W. Newell and D. J. H. Payne, 'An outbreak of typhoid fever associated with canned ox-tongue', *British Medical Journal*, 1956, vol. 1, pp. 1057–9.

Craigie, J., 'Arthur Felix', *Biographical Memoirs of Fellows of the Royal Society*, 1957, vol. 3, pp. 53–82.

Craigie, J. and C. H. Yen, 'Demonstration of types of B. Typhosus by means of preparations of Type II V_i phage: stability and epidemiological significance', *Canadian Journal of Public Health*, 1938, vol. 29, p. 484.

Critchell, J. T. and J. Raymond, *A History of the Frozen Meat Trade*, London, 1969 (first published 1912).

Culley, A. R., 'An account of paratyphoid fever in South Wales, 1952', *Medical Officer*, 1953, vol. 89, pp. 243–9, 257–62.

Deedes, W. F., *'Dear Bill' W. F. Deedes Reports*, London, 1997.

Department of Health and Social Security, *Prevention and Health, Everybody's Business: A Reassessment of Public and Personal Health*, London, 1976.

Department of Health and Social Security, *Report of the Committee of Inquiry into an Outbreak of Food Poisoning at Stanley Royd Hospital*, London, 1986.

Department of Health and Social Security, Ministry of Agriculture, Fisheries and Food, Welsh Office, *Hygiene in the Meat Trades*, London, 1969.

Dewberry, E. B., *Food Poisoning, its Nature, History and Causation: Measures for its Prevention and Control*, London, 1950.

Diack, L., 'Myths of a beleaguered city: Aberdeen and the typhoid outbreak explored through oral history', *Oral History*, 2001, vol. 29, pp. 62–72.

Diack, L. and D. F. Smith, 'Professional strategies of Medical Officers of Health in the post war period (1): 'innovative traditionalism': the case of Dr Ian MacQueen, MOH for Aberdeen 1952–1974', *Journal of Public Health Medicine*, 2002, vol. 24, pp. 123–9.

Diack, L. and D. F. Smith, 'The media and the management of a food crisis: Aberdeen's typhoid outbreak in 1964', in V. Berridge and K. Loughlin, *Medicine, the Market and the Mass Media*, London, forthcoming, 2005.

Diack, L., T. H. Pennington, E. Russell and D. F. Smith, 'Departmental and professional agendas in the implementation of the recommendations of a food crisis enquiry: the Milne report and inspection of overseas meat plants', in D. F. Smith and J. Phillips (eds), *Food, Science, Policy and Regulation in the Twentieth Century: International and Comparative Perspectives*, London, 2000, pp. 189–206.

Drummond, J. C. and A. Wilbraham, *The Englishman's Food. A History of Five Centuries of English Diet*, London, 1939.

Evans, D. J., 'An account of an outbreak of typhoid fever due to infected ice-cream in the Aberystwyth Borough during the summer of 1946', *Medical Officer*, 1947, vol. 77, pp. 39–44.

Felix, A., 'Test for V_i antibody', *British Medical Journal*, 1939, vol. 2, p. 1253.

Felix, A., 'Experiences with typing of typhoid bacilli by means of V_i bacteriophage', *British Medical Journal*, 1943, vol. 1, pp. 435–8.

Felix, A., 'Laboratory control of the enteric fevers', *British Medical Bulletin*, 1951, vol. 7, pp. 153–62.

Folb, P. I., *The Thalidomide Disaster, and its Impact on Modern Medicine*, Cape Town, 1977.

Food Hygiene Advisory Council, 'Food Hygiene Education and Publicity Report to the Minister of Health', *Monthly Bulletin of the Ministry of Health and Public Health Laboratory Service*, 1966, vol. 25, pp. 31–3.

French, M. and J. Phillips, *Cheated not Poisoned? Food Regulation in the United Kingdom 1875–1938*, Manchester, 2000.

French, M. and J. Phillips, 'Windows and barriers in policy-making: food poisoning in Britain, 1945–56', *Social History of Medicine*, 2004, vol. 14, pp. 269–84.

Gebhardt, R. C., 'The River Plate meat industry since c. 1900: technology, ownership, international trade regime and domestic policy', Ph.D. thesis, London School of Economics, 2000.

Geissler, C. and D. J. Oddy, *Food, Diet and Economic Change Past and Present*, Leicester, 1993.

Gilbert, R. J., 'Cross contamination by cooked-meat slicing machines and cleaning cloths', *Journal of Hygiene*, 1969, vol. 67, pp. 449–53.

Gilbert, R. J., 'Comparison of materials used for cleaning equipment in retail food premises, and of two methods for the enumeration of bacteria on cleaned equipment and work surfaces', *Journal of Hygiene*, 1970, vol. 68, pp. 221–32.

Gilbert, R. J. and I. M. Maurer, 'The hygiene of slicing machines, carving knives and can-openers', *Journal of Hygiene*, 1968, vol. 66, pp. 439–50.

Greenwood, M., *Epidemics and Crowd-diseases*, London, 1935.

Greenwood, M., A. B. Hill, W. W. C. Topley and J. Wilson, *Experimental Epidemiology*, Medical Research Council Special Report Series No. 209, London, 1936.

Hammond, R. J., *Food Volume II Studies in Administration and Control*, London, 1956.

Hardy, A., *The Epidemic Streets: Infectious Disease and the Rise of Preventive Medicine, 1856–1900*, Oxford, 1993.

Hardy, A., 'Food, hygiene and the laboratory: a short history of food poisoning in Britain, circa 1850–1959', *Social History of Medicine*, 1999, vol. 12, pp. 293–331.

Hardy, A., 'Methods of outbreak investigation in the "era of bacteriology" 1880–1920', *Sozial- und Präventivmedizin*, 2001, vol. 46, pp. 355–60.

Hay, M., *Report on the Origin and Spread of the Epidemic of Typhoid Fever in 1907*, Peterhead, 1908.

HM Government, *Food Safety: Protecting the Consumer*, London, 1989.

Holden, W. S., *Water Treatment and Examination*, London, 1970.

House of Commons Agriculture Committee, *Salmonella in Eggs*, London, 1989.

House of Commons Social Services Committee, *Listeria and Listeriosis*, London, 1989.

Huckstep, R. L., *Typhoid Fever and other Salmonella Infections*, Edinburgh, 1962.

Hughes, H. L., 'How Harlow tackled its Whitsun typhoid outbreak', *Municipal Engineering*, 1963, vol. 140, p. 1176.

Hughes, H. L., 'Typhoid outbreak showed importance of liaison', *Municipal Engineering*, 1965, vol. 142, p. 59.

International Commission on Microbiological Specifications for Foods, 'Prevention and control of food-borne salmonellosis through application of hazard analysis critical control point', *International Journal of Food Microbiology*, 1987, vol. 4, pp. 227–47.

Kiple, K. F. (ed.), *The Cambridge World History of Disease*, Cambridge, 2003.

Koolmees, P. A., 'The development of veterinary public health in Western Europe, 1850–1940', *Sartoniana*, 1999, vol. 12, pp. 153–79.

Koolmees, P. A., J. R. Fisher and R. Perren, 'The traditional responsibility of veterinarians in meat production and meat inspection', in F. J. M. Smulders (ed.), *Veterinary Aspects of Meat Production, Processing and Inspection. An Update of Recent Developments in Europe*, Utrecht, 1999, pp. 7– 31.

Lang, T., 'Going public: food campaigns during the 1980s and 1990s', in D. F. Smith, (ed.), *Nutrition in Britain: Science, Scientists and Politics in the Twentieth Century*, London, 1997, pp. 238–60.

Leavitt, J. W., ' "Typhoid Mary" strikes back bacteriological theory and practice in early twentieth-century public health', *ISIS*, 1992, vol. 83, pp. 608–29.

LeBaron, C. W. and D. W. Taylor, 'Typhoid fever', in K. F. Kiple (ed.), *The Cambridge World History of Disease*, Cambridge, 2003, pp. 1071–7.

Ledingham, A. and J. C. G. Ledingham, 'Typhoid carriers', *British Medical Journal*, 1908, vol. 1, pp. 15–17.

Ledingham, J. C. G., 'Report on the enteric fever 'carrier': being a review of current knowledge on the subject', *Report of the Local Government Board*, 1909–10, vol. 39, pp. 250–384.

Ledingham, J. C. G. and J. A. Arkwright, *Carrier Problem in Infectious Diseases*, London, 1912.

Lewis, C., 'Anglo–Argentine Trade 1945–1965', in D. Rock (ed.) *Argentina in the Twentieth Century*, London, 1975, pp. 114–34.

Lewis, J., *What Price Community Medicine?*, Brighton, 1986.

Loughlin, K., 'Networks of mass communication: reporting science, health and medicine from the 1950s to the 1970s', in V. Berridge (ed.), *Making Health Policy: Networks in Research and Policy after 1945*, Amsterdam, forthcoming, ch. 11.

Macgregor, I. M., *The Two-year Mass Radiography Campaign in Scotland 1957–1958: A Study of Tuberculosis Case-finding by Community Action*, Edinburgh, 1961.

McKee, M., T. Lang and J. A. Roberts, 'Deregulating health: policy lessons from the BSE affair', *Journal of the Royal Society of Medicine*, 1996, vol. 89, pp. 424–6.

MacQueen, I. A. G., 'Teamwork and leadership in public health', *Public Health*, 1960, April, pp. 244–52.

MacQueen, I. A. G., 'Random reflections on the outbreak', *Health and Welfare*, 1964, No. 23, pp. 1–6.

MacQueen, I. A. G., 'Reflections on the typhoid report', *Medical Officer*, 1965, vol. 113, pp. 31–3.

McNalty, A. S., 'Prefatory note', in W. V. Shaw, *Report on an Outbreak of Enteric Fever in the County Borough of Bournemouth and in the Boroughs of Poole and Christchurch*, Reports on Public Health and Medical Subjects No. 81, London, 1937.

Maurer, D. and J. Sobal (eds), *Eating Agendas: Food and Nutrition as Social Problems*, New York, 1995.

Mendelson, J. A., ' "Typhoid Mary" strikes again: the social and the scientific in the making of modern public health', *ISIS*, 1995, vol. 86, pp. 268–77.

Mepham, B. (ed.), *Food Ethics*, London, 1996.

Miller, D., 'Risk, science and policy: definitions struggles, information management, the media and BSE', *Social Science and Medicine*, 1999, vol. 49, pp. 1239–55.

Miller, D., and J. Reilly, 'Making an issue of food safety: the media, pressure groups and the public sphere', in D. Maurer and J. Sobal (eds), *Eating Agendas: Food and Nutrition as Social Problems*, New York, 1995, pp. 305–36.

Millstone, E., 'Food safety: the ethical dimensions', in B. Mepham (ed.), *Food Ethics*, London, 1996, pp. 84–100.

Ministry of Agriculture, Fisheries and Food, *Fatstock and Carcase Meat Marketing*, London, 1964.

Ministry of Agriculture, Fisheries and Food, *Animal Health A Centenary 1865–1964*, London, 1965.

Ministry of Agriculture, Fisheries and Food, *Marketing of Meat and Livestock*, London, 1965.

Ministry of Agriculture, Fisheries and Food, *Report of the Committee of Inquiry on Foot-and-Mouth Disease 1968, Part one*, London, 1968.

Ministry of Agriculture, Fisheries and Food, *Food Quality and Safety: A Century of Progress*, London, 1976.

Ministry of Agriculture, Fisheries and Food, and Department of Health, *Report of the Working Party on Bovine Spongiform Encephalopathy*, London, 1989.

Ministry of Agriculture, Fisheries and Food, *Salmonella in Eggs – A Progress Report*, London, 1990.

Ministry of Food, *Report of the Manufactured Meat Products Working Party*, London, 1950.

Ministry of Food, *Report of the Inter-departmental Committee on Meat Inspection*, London, 1950.

Ministry of Food, *Hygiene in Catering Establishments*, London, 1951.

Ministry of Health, *Memorandum on Safeguards to be Adopted in the Administration of Water Undertakings*, London, 1939.

Ministry of Health, *Memorandum on Typhoid Fever*, London, 1939.

Ministry of Health, *Report on the Outbreak of Poliomyelitis during 1961 in Kingston-upon-Hull*, Reports on Public Health and Medical Subjects, No. 107, London, 1963.

Ministry of Health, Scottish Health Service Advisory Council, *Memorandum on the Control of Outbreaks of Smallpox*, London, 1964.

Moore, W. B., 'Typhoid fever, with particular reference to the Crowthorne epidemic, 1949', *Journal of the Royal Sanitary Institute*, 1950, vol. lxx, pp. 93–101.

Murcott, A. (ed.), *The Nation's Diet*, London, 1998.

Murphy, H. L., *Report on a Public Local Enquiry into an Outbreak of Typhoid Fever at Croydon*, London, 1939.

Nairn, M., 'Health visitors in the Aberdeen typhoid outbreak', *Nursing Times*, 8 January 1965, pp. 59–60.

Newman, G., 'Prefatory note', in W. V. Shaw, *Report to the Minister of Health on an Epidemic of Enteric Fever at Bolton-upon-Dearne*, Reports on Public Health and Medical Subjects, No. 12, London, 1922.

Newman, G., 'Prefatory note', in W. V. Shaw, *Report on an Outbreak of Paratyphoid Fever in the Borough of Chorley*, Reports on Public Health and Medical Subjects, No. 30, London, 1925.

Newman, G., 'Prefatory note', in W. V. Shaw, *Report on an Outbreak of Enteric Fever in the Malton Urban District*, Reports on Public Health and Medical Subjects, No. 69, London, 1933.

Oddy, D. J. and D. S. Miller, *The Making of the Modern British Diet*, London, 1976.

Oddy, D. J. and D. S. Miller, *Diet and Health in Modern Britain*, London, 1985.

Office of Health Economics, *Progress against Tuberculosis*, London, 1962.

Patton, J. L., 'The future of notification of infectious disease', *Public Health*, 1958, vol. 72, pp. 7–16.

Pennington Group, *Report on the Circumstances Leading to the 1996 Outbreak of Infection with E. coli O157 in Central Scotland*, Edinburgh, 1997.

Pennington, T. H., 'Recent experiences in food poisoning', in D. F. Smith and J. Phillips (eds), *Food, Science, Policy and Regulation in the Twentieth Century: International and Comparative Perspectives*, London, 2000, pp. 223–38.

Pennington, T. H., *When Food Kills, BSE, E. Coli and Disaster Science*, Oxford, 2003.

Penny, W. M., 'Typhoid precautions', *British Medical Journal*, 1937, vol. 2, pp. 1092–3.

Perren, R., *The Meat Trade in Britain*, London, 1978.

Porter, I. A. and M. J. Williams, *Epidemic Diseases in Aberdeen and the History of the City Hospital*, Aberdeen, 2001.

Reid, J., *Origin of the 1967–68 Foot-and-Mouth Disease Epidemic*, London, 1968.

Reilly, J. and D. Miller, 'Scaremonger or scapegoat? The role of the media in the emergence of food as a social issue', in P. Caplan (ed.), *Food, Identity and Health*, London, 1997, pp. 234–50.

Ritchie, J., 'Enteric fever', *British Medical Journal*, 1937, vol. 2, pp. 160–3.

Rock, D. (ed.), *Argentina in the Twentieth Century*, London, 1975.

Rose, H. and S. P. R. Rose, *Science and Society*, London, 1969, p. 93.

Rose, R., *Ministers and Ministries: A Functional Analysis*, Oxford, 1987.

Royal Society of Health, *The Safety of Canned Foods. Report of the Royal Society of Health Conference on the Safety of Canned Foods*, London, 1966.

Russell, E. M., 'Typhoid fever in Aberdeen – a critical analysis', MD thesis, University of Glasgow, 1965.

Russell, E. M., A. Sutherland and W. Walker, 'Ampicillin for persistent typhoid excreters, including a clinical trial in convalescence', *British Medical Journal*, 1966, vol. 2, pp. 555–7.

Savage, W. G., *Food Poisoning and Food Infections*, Cambridge, 1920.

Savage, W. G., 'Acute food poisoning', *Public Health*, 1957, vol. 71, pp. 323–35.

Savage, W. G. and P. Bruce White, *An Investigation of the Salmonella Group*, *with Special Reference to Food Poisoning*, Medical Research Council Special Report Series, No. 91, London, 1925.

Savage W. G. and P. Bruce White, *Food Poisoning: A Study of 100 Recent Outbreaks*, Medical Research Council Special Report Series, No. 92, London, 1925.

Schwabe, C. W., *Veterinary Medicine and Human Health* (3rd edn), Baltimore, 1984.

Schwartz, M. and M. Thompson, *Divided we Stand: Redefining Politics, Technology and Social Choice*, London, 1990.

Scottish Home and Health Department, *The Aberdeen Typhoid Outbreak*, Edinburgh, 1964.

Sharp, J. C., P. P. Brown and G. Sangster, 'Outbreak of paratyphoid in the Edinburgh area', *British Medical Journal*, 1964, vol. 1, pp. 1282–5.

Shaw, W. V., *Report to the Minister of Health on an Epidemic of Enteric Fever at Bolton-upon-Dearne*, Reports on Public Health and Medical Subjects, No. 12, London, 1922.

Shaw, W. V., *Report on an Outbreak of Paratyphoid Fever in the Borough of Chorley*, Reports on Public Health and Medical Subjects, No. 30, London, 1925.

Shaw, W. V., *Report on an Outbreak of Enteric Fever in the Malton Urban District*, Reports on Public Health and Medical Subjects, No. 69, London, 1933.

Shaw, W. V., *Report on an Outbreak of Enteric Fever in the County Borough of Bournemouth and in the Boroughs of Poole and Christchurch*, Reports on Public Health and Medical Subjects, No. 81, London, 1937.

Sheppard, J., *The Big Chill: A Report on the Implications of Cook-chill Catering for the Public Services*, London, 1987.

Skeat, W. O., *Manual of British Water Engineering Practice*, Cambridge, 1969.

Smith, D. F., 'The social construction of dietary standards: The British Medical Association – Ministry of Health Advisory Committee on Nutrition Report of 1934', in D. Maurer and J. Sobal (eds), *Eating Agenda: Food and Nutrition as Social Problems*, New York, 1995, pp. 279–304.

Smith, D. F. (ed.), *Nutrition in Britain: Science, Scientists and Politics in the Twentieth Century*, London, 1997.

Smith, D. F., 'The discourse of scientific knowledge of nutrition and dietary change in the twentieth century', in A. Murcott (ed.), *The Nation's Diet*, London, 1998, pp. 311–31.

Smith, D. F., 'The rise and fall of the Scientific Food Committee during the Second World War', in D. F. Smith and J. Phillips (eds), *Food, Science, Policy and Regulation in the Twentieth Century: International and Comparative Perspectives*, London, 2000, pp. 101–16.

Smith, D. F. and J. Phillips, 'Food policy and regulation: a multiplicity of actors and experts', in D. F. Smith and J. Phillips (eds), *Food, Science, Policy and Regulation in the Twentieth Century: International and Comparative Perspectives*, London, 2000, pp. 1–16.

Smith, D. F. and J. Phillips (eds), *Food, Science, Policy and Regulation in the Twentieth Century: International and Comparative Perspectives*, London, 2000.

Smith, H. G., 'The Bournemouth, Poole and Christchurch typhoid epidemic', *Public Health*, 1937, vol. 50, pp. 295–6.

Smith, M. J., *The Politics of Agricultural Support in Britain*, London, 1990.

Smulders, F. J. M. (ed.), *Veterinary Aspects of Meat Production, Processing and Inspection. An Update of Recent Developments in Europe*, Utrecht, 1999.

Swabe, J., *Animals, Disease and Human Society: Human–Animal Relations and the Rise of Veterinary Medicine*, London, 1999.

van Zwanenberg, P. and E. Millstone, 'Beyond skeptical relativism: evaluating the social constructions of expert risk assessment', *Science, Technology and Human Values*, 2000, vol. 25, pp. 259–82.

van Zwanenberg, P. and E. Millstone, 'BSE: a paradigm of policy failure', *The Political Quarterly*, 2003, vol. 74, pp. 27–37.

Walker, W., 'Cephaloridine in typhoid', *British Medical Journal*, 1964, vol. 2, pp. 1529–30.

Walker, W. (ed.), 'The Aberdeen typhoid outbreak of 1964', *Scottish Medical Journal*, 1965, vol. 10, pp. 466–79.

Watt, J. P., 'Typhoid carriers in Aberdeenshire', *Journal of Hygiene*, 1924, vol. 22, pp. 417–37.

Webb, T., *Food Irradiation in Britain?*, London, 1985.

Webster, C., 'Government policy on school meals and welfare foods 1939–1970', in D. F. Smith (ed.), *Nutrition in Britain: Science, Scientists and Politics in the Twentieth Century*, London, 1997, pp. 190–213.

Wilson, G. S., 'The Public Health Laboratory Service', *British Medical Journal*, 1948, vol. 1, pp. 627–31, 677–82.

Wilson, L. G., 'Fevers', in W. F. Bynum and R. Porter (eds), *Companion Encyclopaedia of the History of Medicine*, London, 1993, pp. 382–411.

Winnifrith, J., *The Minister of Agriculture, Fisheries and Food* (New Whitehall Series No. 11), London, 1962.

Woodward, T. E., J. E. Woodward, H. L. Ley, R. Green and D. S. Mankikar, 'Preliminary report on the beneficial effect of chloromycetin in treatment of typhoid fever', *Archives of Internal Medicine*, 1948, vol. 29, pp. 131–4.

Worth, H., 'Typhoid in Aberdeen', *British Medical Journal*, 1964, vol. 1, p. 1706.

Yellowlees, H., 'Food safety: a century of progress', in Ministry of Agriculture, Fisheries and Food, *Food Quality and Safety a Century of Progress*, London, 1976, pp. 62–7.

Index